FOURTH EDITION

Living a Healthy Life with Long-Term Conditions

Self-Management Skills for Physical and Mental Health Conditions; including Heart Disease, Arthritis, Diabetes, Depression, Asthma, Bronchitis, Emphysema, Coronavirus (COVID-19) and Others

Kate Lorig, DrPH • **David Sobel**, MD, MPH

Diana Laurent, MPH • **Marian Minor**, PT, PhD

Virginia González, MPH • **Maureen Gecht-Silver**, OTD, MPH

Jane Cooper-Neville, MSc (UK 4th Edition)

Bull Publishing Company
Boulder, Colorado

Published by Bull Publishing Company
P.O. Box 1377
Boulder, CO, USA 80306
www.bullpub.com

Library of Congress Cataloging-in-Publication Data

Names: Lorig, Kate, author.
Title: Living a healthy life with long-term conditions: self-management skills for physical and mental health conditions; including heart disease, arthritis, diabetes, depression, asthma, bronchitis, emphysema, coronavirus (COVID-19) and others / Kate Lorig, DrPH [and six others].
Description: UK Fourth edition. | Boulder, Colorado : Bull Publishing Company, [2021] | Includes bibliographical references and index. | Summary: "OUR READERS LEARN HOW TO BECOME ACTIVE SELF-MANAGERS through problem solving, decision making, goal setting, and action planning. This book shares these tools of self-management as well as the basics of healthy eating, exercise, relaxation, communication, and emotional empowerment. Living a Healthy Life with Long-Term Conditions offers readers a unique and exciting opportunity-the chance to take control of their health and enjoy their lives to the fullest extent possible with long-term illness. Originally based on a five-year study at Stanford University, the content of this UK 4th edition draws upon the completely revised US 5th edition and includes the feedback of medical professionals and people with long-term conditions all over the world. Kate Lorig, DrPH, is professor emerita at Stanford University School of Medicine and a partner in the Self-Management Resource Center"-- Provided by publisher.
Identifiers: LCCN 2021005370 | ISBN 9781945188435 (paperback)
Subjects: LCSH: Chronic diseases--Psychological aspects. | Chronically ill--Care. | Long-term care of the sick. | Self-care, Health.
Classification: LCC RC108 .L56512 2021 | DDC 616/.044--dc23
LC record available at https://lccn.loc.gov/2021005370

Fourth Edition
27 26 25 24 23 22 21   10 9 8 7 6 5 4 3 2

Interior design and project management: Dovetail Publishing Services
Cover design and production: Shannon Bodie, Bookwise Design

To David Bull,

> *who made this book possible*

and Lara Noel Borowski

> *who taught us about living and dying*

Acknowledgments

Acknowledgments to the US Fifth Edition

More than a million and a half readers have used the first four editions of *Living a Healthy Life with Chronic Conditions*. Thanks to all of you, self-management has become a common term. Our programs reach more than 30 countries in many languages. This revised fifth edition reflects the efforts of the six authors, each with over thirty years of experience, and five additional contributors, as well as hundreds of comments from workshop leaders and trainers. You are the village – now grown into a large city – that made this possible.

For fear of making this book much too heavy to lift – never mind forgetting someone – we are not going to list all the people we would like to thank individually. All of you have helped, made us think and moved us forward. Know that this edition is for you and by you.

One very special person, Dr. Halsted (Hal) Holman, MD, has served as mentor, friend, and critic to our work. Dr. Holman is Professor Emeritus of Stanford University School of Medicine and served as chair the Department of Medicine, Director of the Robert Wood Johnson Clinical Scholar Program, and Director of the Stanford Arthritis Center. He was creating patient centered health care long before the term existed. Hal believes that healthcare should be effective, efficient, and cost-effective and that the only way to make this possible is to foster informed, active patients. He has supported our self-management programs and this book from its very beginning. Without his support there would be no book and no workshops.

We also owe a debt of gratitude to Dr. Albert Bandura, PhD, Emeritus Professor of Psychology at Stanford University School of Medicine and father of self-efficacy theory. Over many years, Dr. Bandura helped us move theory to practice. The idea of assigning a confidence level of 0–10 in our action planning tool comes directly from him as does so much more.

Finally, thanks to Jim Bull, our publisher, Erin Mulligan, our editor, and Jonathan Peck, the director of production at Dovetail Publishing Services. They have stuck by us for many editions, put up with all the authors, and made this book better for their tireless efforts.

Acknowledgments to the UK Fourth Edition

Thank you to the many people and organisations that have contributed to the development of the UK fourth edition of this handbook. Special thanks to Jim Bull for his support in ensuring that a fourth edition would be made available to people across the UK. Thanks to the editorial team of Jane Cooper-Neville, Jean Thompson, MBE, and Julie Dawson. Thanks to Jon Peck of Dovetail Publishing Services for his advice and support in developing the drafts and final copy.

Thanks to the following people and organisations for their support in developing the content for the UK 4th edition: Judith Andrews, Age UK (Thanet Branch), Brid Cronin, the Enhanced Respiratory Service Team (Bury & Rochdale Care Organisation), Paula Graham, Louise Heron, Mrs Toni Miles, Runa Mishra, Northern Ireland Chest Heart and Stroke (NICHS), Nitin Sharma, and Versus Arthritis,

Special thanks to Jean Thompson, MBE, Patrick Hill, Solutions4Health, Harkesh Verdi, Rachael Thornton and Catherine Washbrook-Davies and for their detailed comments and contributions.

SMRC Programmes in the UK

Structured patient education programmes originally developed by Professor Kate Lorig and her colleagues at Stanford University were introduced to the UK during the 1990's. The Long-term Medical Conditions Alliance (LMCA) built upon the efforts of Arthritis Care and others to increase knowledge about and use of lay led self-management programmes among people living with a range of long-term conditions. The work of LMCA and its voluntary sector partners laid the foundations for the development of the NHS Expert Patients Programme which was launched in 2002.

Over the intervening 18 years the evidence base demonstrating the benefits of self-management to the individual, families, communities, the health care system and wider economy has grown. Consequently, self-management has gained increasing relevance within the vision and planning for a twenty-first century health care service. In 2019 Supported Self-management (SSM) was included as part of NHS England's commitment to make personalised care services business as usual across the health and care system.

Today there are many different types of self-management interventions available to people living with long-term conditions across the UK. However, the central messages of the programmes developed by Kate Lorig – that people are active partners in their own care; that individuals are experts in their own condition; that goal setting and action planning is key to individual change; that people can become active resource finders and work in partnership with professionals to find the solutions that are right for them; that peer support from others with similar experiences can help people take control of their daily lives – are at the core of what is recognised by NHS England as good supported self-management.

This handbook provides road map for anyone on their journey of becoming an active self-manager and is an invaluable tool to support people living with long-term conditions to lead more fruitful and enabled lives. At the time of writing we are in the midst of a global coronavirus pandemic and it is clear that the ethos and content of the Chronic Disease Self-Management Programme provides the building blocks for self-managing the emrging symptoms of Long Covid. Positive thinking, goal setting and action planning, living a healthy lifestyle, having an active daily routine, medical management of your condition and effective communication with healthcare professionals, family and friends are all essential to living a healthy life with long-term conditions.

The written words in this book are important but only you can make them jump from the page and effect the change you want! So Always keep it close ….

Contents

Disclaimer

This book is not intended to replace common sense, professional medical or psychological advice. You should seek and get appropriate professional evaluation and treatment for problems – especially unusual, unexplained, severe, or persistent symptoms. Many symptoms and diseases require and benefit from specific medical or psychological evaluation and treatment. Don't deny yourself proper professional care.

- If your symptoms or problems persist beyond a reasonable period despite using self-care recommendations, you should consult a health professional. What is a reasonable period will vary; if you're not sure and you're feeling anxious, consult a healthcare professional.

- If you receive professional advice in conflict with this book, you should rely upon the guidance provided by your healthcare professional. He or she is likely to be able to take your specific situation, history and needs into consideration.

- If you are having thoughts of harming yourself in any way, please seek professional care immediately.

This book is as accurate as its publisher and authors can make it, but we cannot guarantee that it will work for you in every case. The authors and publisher disclaim any and all liability for any claims or injuries that you may believe arose from following the recommendations set forth in this book. This book is only a guide; your common sense, good judgment, and partnership with health professionals are also needed.

Finally, this book was written during the Brexit transition period and some of the advice contained within might change as of 1st January 2021.

Editor's Notes

This handbook draws on the material in the US 5th edition of Living a Healthy Life with Chronic Conditions, by Kate Lorig, Halsted Holman, David Sobel, Diana Laurent, Virginia Gonzalez, Marian Minor, Maureen Gecht-Silver, and Peg Harrison. While keeping to the integrity of the US edition some text has been revised for UK users of the handbook, taking into account UK guidance and feedback from practitioners in the field.

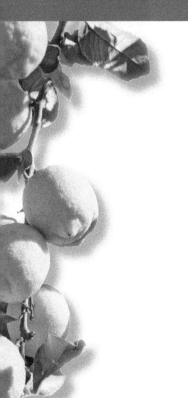

CHAPTER 1

Self-Management: What Is It and How Can You Do It?

Nobody wants to have a long-term illness. Unfortunately, most of us will have two or more of these conditions during our lives. The goal of this book is to help people with long-term illness explore healthy ways to live with challenging physical or mental health conditions. This may seem like a strange statement. How can you have an illness and live a healthy life?

To answer this, let's look at what happens with most long-term health problems. It is true that these conditions, such as heart disease, diabetes, depression, liver disease, bipolar disorder, emphysema and other breathing issues, or other conditions often cause fatigue. They can also result in decreased physical strength and endurance. In addition, long-term conditions may cause emotional distress, such as frustration, anger, anxiety, or a sense of helplessness.

1

So how can you be healthy when these things may be happening to you? Health is soundness of body and mind, and a healthy life is one that seeks that soundness. A healthy way to live with a long-term condition is to seek soundness of body and mind and work to overcome the physical and emotional issues caused by long-term conditions. The challenge is to learn how to function at your best regardless of the difficulties life presents. The goal is to achieve the things you want to do and to get pleasure from life. That is what this book is all about.

How to Use This Book

Before we go any further, let's talk about how to use this book. At the end of this chapter on page 17, you will find a self-test. After you read this chapter, take the test and score it. Then read the suggestions in this book that can be most helpful to you. You do not need to read every word in every chapter. Instead, read the first two chapters and then use your self-test results and the table of contents to find the information you need from the other chapters. In every chapter and every section of this book, you will find information to help you learn and practice self-management skills. This is not a textbook. It is more like a workbook. Feel free to skip around and to make notes in the book. This will help you learn the skills you need to follow your own path.

You will not find any miracles or cures in the book. But you will find hundreds of tips and ideas to make your life easier. The advice comes from doctors and other healthcare professionals, as well as people like you who have learned to actively manage their long-term health problems. Please note that we said 'actively manage'. We use the word *manage* on purpose. Management is the key to the tools this book gives you. There is no way to avoid managing a long-term condition. If you choose to do nothing, that is one way of managing. If you only take medication, that is another management approach. But if you choose to be an active self-manager, follow the best treatments that healthcare professionals have to offer, and are actively involved in your own day-to-day management, you will live a healthier life.

In this chapter, we discuss long-term conditions in general in the context of self-management. We also introduce the most common problems people with long-term conditions face. The problems for most conditions have much more in common than you might think, and the self-management skills to address those problems are also similar. It does not matter what conditions you have. This can be good news because most people have more than one long-term condition. Therefore, learning the common life-management skills allows you to successfully manage your life, not just a single condition. The rest of the chapters in the book give you the tools needed to become a great manager of both your long-term conditions and the other parts of your life. At the end of each chapter you will find a list of useful websites where you can obtain additional information and support.

What Is a Long-Term Health Condition?

Health problems can be either 'acute' or 'chronic' (that is, 'long-term'). Acute health problems usually begin suddenly, have a single cause, are often easily diagnosed, last a short time, and get better with medication, surgery, rest, and time. Most people with acute illnesses are cured and return to normal health. Both the patient and the doctor usually know what to expect. An acute illness typically follows a cycle of getting worse for a while, carefully treating or observing the symptoms, and then getting better. The care of acute illness depends on the body's ability to heal itself and sometimes on a health professional's knowledge and experience in finding and giving the correct treatment.

For example, appendicitis is an acute illness. It typically begins rapidly, signalled by nausea and pain in the abdomen. A diagnosis of appendicitis usually leads to removal of the appendix. There follows a period of recovery and then a return to normal health.

Long-term conditions differ from acute illnesses (see Table 1.1). Long-term conditions usually begin slowly and proceed slowly. Because long-term conditions start with problems at the cellular level, you may not notice the condition until it causes symptoms or shows up as an abnormal test result. For example, a person may slowly develop blockage of the arteries over decades and then might have a heart attack or a stroke. Or arthritis will start with brief annoying twinges that gradually increase. Unlike acute illness, long-term conditions usually have multiple causes that vary over time. These causes may be heredity or lifestyle-related (smoking, lack of exercise, poor diet, stress, etc.). Long-term conditions can also result from exposure to environmental factors, such as second-hand smoke or air pollution, or physiological factors, such as low levels of thyroid hormone or changes in brain chemistry that may cause depression.

Table 1.1 **Differences Between Acute and Long-Term Conditions**

	Acute Illness	**Long-Term Condition**
Beginning	Usually rapid	Slow
Cause	Usually one, sometimes uncertain	Often uncertain, especially early on
Duration	Short	Usually for life
Diagnosis	Commonly accurate	Sometimes difficult
Tests	Give good answers	Often of limited value
Role of professional	Select and conduct treatment	Teach and partner
Role of patient	Follow orders	Partner with healthcare professionals; responsible for daily management

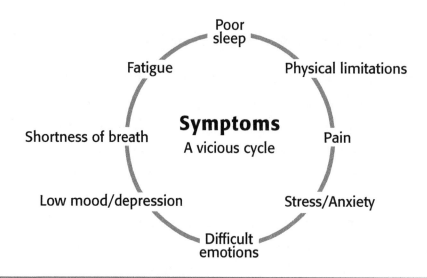

Figure 1.1 **The Vicious Cycle of Symptoms**

Long-term conditions can be frustrating. It is difficult for both the doctor and the patient when there are not clear answers. In some cases, even when diagnosis is rapid, as in the case of a stroke or heart attack, the long-term effects may be hard to predict. The lack of a regular or predictable pattern is a major characteristic of most long-term conditions.

For acute illness, a full recovery is usually the expectation. In contrast, a long-term condition usually leads to more symptoms and loss of physical or mental functioning. Many people assume that the symptoms of long-term conditions are due to the condition. This is only partly true. Although the condition can certainly cause

pain, shortness of breath, fatigue, and the like, the condition is not the only cause. Each of these symptoms can make other symptoms worse, and all of these symptoms can trigger and feed on each other. For example, depression causes fatigue and pain causes physical limitations, and depression and pain can lead to poor sleep and more fatigue. The interactions of symptoms make the condition worse. It becomes a vicious cycle that only gets worse unless you find a way to break the cycle (see Figure 1.1).

Throughout this book we examine ways of breaking the cycle and getting away from the problems of physical and emotional helplessness by using self-management tools and skills.

What Causes a Long-Term Condition?

To understand why a long-term condition happens, you need to understand something about how your body works. Your organs include your heart, lungs, brain, blood, blood vessels, bones,

and muscles. Cells are the building blocks of tissues and organs – in fact, everything in your body. For a cell to remain alive and function normally, three things must happen: it must be nourished, receive oxygen, and get rid of waste products. If anything goes wrong with any of these functions, the cell becomes diseased. If cells are diseased, your organ or tissue suffers. Organ or tissue damage can limit your ability to be active in daily life.

The differences among long-term conditions depend on which cells and organs are affected and how the disruption occurs.

■ If you have a stroke, a blood vessel in the brain becomes blocked or bursts. Oxygen and nutrition are cut off from the part of the brain supplied by that artery. As a result, the part of your body controlled by the damaged brain cells, such an arm, a leg, or a portion of your face, loses function.

■ If you have heart disease, heart attacks occur when the vessels supplying blood to the heart muscle become blocked. When this happens, oxygen is cut off, the heart muscle is injured, and pain results. After the injury, the heart may not work as well. It may not be as good at supplying your body with oxygen-carrying blood. Because the heart is pumping blood less efficiently through the body, fluid accumulates in tissues. You may have shortness of breath and fatigue.

■ With diseases of the lungs, either there is a problem getting oxygen to your lungs, as with bronchitis or asthma, or the lungs cannot effectively transfer oxygen to the blood, as with emphysema. In both cases, your body does not get all the oxygen it needs.

■ With diabetes, the pancreas does not produce enough insulin or produces insulin that cannot be used efficiently by your body. Without this insulin, your body's cells are not able to use the glucose (sugar) in the blood for energy.

■ With liver and kidney disease, the cells of these organs do not work properly, making it difficult for your body to get rid of waste products.

The results of these diseases are similar: loss of function due to a reduction in oxygen, accumulation of waste products, or inability of the body to use glucose for energy. (By 'loss of function', we mean your ability to go about your daily activities normally and without discomfort.)

Loss of function also occurs in arthritis, but for different reasons. With osteoarthritis, cartilage (the cushioning material found on the ends of bones and as the 'disks' between the vertebrae of the back) becomes worn, frayed, or displaced, causing pain. Healthcare professionals often do not know exactly why the cartilage cells begin to weaken or die. But the results are pain and disability.

There is evidence to suggest that mental health issues may be linked to a variation in certain brain chemicals. Too much or too little of various chemicals in the brain can affect our moods, thoughts, and behaviours. Some psychiatric medications work by acting on chemicals in the brain, and there's lots of evidence to show that medication can be effective in treating some symptoms of mental health problems. Treatment of such conditions as depression, bipolar disorder, and schizophrenia often includes restoring chemical balance with medications as well as changes in the environment or self-management practices to support effective coping.

Different Conditions, Similar Symptoms

Although the biological causes of long-term conditions differ, the problems they cause are similar. For example, most people with long-term conditions experience fatigue and loss of energy. Sleeping problems are also common. One illness may cause pain, while with another illness there may be trouble breathing. Disability, to some extent, is a part of most long-term conditions. You may be unable to use your hands well because of arthritis or stroke, or you may have difficulty walking due to shortness of breath, stroke, arthritis, or diabetes. Sometimes disability is caused by lack of energy, extreme fatigue, or change in mood.

Depression is another common problem that is associated with many long-term conditions. It can be caused by a disease-related imbalance in brain chemicals. Depression can also simply be the 'feeling down' or ' low mood' that results from having long-term conditions. It is hard to maintain a cheerful disposition when your condition causes annoying problems that are unlikely to go away. Fear and concern for the future also cause depression. Will I be able to remain independent? If I can't care for myself, who will care for me? Will I get worse? How bad will it get? Both disability and depression may bring loss of self-esteem. Because there are similarities among

long-term conditions, the key management tasks and skills needed to live with different long-term conditions are also similar.

Perhaps the most important skill is responding to any problems on a day-to-day basis. You live with your condition 24 hours a day; your healthcare professional sees you only a tiny portion of this time. This means that you must manage your condition daily. Table 1.2 on page 7 lists some of the self-management challenges of long-term conditions. Although there are some differences among conditions, the problems and symptoms overlap across conditions.

As you can see, long-term conditions have much in common. In this book we sometimes discuss managing specific conditions. In most of the book, however, you will find information about the management tasks that are common across many conditions. If you have more than one health problem, you need not be confused about how to start. Self-management tools for heart disease will often also help with lung disease, arthritis, depression, or a stroke. Start with the problem or condition that bothers you most. Table 1.3 on pages 10–12 lists some of the management skills for condition-specific problems. We also discuss some of these skills in various chapters later in the book.

Understanding the Long-Term Condition Path

The first responsibility of any long-term condition self-manager is to understand the condition. This means more than learning about

what causes the condition, what symptoms it may cause, and what you can do. It also means observing how the condition and its treatment

Table 1.2 **Self-Management Problems for Long-Term Conditions**

Long-Term Condition	Possible Problems Caused by Long-Term Conditions				
	Pain	Fatigue	Shortness of Breath	Physical Function	Difficult Emotions
Anxiety/Panic Disorder		✔	✔	✔	✔
Arthritis	✔	✔		✔	✔
Asthma and Lung Disease		✔	✔	✔	✔
Cancer	✔	✔	✔	✔	✔
Long-Term Heartburn and Acid Reflux	✔				✔
Long-Term Pain	✔	✔		✔	✔
Congestive Heart Failure		✔	✔	✔	✔
Depression		✔		✔	✔
Diabetes	✔	✔		✔	✔
Heart Disease	✔	✔	✔	✔	✔
Hepatitis	✔	✔			✔
High Blood Pressure					✔
HIV Disease (AIDS)	✔	✔	✔	✔	✔
Inflammatory Bowel Disease	✔				✔
Irritable Bowel Syndrome	✔				✔
Kidney Disease and Renal Failure		✔		✔	✔
Kidney Stones	✔				
Multiple Sclerosis	✔	✔		✔	✔
Parkinson's Disease	✔	✔		✔	✔
Peptic Ulcer Disease	✔				✔
Stroke		✔		✔	✔

affect you. An illness is different for each person. With experience, you will become an expert at knowing the effects of the condition and its treatment. In fact, you are the only person who lives with your health problem(s) every minute of every day. Watching how it affects you and making accurate reports to your healthcare professionals are key parts of being a good manager.

When you develop a long-term condition, you become more aware of your body. Minor symptoms that were ignored may now cause concerns. For example, is your chest pain a signal of a heart attack? Is the new pain in your knee a sign that the arthritis has gotten worse? There are no simple reassuring answers. Nor is there a fail-safe way to sort out serious signals from minor temporary symptoms that can be ignored. But it is helpful to understand the natural rhythms of your long-term condition. In general, symptoms should be checked out with your doctor if they are unusual, severe, last a long time, or if they occur after starting a new medication or treatment plan.

Throughout this book, we give some specific examples of what actions to take if you have certain symptoms. Deciding when to take action when you experience symptoms is where your partnership with your healthcare professional becomes critical. Self-management does not mean managing your long-term condition alone. Get help or advice when you are concerned or uncertain.

Most long-term conditions follow an up-and-down path. They do not follow a steady path. Good treatment depends on good communication with healthcare professionals. Let's look at an example: Jessica, Sandra, and Julie all have a blood pressure of 160/100, which is too high. They have all already been prescribed medicine for this condition, but so far there have been no improvements.

■ Julie tells her doctor that she sometimes forgets her medications and is not getting much exercise. She is also overweight. Her doctor talks with her, and together they work out a plan to help her remember her medications, start an exercise programme, and cut down on the amount of food she eats.

■ Jessica says she is taking her medications, exercising, and eating well. The doctor decides to change her medications, because what she is currently taking is probably not working.

■ Sandra does not want to take the prescribed medication. She is doing everything she can to lower her blood pressure: eating well, losing weight, and exercising. Though her blood pressure has improved a bit, it is not good enough. The doctor talks to her about the dangers of high blood pressure and advises continuing the medication. In the end Sandra decides that this might be best.

The successful management of high blood pressure varied for each of these patients. Their treatments were different and depended on what each person was doing and what they told the doctor. Effective control of the illness in each of these cases involved an observant patient talking openly and truthfully with the healthcare professional.

What Is Self-Management?

Self-management is the use of skills (tools) to manage the work of living with your long-term condition, continuing your daily activities, and dealing with emotions brought about by the illness.

Both at home and in the business world, managers are in charge. They don't do everything themselves; they work with others, including consultants, to get the job done. What makes them managers is that they are responsible for making decisions and making sure that their decisions are carried out.

As the manager of your condition, your job is much the same. You gather information and work with a consultant or team of consultants consisting of your GP and other healthcare professionals. Once they have given you their best advice, it is up to you to follow through. All long-term conditions need day-to-day management.

Managing a long-term condition, like managing a family or a business, is a complex undertaking. There are many twists, turns, and midcourse corrections. By learning self-management skills, you can ease the problems of living with your condition.

The key to success in any undertaking is (1) defining the problem, (2) deciding what you want to do, (3) deciding how you are going to do it, and (4) learning a set of skills and practicing them until you master them. Success in long-term condition self-management is the same. In fact, mastering such skills is one of the most important tasks of life.

What Are Self-Management Skills?

This book is about self-management skills. You do not have to learn and use all these self-management skills. You can just learn and practice the ones that are most useful for you. Also, you do not have to learn all these skills at once. Slow and steady wins the race. A list of some of the major skills follows:

- problem solving and action planning to make positive changes in your life

- making decisions about your health, such as when to seek medical help and what treatments to try

- maintaining a healthy lifestyle with regular exercise, healthy eating, good sleep habits, and stress management

- finding and using community resources

- understanding and managing your condition

- understanding and managing your symptoms

- working effectively with your healthcare team

- using medications and assistive devices safely and effectively

- talking about your condition with family and friends

- adapting social activities

- managing your work-life balance

Using Self-Management Skills and Tools

In this book, we describe many skills and tools to help relieve the problems caused by long-term conditions. We do not expect you to use all of them. Pick and choose. Experiment. Set your own goals. What you do may not be as important as the sense of confidence and control that comes from successfully doing something you want to do. We have learned that knowing the

Table 1.3 **Management Skills for Dealing with Long-Term Conditions**

Long-Term Condition	Management Skills							Other Management Tools
	Pain Management	Fatigue Management	Breathing Techniques	Relaxation and Emotion Management	Nutrition	Exercise	Medications	
Anxiety/Panic Disorder		✓	✓	✓	✓	✓	✓	• behavioural techniques to manage triggers
Arthritis	✓	✓	✓	✓	✓	✓	✓	• Assistive devices • Appropriate movement of joints • Cold/heat • Pacing of activities
Asthma and Lung Disease		✓		✓		✓	✓	• Inhalers and peak flow meters • Avoiding triggers • Not smoking
Cancer	✓	✓		✓	✓	✓	✓	• Varies with site of the cancer • Managing effects of surgery, radiation, chemotherapy, and other treatments
Long-term Heartburn and Acid Reflux					✓		✓	• Avoiding stomach irritants (e.g., coffee, alcohol, aspirin, nonsteroidal anti-inflammatory medications) • Elevating head of bed
Long-Term Pain	✓	✓		✓		✓	✓	• Pacing of activities • Specific exercises • behavioural pain management techniques
Congestive Heart Failure		✓	✓	✓	✓	✓	✓	• Monitoring of daily weight • Salt (sodium) and fluid restriction

Table 1.3 **Management Skills for Dealing with Long-Term Conditions** (*continued*)

Long-Term Condition	Management Skills							Other Management Tools
	Pain Management	Fatigue Management	Breathing Techniques	Relaxation and Emotion Management	Nutrition	Exercise	Medications	
Depression		✓		✓	✓	✓	✓	• Engaging in pleasant activities • Exposure to light (phototherapy)
Diabetes	✓	✓		✓	✓	✓	✓	• Home blood glucose monitoring • Insulin injection • Foot care • Regular eye (retinal) exams
Heart Disease	✓	✓	✓	✓	✓	✓	✓	• Knowing and watching for warning signs of heart attack
Hepatitis	✓	✓		✓	✓		✓	• Avoiding alcohol, IV drugs, and medications toxic to liver • Preventing spread of infection (e.g., for hepatitis B and C, safer sex practices, hygiene)
High Blood Pressure				✓	✓	✓	✓	• Home blood pressure monitoring • Salt (sodium) restriction
HIV Disease (AIDS)	✓	✓	✓	✓	✓	✓	✓	• Preventing spread of infection (e.g., safer sex practices, hygiene) • Watching for signs of early infection • Avoiding IV drugs

Continues ▲

11

Table 1.3 **Management Skills for Dealing with Long-Term Conditions (*continued*)**

Long-Term Condition	Management Skills							Other Management Tools
	Pain Management	Fatigue Management	Breathing Techniques	Relaxation and Emotion Management	Nutrition	Exercise	Medications	
Inflammatory Bowel Disease	✓			✓	✓		✓	
Irritable Bowel Syndrome	✓			✓	✓		✓	
Kidney Disease and Renal Failure		✓		✓	✓	✓	✓	• Restricting salt (sodium) potassium, phosphorous, protein, and fluid as needed • Avoiding NSAIDs* • Diabetes and blood pressure control • Undergoing dialysis
Kidney Stones	✓				✓		✓	• Maintaining fluid intake • Avoiding calcium or oxalates, as needed depending on type of stones
Multiple Sclerosis	✓	✓		✓	✓	✓	✓	• Managing incontinence • Managing mobility
Parkinson's Disease		✓		✓	✓	✓	✓	• Managing mobility
Peptic Ulcer Disease	✓			✓	✓	✓	✓	• Avoiding stomach irritants (e.g., coffee, alcohol, aspirin, NSAIDs*) and early infection
Stroke		✓		✓		✓	✓	• Using assistive devices

*Nonsteroidal anti-inflammatory drugs, e.g., aspirin, ibuprofen, naproxen skills is not enough. You need a way of using these skills in your daily life. Whenever you try a new skill, the first attempts may be clumsy, slow, and show few results. It is easier to return to old ways than to continue trying to master new, and sometimes difficult, tasks. The best way to master new skills is to go slow, practice, and evaluate the results.

What you do about something is largely determined by how you think about it. For example, if you think that having a long-term condition is like falling into a deep pit, you may have a hard time motivating yourself to crawl out, or you may even think the task is impossible. The thoughts you have can greatly determine what happens to you and how you handle your health problems.

Some of the most successful self-managers are people who think of their condition as a path. This path, like any path, goes up and down. Sometimes it is flat and smooth. At other times, the way is rough. To negotiate this path, you have to use many strategies. Sometimes you can go fast; other times you must slow down when there are obstacles to negotiate.

Good self-managers are people who have learned three types of skills to negotiate this path:

■ **Skills to deal with the condition.** Any illness requires that you do new things. These may include taking medicine, using an inhaler, or using oxygen. It means more frequent interactions with your GP and the healthcare system. Sometimes you need to adopt new exercises or a new diet. Even conditions such as cancer require self-management. Chemotherapy, radiation,

and surgery can all be made easier through good day-to-day self-management. All of these are examples of the work you must do just to manage your condition.

■ **Skills to continue your normal life.** Just because you have a long-term condition does not mean that life does not go on. There are still chores to do, friendships to maintain, jobs to perform, and relationships to continue. In the face of a long-term condition, things that you once took for granted can become much more complicated. You may need to learn new skills or adapt the way you do things in order to keep doing the things you need and want to do.

■ **Skills to deal with emotions.** When you are diagnosed with a long-term condition, your future changes, and with this come changes in plans and changes in emotions. Many of the new emotions are negative. They may include anger ('Why me? It's not fair'), fear ('I am afraid of becoming dependent on others'), depression ('I can't do anything anymore, so what's the use?'), frustration ('No matter what I do, it doesn't make any difference. I can't do what I want to do'), isolation ('No one understands, no one wants to be around someone who is sick'), or thinking the worst ('I have cancer and am going to die'). Negotiating the path of a long-term condition means learning skills to work with these negative emotions. This book will introduce you to some emotional management skills in Chapter 5, *Understanding and Managing Common Symptoms and Emotions*, and Chapter 6, *Using Your Mind to Manage Symptoms*.

Same Condition, Different Responses

Ali has severe arthritis. He is in pain most of the time and can't sleep. He took early retirement because of his arthritis and now, at age 55, he spends his days sitting at home bored. He seldom takes his medications because he does not like the side effects. He avoids most physical activity because of pain, weakness, and shortness of breath. Ali has become very irritable. Most people, including his family, don't enjoy his company. It even seems like too much trouble when the grandchildren he adores come to visit.

Isabel, age 66, also has severe arthritis. She takes her medications and plans for the side effects. Every day she manages to walk to the local library or the park. When the pain is severe, she practices relaxation techniques and tries to distract herself. She works several hours a week as a volunteer at a local hospital. She also loves going to see her young grandchildren and even manages to take care of them for a while if her daughter has to run errands. Her husband is amazed at how much zest she has for life.

Ali and Isabel both live with the same condition with similar physical problems. Yet their abilities to function and enjoy life are very different. Why? The difference is in their attitudes toward the condition and their lives. Ali has allowed his quality of life and physical abilities to decline. Isabel has learned to take an active role in managing her long-term condition. Even though she has limitations, Isabel controls her life instead of letting the condition take control.

Why is it that two people with similar long-term conditions live their lives so differently? One may be able to minimise the effect of symptoms, while the other is always thinking about the worst and is extremely disabled. One may focus on healthy living, while the other is completely concentrated on the condition. We have all noticed that some people with severe physical problems get on well while others with lesser problems seem to give up on life. The difference often lies in their management style. One of the keys that affects the impact of any condition is how effective and engaged the person is in self-management.

Attitude cannot cure a long-term condition. But a positive attitude and certain self-management skills can make it much easier to live a healthy life with a long-term condition. Research shows that pain, discomfort, and disability can be modified by beliefs, mood, and the attention paid to symptoms. For example, with arthritis of the knee, a person's degree of depression has been found to be a better predictor of how disabled, limited, and uncomfortable the person will be than the evidence of physical damage to the knee visible on X-rays. What goes on in a person's mind is at least as important as what is going on in the person's body. This is not to say your condition is all in your head. A long-term condition is real, but so are your thoughts about your condition. As one self-manager from our programme says, 'It is not mind over matter. It is that mind matters!'

Heart attacks, for example, sometimes make people decide to slow down at work and focus on their home life. They would rather have more time to deepen relationships with family and friends than pursue success at work. A long-term condition that restricts movement may lead some to think again about their unused intellectual talents. Megan learned a new language and found an overseas pen pal; Fred dared to sit down and compose the novel he had always wanted to write. Though a long-term condition may close some doors, you can choose to open new ones.

Jill has breast cancer. Since her diagnosis, she lives more fully than ever: 'I was a housewife – lost and aimless after my children grew up and left home. One of the first things I did after the diagnosis was go and teach myself to swim with my head in the water. I had always kept it above, too scared to put my whole self in. That had been the story of my life. Now I do whatever I want. I don't think about how much time there is, just what I want to do with my time. Surprisingly, I feel less afraid.'

Additional Important Points to Ponder

- **You're not to blame.** Long-term conditions are caused by a combination of genetic, biological, environmental, and psychological factors. For example, stress alone does not cause most long-term conditions. Mind matters, but mind cannot always triumph over matter. If you have trouble recovering, it is not because of lack of the right mental attitude. There are many things you can control that will help you cope with long-term conditions. Remember, you are not responsible for causing the condition or failing to cure it, but you are responsible for acting to manage it.

- **Don't do it alone.** One of the side effects of a long-term condition is a feeling of isolation. As supportive as friends and family members may be, they often cannot understand what you feel as you struggle to cope with a long-term condition. However, there most likely are others who know first-hand what it is like to live with a long-term

condition just like yours. Connecting with other people with similar conditions can reduce your sense of isolation and help you understand what to expect. Someone who is like you can offer practical tips on how to manage symptoms and feelings on a day-to-day basis. Additional benefits of reaching out to others include having the experience of helping them cope with *their* condition, which can help you appreciate your strengths and inspire you to take a more active role in managing your own condition. Support can also come from reading a book, website, or newsletter about how someone else lives with a long-term condition. Or it can come from talking with others on the telephone, in support groups, or online in computer and electronic support groups.

- **You're more than your condition.** When you have a long-term condition, too often your condition becomes the centre of your life. But you are more than your condition – more than a 'diabetic', 'heart patient', or 'lung patient'. And life is more than trips to the GP and managing symptoms. It is important to do the things you enjoy. Small daily pleasures can help balance the other parts of your life in which you have to manage uncomfortable symptoms or emotions. Find ways to enjoy nature by growing a plant or watching a sunset, or indulge in the pleasure of human touch or a tasty meal. Celebrate companionship with family or friends. Finding ways to introduce moments of pleasure is vital to long-term condition self-management. Focus on your abilities and strengths rather than disabilities and problems. Helping others is one way to increase your own sense of what you can do instead of focusing on what you can't. Celebrate small improvements. If a long-term condition teaches anything, it is to live each moment more fully. Within the true limits of whatever condition you have, there are ways to enhance your function, sense of control, and enjoyment of life.

■ **A long-term condition can be an opportunity.** A long-term condition, even with its pain and disability, can enrich our lives. It can make us re-evaluate what is important, shift priorities, and move in exciting new directions that we may never have considered before.

Long-Term Conditions Self-Test

Now that you have the basics, take this self-test and score your responses. At the end of the test, you will find suggestions about what parts of this book will be most helpful to you based on your scores. Use the book as a workbook – skip around and take notes right in the book as you follow your own path. You don't need to read every word in every chapter, but we suggest you read the first two chapters. Then use your self-test results and the table of contents to locate any additional information that you feel can help you.

Long-Term Conditions Self-Test

To help you figure out where you are with your long-term condition, please take this self-test. Score each section and write your score in the appropriate box. After you take the test, look at the instructions starting on page 19 for ideas about where to find some help.

Eating

1. In the past week, how often did you eat a variety of foods (especially fruits, vegetables, and grains)?	Nearly all the time ☐	Most of the time ☐	Some of the time ☐	A little of the time ☐	Seldom ☐
2. In the past week, how often were you aware of how much and what types of food you ate?	Nearly all the time ☐	Most of the time ☐	Some of the time ☐	A little of the time ☐	Seldom ☐
3. In the past week, how often did you drink sweetened and sugary drinks (fizzy drinks, energy drinks, fruit drinks, etc.)?	More than once a day ☐	Once a day ☐	Nearly every day ☐	A few times ☐	Seldom ☐
4. In the past week, how often did you check that the fat you ate (including fat in baked goods and packaged foods) was heart healthy (such as fats that come from plants)?	Nearly all the time ☐	Most of the time ☐	Some of the time ☐	A little of the time ☐	Seldom ☐
5. In the past week, how often did you limit eating processed foods (such as microwaved meals, snack foods, bacon and cooked meats, and most fast food)?	Nearly all the time ☐	Most of the time ☐	Some of the time ☐	A little of the time ☐	Seldom ☐

Pain

Circle the number that describes your pain in the past two weeks.

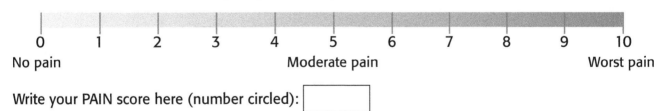

0 1 2 3 4 5 6 7 8 9 10
No pain   Moderate pain   Worst pain

Write your PAIN score here (number circled): ☐

Fatigue

Circle the number that describes your fatigue in the past two weeks.

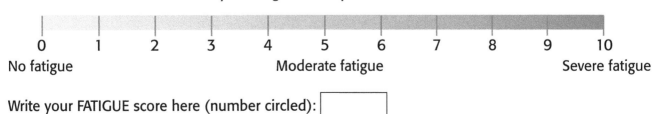

0 1 2 3 4 5 6 7 8 9 10
No fatigue   Moderate fatigue   Severe fatigue

Write your FATIGUE score here (number circled): ☐

Physical limitations

Please circle the number on each line that best describes your abilities.

At this moment, are you able to:	Without ANY difficulty	With SOME difficulty	With MUCH difficulty	UNABLE to do
1. Dress yourself, including tying shoelaces and doing buttons?	0	1	2	3
2. Get in and out of bed?	0	1	2	3
3. Lift a full cup or glass to your mouth?	0	1	2	3
4. Walk outdoors on flat ground?	0	1	2	3
5. Wash and dry your entire body?	0	1	2	3
6. Bend down to pick up clothing from the floor?	0	1	2	3
7. Turn taps on and off?	0	1	2	3
8. Get in and out of a car?	0	1	2	3

Write your PHYSICAL LIMITATIONS score here. Add all the numbers you circled.

Health worries

Please circle the number on each line that best describes your worries

How much time during the past two weeks (circle one number on each line) . . .	None of the time	A little of the time	Some of the time	A good bit of the time	Most of the time	All of the time
1. Were you discouraged by your health problems?	0	1	2	3	4	5
2. Were you fearful about your future health?	0	1	2	3	4	5
3. Was your health a worry in your life?	0	1	2	3	4	5
4. Were you frustrated by your health problems?	0	1	2	3	4	5

Write your HEALTH WORRIES score here. Add all the numbers you circled.

What do you do for fun?

Write your answer here:

_____

_____

_____

_____

_____

_____

Self-Test Scoring Instructions

Eating

There is no overall score. Here are some suggestions for each item.

If your answer is:

Question 1: Nearly all the time or most of the time, you are probably getting enough fruits and vegetables. If you marked any of the other answers, consider slowly adding more fruits and vegetables to your diet. See Chapter 10, *Healthy Eating*, for more information.

Question 2: Nearly all the time or most of the time, you are probably aware of how much you are eating. This is a key self-management skill. Eating more than you need and often want can lead to weight gain and being overweight. Even if you are doing well, you might be interested in learning more about portion sizes and how this affects healthy eating. See pages 237–239. If you marked any of the other answers, consider learning more about how much you are eating and how this can affect your health. For more information, read pages 237, 252 and 253.

Question 3: Seldom – good for you. Sugary drinks add weight and calories. If you marked any of the other answers, you might consider cutting down on the number of sugary drinks and the amount you drink when you have these drinks. To learn more about sugary drinks, see pages 246 and 248.

Question 4: Nearly all the time or most of the time, you have taken the first step toward eating healthy fats and avoiding unhealthy fats. If you marked any of the other answers, consider learning more about fats, such as how much fat to eat and how to tell healthy from unhealthy fats. See pages 243–244.

Question 5: Nearly all the time or most of the time, you are doing well and know that processed foods are often unhealthy foods. If you marked any of the other answers, consider reading page 239–241 about food labels so that you can make better decisions and avoid processed foods.

Pain

Enter your score from the self-test here: ☐

If your score is:

1–4 Pain is probably not your main concern. Although you may want to work on pain management, you may want to address other concerns first. Even if you start with a topic other than pain management, the good news is that almost all of the tools in this book will help your pain when used regularly.

5–7 Pain is probably an important concern for you. You might want to start with the pain management tools on pages 101–104. There are things you can do to help pain, including relaxation and exercise. The good news is by working on pain management day by day, you can do a lot to reduce your pain.

8–10 For you, pain is probably a major problem. A good place to start is with the pain self-management tools on pages 101–104. You should also let your doctor know about your pain level. You may need some medication or a change in medication. By the way, are you taking your medication as prescribed? If not, this might help. The good news is that by working on pain management day by day, you can do a lot to reduce your pain and your need for pain medication.

Fatigue

Enter your score from the self-test here: ☐

If your score is:

1–4 Fatigue is probably not your main concern. Although you may want to work on fatigue management, you may want to address other concerns first. Even if you start with a topic other than fatigue management, the good news is that almost all of the tools in this book will help your fatigue when used regularly.

5–7 Fatigue is probably an important concern for you. You might want to start with the fatigue management tools on page 98. The good news is by working on fatigue management day by day, you can do a lot to reduce your fatigue.

8–10 For you, fatigue is probably a major problem. A good place to start is with the fatigue self-management tools on page 98. You should also let your doctor know about your fatigue level. Some medications can cause fatigue, so you might want to check with your pharmacist. You might need to change your medications. By the way, are you taking your medication as prescribed? If not, this might help. The good news is that by working on fatigue management day by day, you can do a lot to reduce your fatigue.

Physical Limitations

Enter your score from the self-test here ☐

If your score is:

0–9 You have a few problems with physical limitations. Learn more about exercises that are suggested for people with your specific condition in Chapter 4, *Understanding and Managing Common Conditions*. Remember that endurance exercise is also important.

10–19 You have some physical limitations. Learn more about exercises that are suggested for people with your specific condition in Chapter 4, *Understanding and Managing Common Conditions*.

20–27 You have many physical limitations. The good news is that consistent exercise can probably help you. First, decide which limitations are most important to you, and then start the appropriate exercise to address that specific issue.

Exercises for Specific Limitations

Exercises if you have trouble dressing.

- If you have trouble reaching your feet, try: Knee-to-Chest Stretch, page 190; Low-Back Rock and Roll, page 192; Hip Hooray, page 194; Achilles Stretch, page 197

- If you have trouble using your arms and hands for buttons and zips, try: Thumb Walk, page 186; Pat and Reach, page 189

Exercises if you have trouble getting in and out of bed.

Pelvic Tilt, page 191; Low-Back Rock and Roll, page 192; either Curl-Up or Roll-Out for abdominal strengthening on pages 192 and 193

Exercises if you have trouble lifting a full cup or glass to your mouth.

- If you have trouble gripping the cup or glass, try: Thumb Walk, page 186

- If you have trouble lifting the cup or glass, try: Wand Exercise, page 188

Exercises if you have trouble walking.

Back Kick, page 195; Hamstring Stretch, page 197; Achilles Stretch, page 197; Towel Grabber, page 198

Exercises if you have trouble washing and drying your body.

- If you have trouble reaching your feet, try: Knee-to-Chest Stretch, page 190; Low-Back Rock and Roll, page 192; Hip Hooray, page 194; Achilles Stretch, page 197

- If you have trouble using your arms and hands, try: Thumb Walk, page 186; Pat and Reach, page 189

Exercises if you have trouble bending down to pick something up from the floor.

Good Morning, page 188; Knee-to-Chest Stretch, page 190; Power Knees, page 195; Hamstring Stretch, page 197; Achilles Stretch, page 197

Exercises if you have trouble turning taps on and off.

Thumb Walk, page 186; Wand Exercise, page 188; Pat and Reach, page 189

Exercises if you have some trouble getting in and out of the car.

Low-Back Rock and Roll, page 192; Hip Hooray, page 194; Back Kick, page 195; Power Knees, page 195

For most people with long-term conditions, endurance exercise such as walking, swimming, and dancing should be part of their physical activity plan. Learn more in Chapter 7, *Being Physically Active*, and Chapter 8, *Exercising to Make Life Easier*.

Health Worries

Enter your score from the self-test here: ☐

If your score is:

0–4 You are not very worried about your long-term health conditions. You might want to start with a tool other than the one dealing with troubling emotions. The good news is that no matter where you start, your worries will probably become less.

5–12 You have some worries about your long-term health conditions. This is not unusual. You might want to start by reading Chapter 5, *Understanding and Managing Common Symptoms and Emotions*. No matter where you decide to start in the book, almost all self-management activities help you to address your worries.

13–20 You are worried about your long-term health conditions. This is not at all unusual, but you may be worrying more than you need. Read Chapter 5, *Understanding and Managing Common Symptoms and Emotions*. You might also want to discuss your worries with your GP or a counsellor such as a psychologist or social worker. The good news is that most people's worries become less as they learn about their condition and start to take an active part in self-management.

What Do You Do for Fun?

If you answered this question positively, go on to the next chapter.

If you had a very difficult time answering this question or did not answer it at all, it may be that you are experiencing some depression. This is not at all unusual for someone with one or more long-term conditions. Start by reading about depression on pages 117–122. It is also a good idea to discuss your worries with your GP or a counsellor such as a psychologist or social worker. The good news is that most people's worries become less as they learn about their condition and start to take an active part in self-management.

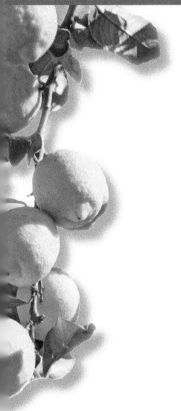

CHAPTER 2

Becoming an Active Self-Manager

IT IS IMPOSSIBLE TO HAVE A LONG-TERM CONDITION without becoming a self-manager. How you live each day and the decisions you make affect you, your symptoms, and the quality of your health and life. For example, some people with long-term conditions manage by withdrawing from life. They may stop doing their favourite activities, stay in bed, or socialise less. The condition becomes the centre of their existence. Other people with the same condition and symptoms somehow manage to get on with life. They may have to change some of the things they do or the way they do them. Nevertheless, life continues to be full and active. The difference between these two examples is not the condition but rather how the person with the long-term condition has decided to manage it. Please note the word *decided*. Self-management is always a decision: a decision to be active or a decision to do nothing, a decision to seek help or a decision to suffer in silence.

Self-Management Tasks and a Self-Management Plan

The information and skills in this book are the tools you need to become an active manager. Being an active self-manager means you are ready and willing to take on the following tasks:

1. **Take care of your health condition.** When you are taking care of your health, you are following a treatment plan, such as taking medicine and adopting new behaviours, including exercising and healthy eating. You are also keeping informed about your health status, asking questions, and sharing this information with other healthcare professionals, family, and friends. You actively take part in planning your treatment by monitoring and reporting on your condition, as well as sharing your preferences and goals with all the members of your health care team.

2. **Carry out your normal activities.** These are the activities of life that are important and meaningful to you, including work, hobbies, socialising, volunteering, and being with family. Sometimes you may need to adjust the way you do these activities, but you continue to do them. As a self-manager, you are also willing to add new healthy activities into your daily life, such as exercising, eating more healthy foods, and taking medications. You are also willing to eliminate unhealthy habits such as smoking.

3. **Manage your emotions.** Emotional changes are brought on by the condition. You may experience anger, uncertainty about the future, sadness due to changed expectations and unmet goals, and sometimes even depression. Having a long-term condition and going through these emotions can also affect your relationships with family and friends. These feelings are a part of the natural 'ups and downs' in life that everyone experiences. A self-manager knows this and is committed to learning how to deal with emotions.

Self-Management Tasks

1. Take care of your health condition.
2. Carry out your normal activities.
3. Manage your emotions.

Remember: you are the manager of your life, and like the manager of an organisation or a household, you need information, a variety of helpful tools or skills, and an overall plan to take on these self-management tasks. This book is designed to give you these things. A self-management plan features the steps shown in the box at the top of page 25.

Although many self-management tools are discussed throughout this book, in this chapter we start by presenting the three most important tools: problem solving, decision making, and action planning. These are the tools that help you to decide which of the other tools work best for you, as well as when and how to use the tools successfully.

Self-Management Plan

1. Decide what you want to accomplish (your goal).
2. Look for various ways to accomplish your goal.
3. Draft a short-term action plan or agreement with yourself.
4. Carry out your action plan.
5. Check the results.
6. Make changes as needed.
7. Reward yourself for your success.

Solving Problems

Problems sometimes start with a general feeling of uneasiness. Let's say you are unhappy but not sure why. Upon closer examination, you find that you miss contact with some relatives who live far away. With the problem identified, you decide to take a trip to visit these relatives. You know what you want to accomplish, but now you need to make a list of ways to solve the problem.

In the past you have always driven to see them, but now making the trip in one day of driving is too tiring, so you consider other options. You consider leaving at noon instead of early in the morning and making the trip in two days instead of one. You consider asking a friend along to share the driving. There is also a train that stops within 20 miles of your destination. Or you could travel by air. You decide to take the train.

The trip still seems overwhelming because there is so much to do to prepare. You decide to write down all your ideas for steps to take to make the trip a reality. These include finding a good time to go, buying your ticket, figuring out

how to handle luggage, figuring out how you will get to and from the station, deciding if you can make it up and down the stairs to get on the train, and determining if you can walk on a moving train to get food or go to the toilet.

You come up with a few problem-solving ideas to get started. You decide that you will call the National Rail Enquiries helpline. You also decide to start taking a short walk each day, including walking up and down a few steps so that you will be steadier on your feet. The next day, you call National Rail Enquiries and start your walking programme.

A week later you check the results of your actions. Looking back at all the steps to be accomplished, you see that a single call answered many questions. You discovered that National Rail Enquiries can help people who have mobility problems and has ways of dealing with many of your concerns. However, you are still worried about walking. Even though you are walking daily and doing better, you are still unsteady. You make a change in your plan after asking your GP to refer you to a physiotherapist, who suggests using a walking stick. Although you don't like using it, you realise that a walking stick will give you the extra security you need on a moving train.

You have just engaged in problem solving to achieve your goal of taking a trip. Let's review the specific steps in problem solving.

1. **Identify the problem.** This is the first and most important step in problem solving—and usually the most difficult step. You may know, for example, that stairs are a problem, but with a little more effort, you can determine that the real problem is your fear of falling.

2. **List ideas to solve the problem.** You may be able to come up with a good list yourself. You may also want to call on friends, family, members of your health care team, or community resources. These are your 'consultants'. One note about using consultants: these people cannot help you if you do not describe the problem well. For example, there is a big difference between saying that you can't walk because your feet hurt and saying that your feet hurt because you cannot find walking shoes that fit properly.

3. **Pick an idea to try.** As you try something new, remember that new activities are usually difficult. Be sure to give your potential solution a fair chance before deciding it won't work.

4. **Check the results.** After you've given your idea a fair trial, figure out how you are doing with your problem. If all goes well, your problem will be solved.

5. If you still have the problem, **pick another idea from your list and try again.**

6. **Use other resources.** Ask your consultants for more ideas if you still do not have a good solution.

7. Finally, if you have gone through all the steps until all ideas have been exhausted and the problem is still unsolved, you may have to **accept that your problem may not be solvable right now.** This is sometimes hard to do. If a problem can't be solved right now, that doesn't mean that it won't be solvable later. That also doesn't mean that other problems you have cannot be solved now. Even if your path is blocked, there are probably alternative paths. Don't give up. Keep going.

Problem-Solving Steps

1. Identify the problem.
2. List ideas to solve the problem.
3. Pick one idea to try.
4. Check the results.
5. Pick another idea if the first didn't work.
6. Use other resources.
7. Accept that the problem may not be solvable now.

Living with Uncertainty

Living with uncertainty can be hard. However, it is something that most people cannot avoid. Uncertainty is one of the causes of emotional ups and downs. A diagnosis of a long-term condition takes away some of our sense of security and control. It can be frightening. We are following our life path, and suddenly we are forced to detour to a different, unwanted path. And even as we work with healthcare professionals and start new treatments, this uncertainty continues. Of course, everyone has an uncertain future, but most people do not think about this. When you have a long-term condition, however, this becomes an important part of your life. You are uncertain about your future health, and perhaps about your ability to continue to do the things you want, need, and like to do. Many people find it very challenging to make decisions while accepting uncertainty.

Making Decisions: Weighing the Pros and Cons

Making decisions is another important tool in our self-management toolbox. Some of the steps in decision making are like the problem-solving steps we just discussed. These steps can help you solve problems and make decisions.

1. **Identify the options.** For example, you may have to make a decision about getting help around the house or continuing to do all the work yourself. Sometimes the options are to change a behaviour or to not change at all.

2. **Identify what you want.** It may be important for you to continue your life as normally as possible, to have more time with your family, or not have to sweep the path, cut the grass, or clean the house. Sometimes identifying your deepest, most important values (such as spending time with family) helps you set priorities and increases your motivation to change.

3. **Write down pros and cons for each option.** List as many items as you can for each side. Don't forget the emotional and social effects of each option.

4. **Rate each item on the pros and cons list** on a 5-point scale, with 1 indicating 'not important' and 5 indicating 'extremely important'.

5. **Add up the ratings for each column** and compare the pros and the cons. The column with the higher total should give you your decision. If the totals are close or you are still not sure, go to the next step.

6. **Apply the 'gut test'.** For example, does going back to work part-time feel right to you? If so, you have probably reached a decision. If not, the way you feel should probably win out over the maths. When your feelings don't agree with the score,

it helps you understand that the reasons for your decision are emotional. Also, you may decide that you need to explore these feelings more, gather more information, or perhaps discuss this with someone else, such as your healthcare team, family, or a friend.

Here is an example of how to do this yourself:

Decision-Making Example

Should I get help around the house?

Pro	Rating	Con	Rating
I'll have more time.	4	It's expensive.	3
I'll be less tired.	4	It's hard to find good help.	1
I'll have a clean house.	3	They won't do things my way.	2
		I don't want a stranger in the house.	1
Total	11		7

Add the points for the pro column and then add the points for the con column. Your decision in this example would be to get help because the pro score (11) is significantly higher than the con score (7). If this feels right in your gut, you have the answer.

Now it's your turn! Try making a decision using the following chart. It's OK to write in your book.

Decision to be made: _____

Pro	Rating	Con	Rating

The key to successful problem solving and decision making is to take action. We talk about this next.

Taking Action

So far in this chapter we have introduced the steps to both problem solving and decision making. But knowing what to do is not enough. You now have to take action. We suggest that you start by doing one thing at a time.

Setting Goals

Before you can take action, you must decide what you want to do first. Be realistic and specific when stating your goal. Think about what you would really like to do. One self-manager wanted to climb 20 steps to her daughter's home so that she could join her family for a special meal. Another wanted to overcome anxiety and attend social events. Still another wanted to continue to ride his motorbike even though he could no longer lift his 1,000-pound (450 kg) bike.

One of the problems with goals is that they often seem like dreams. They are so far off, big, or difficult that it is easy to be overwhelmed and not even try to accomplish them. We discuss this problem next. For now, take a few minutes and write your goals below (add more lines if you need to).

Goals

_____

_____

_____

_____

Put a star (☆) next to the goal you would like to work on first.

Don't reject a goal until you have thought about possible alternatives to achieve it.

Sometimes we reject options without knowing much about them. In the earlier example, our traveller was unable to make a long driving trip but wrote a list of alternative travel arrangements and then chose the train.

Exploring Options

There are many ways to reach any specific goal. For example, our self-manager who wanted to climb 20 steps could start off with a slow walking programme and climb just a few steps each day, or she could ask to have the family gathering at a different place. The man who wanted to attend social events could start by going on very short outings, or he could ask a friend to go along to help, use distraction techniques when feeling anxious, or talk to his healthcare team about therapy or medication. Our motorbike rider could buy a lighter motorbike, use a sidecar, put 'training wheels' on his bike, or buy a three-wheeled motorbike.

As you can see, there are many options for reaching each goal. List all the options you can think of and then choose one or two to try out.

Sometimes it is hard to think of all the options yourself. If you are having problems, it is time to use a consultant, just as you do in problem solving. Share your goal with family, friends, or healthcare professionals. Call organisations such as Diabetes UK, one of the many UK cancer charities, or your local social prescribing service (social prescribing is a way for people to be referred to a link worker who can connect people to community groups and statutory services for practical and emotional support). Use the Internet. Don't ask someone else to decide what you should do. Rather, ask for suggestions. It is always good to add to your list of options by getting fresh ideas from someone new.

A note of caution: many options are never seriously considered because people assume they don't exist or are unworkable. Never make this assumption until you have thoroughly investigated the option. One woman we know had lived in the same town all her life and felt that she knew about all the community resources. When she was having problems with her welfare benefits, a friend from another town suggested contacting a local financial advice service. The woman dismissed this suggestion because she was certain that this service did not exist in her town. It was only when, months later, the friend came to visit and called the local branch of Age UK that the woman learned that Age UK and three other local organisations all offered advice on benefits. Our motorbike rider thought that training wheels on a Harley was a crackpot idea but investigated the idea when a worker at a bike shop suggested it. He added 15 years to his riding life using training wheels. In short, never assume anything. Assumptions are the enemies of good problem solving and decision making.

Write the list of options for your main goal here. Put a star (☆) next to the two or three options you want to research further and pursue.

Options

_____

_____

_____

_____

Making Short-Term Plans: Action Planning

Once a decision has been made, we have a pretty good idea of where we are going. However, your goal may still seem overwhelming. How will I ever move, how will I ever be able to paint again, how will I ever be able to _____ (you fill in the blank)? The secret to succeeding is to *not* try to do everything at once. Instead, look at one thing you can realistically expect to accomplish within *the next week*.

This approach to moving toward your goal is *action planning*. An action plan is short-term and doable, and it sets you on the road toward achieving your goal. Your action plan should be about something you *want* to do or accomplish. It should help you solve a problem or reach a goal. It is a tool to help you do what *you* wish. Do not make action plans to please your friends, family, or doctor.

Action plans are probably your most important self-management tool. Most of us are able to do things that will make us healthier, but we fail to do them. For example, most people with long-term conditions can walk—some just across the room, others across the street. Most can walk several streets, and some can walk a mile or more. However, few people have a regular walking exercise programme.

An action plan can help you do the things you know you *should* do. But to create a successful action plan, it is better to start with what you *want* to do. It can be *anything*! Let's go through the steps for making a realistic action plan.

Creating a Realistic Action Plan

First, decide what you will do this week. For a person who wants to be a better step climber, this might be climbing three steps on four consecutive days. A person who wants to continue riding a motorbike might spend half an hour on two days researching lighter motorbikes and motorbike training wheels.

Make very sure that your plans are 'action-specific'. Don't decide 'to lose weight' (which is not an action but the result of an action). Instead, decide to 'drink tea instead of a fizzy drink' (which is an action).

Next, make a specific plan. Deciding what you want to do will get you nowhere without a plan to do it. The plan should answer the following questions:

■ Exactly *what* are you going to do? Are you going to walk? How will you eat less? Which distraction technique will you practice?

■ *How much* will you do? This question is answered with details about time, distance, portions, or repetitions. Will you walk one street, walk without sitting down for 15 minutes, eat half portions at lunch and dinner, or do relaxation exercises for 15 minutes five days this week?

■ *When* will you do this? Again, this must be specific: before lunch, in the shower, as soon as you come home from work. Connecting a new activity with an old habit is a good way to make sure it gets done. Consider what comes right before your action plan that could prompt the new behaviour.

For example, brushing your teeth can remind you to take your medication. Or decide you will do a 15-minute relaxation exercise in the evening after washing up. Another trick is to incorporate your new activity right before an old favourite activity. You may decide to walk round the block before reading the paper or watching your favourite TV programme.

■ *How often* will you do it? This is a bit tricky. We would all like to do the things we want every day, but that is not always possible. It is usually best to decide to do an activity three or four times a week to give yourself 'wriggle room' in case something comes up. If you do it more often, that's even better. However, if you are like most people, you will feel less pressure if you complete your activity three or four times a week and still feel successful. (Note that taking medications is an exception. This must be done exactly as directed by your doctor.)

Take the following steps when creating your action plan:

1. First, *start where you are*. In other words, start small or start slowly. If you can walk for only 1 minute, start your walking programme by walking 1 minute every hour or two, not by trying to walk a couple of streets. If you have never done any exercise, start with just a few minutes of warm-up. A total of 5 or 10 minutes is enough. If you want to lose weight, set a goal based on your existing eating behaviours, such as eating half portions. For example, 'losing a pound (about half a kilogram) this week'

is not an action plan because it does not involve a specific action. 'Not eating after dinner for four days this week', by contrast, is a fine action plan.

2. Second, *give yourself some time off*. All people have days when they don't feel like doing anything. That is a good reason for saying that you will do something three times a week instead of every day.

3. Third, once you've made your action plan, *ask yourself* the following question: 'On a scale of 0 to 10, with 0 being not at all sure and 10 being absolutely sure, how sure am I that I can complete this entire plan?' If your answer is 7 or above, your action plan is probably reasonable. If your answer is below 7, you should revisit your action plan. Ask yourself why you are unsure. What problems do you expect to encounter? Then see if you can change your plan to make yourself more confident of success.

4. Once you have made a plan you are happy with, write it down and post it where you will see it every day. Thinking through a weekly action plan is one thing. Writing it down makes it more likely you will take action. Keep track of how you are doing and the problems you encounter. (There is a blank action-planning form at the end of this chapter. Make photocopies so you can use them weekly.)

Carrying Out Your Action Plan

If your weekly action plan is well written and realistically achievable, completing it should be fairly easy. The following are a few extra

steps you can take to make completing the plan easier:

■ Ask family or friends to check in with you on how you are doing. Having to report your progress is good motivation.

■ Keep track of your daily activities while carrying out your plan. Many good managers make lists of what they want to accomplish.

■ Check things off as you complete them. This will tell you how realistic your planning was and will be useful in making future plans.

■ Make daily notes, even of the things you don't understand at the time. Later these notes may be helpful in adopting the regular use of problem solving.

Parts of a Successful Action Plan

A good action plan:

■ is something *you* want to do

■ is achievable (something you can expect to be able to accomplish in a week)

■ is action-specific

■ answers the questions *What? How much? When?* and *How often?*

■ is something you are sure that you will complete entirely with a confidence level of 7 or higher on a scale from 0 = not at all sure to 10 = absolutely sure

Checking the Results

At the end of each week, check to see if you completed your action plan and if you are any nearer to accomplishing your goal. Are you

Success Improves Health

The benefits of lifestyle change go beyond the rewards of adopting healthier habits. Yes, you feel better when you exercise, eat well, keep regular sleeping hours, stop smoking, and take time to relax. But there's also evidence that the feelings of self-confidence and control over your life that come from making any successful change improve your health as well.

As people age or develop a long-term illness, physical abilities and self-image may decline. For many people, it is discouraging to find that they can't do what they used to do or want to do. By changing and improving one area of your life, whether it is boosting your physical fitness or learning a new skill, you regain a sense of optimism and energy. By focusing on what you can do rather than what you can't do, you're more likely to lead a more positive and happier life.

able to walk further? Have you lost weight? Are you less anxious? Monitoring your progress is important. You may not see progress day by day, but you should see little positive changes each week. If you are having problems, this is the time to use the problem-solving tool.

For example, our stair-climbing friend didn't do her climbing for the first few weeks of her plan. Each day something stopped her from taking action: not enough time, being tired, cold weather, and similar things. When she looked back at her notes, she began to realise that the real problem was her fear of falling with no one around to help her. She then decided to use a walking stick while climbing stairs and to do it when a friend or neighbour was around. This midcourse correction got her back on track and helped her complete her action plan.

Making Midcourse Corrections (Back to Problem Solving)

When you are trying to overcome obstacles, your first action plan may not always be a workable plan. If something doesn't work, don't give up—try something else. Modify your short-term plans so that your steps are easier, give yourself more time to accomplish difficult tasks, choose new steps to get you to your goal, or check with your consultants for advice and assistance. If you are not sure how to go about this, go back and read pages 25–26.

One last note to consider: not all goals are achievable. Having a long-term condition may mean having to give up some options. If this is true for you, don't dwell too much on what you can't do. Rather, start working on another goal that you can and would like to accomplish. One self-manager we know who uses a wheelchair talks about the 90% of things he *can* do. He devotes his life to developing this 90% to the fullest.

How People Change

Thousands of studies have been done to learn how people change—or why they don't change. Here's what we have learned:

■ **Most people change by themselves, when they are ready.** Yes, doctors, counsellors, partners, and self-help groups coax, persuade, nag, and otherwise try to assist people to change their lifestyle and habits. But most people change when they are ready, and without much help from others.

■ **Change is not an all-or-nothing process.** Change happens in stages. Most of us think of change as occurring one step at a time. Each step is an improvement over the one before it. Although a few people do make changes this way, it is rare. For example, more than 95% of people who successfully quit smoking do so only after a series of setbacks and relapses. (For more on smoking, see pages 109–113.) In most cases, the path to change resembles a spiral more than a straight line. People often return to previous stages before moving forward ('two steps forward, one step back'). Relapses are not failures but setbacks, which are a normal part of change. Dealing with relapse helps people learn how to maintain change; it provides feedback about what doesn't work.

■ **Making changes often depends on doing the right things at the right time.** People who are given strategies to change that do not match their readiness to change are less successful at changing than people who receive no assistance at all. For example, making an elaborate written plan of action when you really haven't decided you want to change is a prescription for failure. You're likely to get bored, discouraged, or frustrated before you even start.

■ **Confidence in your ability to change is the key ingredient for success.** Your belief in your own ability to succeed is important. It predicts whether you will attempt change in the first place, whether you will persist if you relapse, and whether you will ultimately be successful in making the desired change.

Rewarding Yourself

The best part of becoming a good self-manager is the reward that comes from accomplishing your goals and living a fuller and more comfortable life. However, you don't have to wait until your goal is reached. You can reward yourself frequently for your short-term successes. For example, decide that you won't read the newspaper or visit your favourite social media site until after you exercise. Thus, reading the paper or scrolling through new posts becomes your reward. One self-manager buys only one or two pieces of fruit at a time and walks the half mile (0.8 kilometre) to the supermarket every day or two to get more fruit. Another self-manager, who stopped smoking, used the money he would have spent on cigarettes to have his house professionally cleaned. There was even money left over to go to a football match with a friend. Rewards don't have to be fancy, expensive, or high in calories. There are many healthy pleasures that can add enjoyment to your life.

The Self-Management Toolbox

You can accomplish a lot with problem solving, decision making, and action planning. Now that you understand the meaning of self-management, the tasks involved with it, and these three key self-management tools, you are ready to learn about the other tools that will make you a successful self-manager. Most self-management tools work for all long-term conditions, and the chapters in this book contain a lot of information about the more common long-term conditions. Because diabetes requires many self-management skills, Chapter 14, *Managing Diabetes*, is all about this condition. Other important self-management tools discussed in the book include medication; exercise; using assistive devices to stay safe; nutrition; symptom management; communicating with family, friends, and healthcare professionals; sex and intimacy; the workplace; finding resources; and planning for the future.

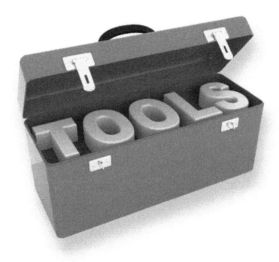

Useful Websites

Age UK: http://www.ageuk.org.uk/

Charity Choice (Provides a list of all UK cancer charities):
    https://www.charitychoice.co.uk/charities/health/cancer/

Diabetes UK: http://www.diabetes.org.uk/

National Rail Enquiries: https://www.nationalrail.co.uk/

My Action Plan

When you write your action plan, be sure it includes the following:

1. What you are going to do (a specific action)
2. How much you are going to do (time, distance, portions, repetitions, etc.)
3. When you are going to do it (time of the day, day of the week)
4. How often or how many days a week you are going to do it

Example: This week, I will walk (what) around the block (how much) before lunch (when) three times (how many).

This week I will _____ (what)

_____ (how much)

_____ (when)

_____ (how often)

How sure are you that you can complete this plan?

0	1	2	3	4	5	6	7	8	9	10

Not at
all sure

Absolutely
sure

Comments

Monday _____

Tuesday _____

Wednesday _____

Thursday _____

Friday _____

Saturday _____

Sunday _____

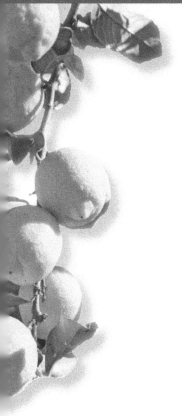

CHAPTER 3

Finding Resources

A MAJOR PART OF BECOMING A SELF-MANAGER is knowing how to find resources and get help when you need it. Asking for help is a strength. Being able to find and get help makes you a good self-manager. In this chapter we offer some tools for finding resources and getting help.

When you first begin to think about getting help, take the following steps:

1. Decide what you want to do to improve your condition or situation.

2. If you cannot do something you want to do, figure out what is getting in your way.

You may find that there is a difference between what you can do and what you want to do (or have done). It is sometimes not easy to know what is getting in the way. If either of these are problems, then it might be time to get help. Don't assume that nothing can be done. This is seldom true. It is important to do the things you need and want to do. Finding a way to do them is worthwhile and rewarding.

Most of us start looking for help by asking family or friends. Sometimes this can be difficult. You might be afraid that others will see you as weak. Sometimes pride gets in the way. The truth is that most people want to be helpful but do not know how. Your job is to tell them what you need. Asking for help is discussed in Chapter 11, *Communicating with Family, Friends, and Healthcare Professionals*. Unfortunately, some people do not have family or close friends. Sometimes, even if you have close people in your life, you cannot bring yourself to ask. Sometimes family or friends are not able to give the needed help. Thankfully, there are many wonderful resources in our communities and on the Internet.

Finding What You Need: Treasure Hunting

Finding resources can be a little like a treasure hunt. As in a treasure hunt, creative thinking wins the game. Finding what you need may be as simple as making a couple of phone calls or searching the Internet. Other times it may require you to investigate like a detective. The community resource detective must find clues and follow leads. Sometimes this means starting over when a clue leads to a dead end.

The first step is defining the problem and the cause of the problem and then deciding what you want. Evaluate your condition or situation. Then ask what you *can* do to improve your condition or situation and ask what you *want* to do to improve your condition or situation. If you cannot do something you want to do, figure out what is getting in your way.

For example, suppose you find it difficult to prepare meals. Standing for a long time is painful for you. After some thought, you decide that you want to continue cooking, but standing is getting in the way. You think that you could continue cooking if you could cook while sitting. Someone else with the same problem might decide that they want food delivered. But the goal of your personal treasure hunt is figuring out how to cook without having to stand.

You look at kitchen stools and do not think they will work for you. So, you decide that you need to redesign your kitchen. The hunt is on. Where can you find an architect or contractor who has experience in kitchen alterations for people with physical limitations? You need a starting point for your treasure hunt. You type the words 'kitchen redesign' into a search engine. The Internet has pages and pages of ads and listings for architects and contractors. It is overwhelming. Maybe you need to narrow your search.

Typing 'kitchen design for physical disabilities' into the search box results in lots of tips from consumers and businesses, and there are also pictures to give you ideas. The first few contractors you contact are not experienced with your problem. You finally find a company that seems to be just what you need, but it is located more than 100 miles (160 kilometres) away.

Now what? You have a couple of choices. You can contact every contractor that turned up in your search until you find what you need. This could be time-consuming. And even if you find someone suitable, you would still have to check references.

Where else could you find the information you need? Maybe someone who works with people with physical disabilities would know. This opens a long list of possibilities: occupational therapists and physiotherapists, organisations supporting people with disabilities and social prescribing services. You decide to ask a friend who is a physiotherapist.

Your friend does not have the answer but says, 'Gosh, Jack So-and-So just had his kitchen remodelled to accommodate his wheelchair.' This is an excellent lead. Jack will almost certainly be able to give you the name of someone who does the kind of work you are seeking. He can also probably give you some ideas about the cost and hassle before you go any further. Unfortunately, though, Jack turns out to be not much help. He didn't have a great experience, so he doesn't have much information that can help you. Now what?

Your next step might be trying to find a person in your community who is a 'natural resource'. There are people like this in every community. These 'naturals' or 'connectors' seem to know everyone and everything about their community. They tend to be people who have lived a long time in the community. And they are very involved in it. They are also natural problem solvers. This is the person who other people turn to for advice. And they always seem to be helpful and have useful information.

The natural in your community could be a friend, a business associate, the postman, your GP, your pet's vet, the assistant in the local shop, the pharmacist, a bus or taxi driver, the school secretary, an estate agent, or the local librarian. Think of this person as an information resource.

Sometimes the natural will taste the thrill of the hunt and, like a modern-day Sherlock Holmes, announce 'the game is afoot!' and promptly join you in your search. For example, you ask the postman, and he tells you about a contractor whose wife uses a wheelchair. He knows this because the man just did a great job on a kitchen that is on his delivery route. You contact the contractor and find everything you need.

Let's review the lessons from this example. The most important steps in finding the resources you need are these:

1. **Evaluate your condition or situation and identify the problem.**

2. **Identify what you want or need.** Ask what you can do to improve your condition or situation and ask what you want to do to improve your condition or situation.

3. **Look for resources.**

4. **Ask friends, family, and neighbours for ideas.** (If you belong to online groups, ask members of those groups too.)

5. **Contact organisations that might deal with similar issues.**

6. **Identify and ask naturals.**

One last note: the best investigator follows several clues at the same time. This will save you lots of time and shorten the hunt. Watch out, though—once you get good at thinking about community resources creatively, you may become a natural in your own right!

Resources for Resources

When you need to find goods or services, there are certain resources you can call on. One resource often leads to another. The natural is one of those resources, but a community resource 'detective's kit' needs a variety of useful tools.

Internet search engines (Google, Bing, Yahoo, etc.) are the most frequently used tools. These are particularly helpful if you are looking for someone to employ. For most searches, this is where you will start.

Organisations and Referral Services

Almost every community has one or more information and referral service. Sometimes these are related to a geographic area such as a town or county. For example, Kent County Council has a comprehensive website where people can access information about local services for people with specific health needs. Other times they are specific to a group, such as Carers UK. Sometimes they are specific to a particular disability or condition, such as Versus Arthritis. Several types of organisations operate these services. Your local social prescribing service (which you can access via the Internet or your GP) will be able to tell you about the range of organisations operating in your area. Use search terms such as 'local care organisation' and 'adult care services'. If you are using a telephone directory, be sure to check your county or town or borough or area listings.

Once you have the telephone number of a reliable information and referral service, your searches will become much easier. These services maintain huge files of referral addresses and telephone numbers. They can help you find information about almost any issue you might have. Even if they don't have the answer you seek, they will almost always be able to refer you to another service that can help.

Charitable organisations such as the British Heart Foundation and Macmillan Cancer Support are great resources. They provide up-to-date information about health issues, as well as support and direct services. They also fund research intended to help people live better with their condition and to some day lead to a cure. For a small fee, you can generally become a member of one of these organisations. Often, this puts you on the list to receive regular bulletins by post or email. But you do not have to be a member to qualify for their services. They are here to help the public. Many of these organisations have wonderful websites. Websites can be accessed anywhere at any time if you have Internet access. In cyberspace, you can live in rural Wales or the Highlands of Scotland and get help on the web from the Stroke Association.

There are other organisations in your community offering information and referral services along with direct services. These include Citizens Advice, local community health and well-being services, advicelocal.uk (for questions about benefits, work, money, housing problems, etc), adult care services, community centres, and social service agencies. These organisations offer information, classes, recreational opportunities, nutrition programmes, legal and tax help, and social programmes.

Most religious groups also offer information and social services to people who need them.

They provide services directly through a place of worship or through groups such as the Salvation Army. To get help from religious organisations, start with the local place of worship. People there can help you or refer you to someone who can help you. You usually do not need to be a member of the congregation or even of the religion to receive help.

Another option is to contact your local GP surgery or hospital. Healthcare professionals and social prescribing link workers are good resources and know about the physical and mental health services available through healthcare organisations.

At a national level GOV.UK is the United Kingdom public sector information website, which provides a single point of access to HM Government services, such as vehicle licencing.

The NHS England website is an excellent resource for people needing information about long-term conditions. It provides information about the full range of services available through the NHS, and also provides advice, tips, and tools to help you make the best choices about your health and well-being. There are equivalent NHS websites available in Northern Ireland, Scotland, and Wales.

Freephone NHS 111 (landline or mobile phone) and 111.NHS.uk (online) are available 24 hours a day, seven days a week. They help people get the right advice or treatment they need for their physical or mental health. In many cases NHS 111 clinicians and call advisers can give people the advice they need without using another service such as their GP or A&E. NHS 111 can also make direct appointments at GP surgeries, pharmacies, and Urgent Treatment Centres (UTCs), as well as sending an ambulance should your condition be serious or life-threatening.

Libraries

Your public library is a particularly good resource if you are looking for information about your long-term condition. Libraries are not just collections of books. The resources your library can connect you to are vast and varied. Even if you are an experienced library detective, it's a good idea to ask the librarian to make sure you haven't overlooked something. Librarians see volumes of material cross their desks daily and are knowledgeable about the community (they may even be local naturals). If you cannot get to the library, you can call or contact them online via your local authority website.

Books

Books can be useful (indeed, you are reading a book now!). Many condition-related books contain reading and resource lists either at the ends of chapters or at the back of the book. These lists can be very helpful.

The Reading Agency is a national charity that provides the Reading Well website, which aims to support people in understanding and managing their health using helpful reading. The Reading Well for long-term conditions section of the website provides information and support for people living with a long-term health condition and their carers. The booklist covers general advice and information about living with a long-term condition, common symptoms, and titles focused on specific conditions such as arthritis, bowel conditions, diabetes, heart disease, and stroke. The books have all been recommended by people with lived experience of long-term conditions and healthcare professionals and are available to borrow for free from public libraries.

Newspapers and Magazines

Your local newspaper, especially if you live in a smaller community, can be an excellent resource. Most newspapers publish both paper and online versions. Be sure to look for your local calendar of events page. On this page you can get an idea of the organisations that are active in your community. Even if you are not interested in a featured event, calling the contact telephone number may help you find what you are looking for. News stories might also be of interest, especially the local stories in the pages around the calendar section. If you are looking for an exercise programme for people with your health problem, for example, look in the local activities section.

Sometimes you can find clues in the classified section. Look under 'announcements', 'health', or any other heading that seems promising. Review the index of classified headings to see which headings your newspaper uses.

At a local bookshop or newsagents you can find a variety of general health magazines that can be useful. For example, some publications focus on specific health conditions such as diabetes or arthritis. You can also find many of these on the Internet.

See the Useful Websites section at the end of this chapter for information about how to contact the organisations we have referred to in this section.

The Internet

Today most people have access to the Internet. If you are not an Internet user, you probably know an Internet user. Even if you do not have a computer, smartphone, or tablet, you can use one in your local library or ask a friend for help. The Internet is the fastest-growing source of information. New information is being added every second of every day. The Internet offers information about health and anything else you can imagine. It also provides several ways in which you can interact with people all over the world. For example, someone who has Gaucher disease, a rare health condition, might find it difficult to find others locally who have the same condition. The Internet can put the person in touch with a whole group of such people; it doesn't matter whether they are across the street or on the other side of the world.

The good thing about the Internet is that anyone can maintain a website, a Facebook or other social networking page, a blog, or a group. That is also the bad thing about the Internet. There are virtually no controls over who is posting information or whether the information is accurate or even safe. This can mean that even though there is a lot of information out there that might be very useful, you may see incorrect or even dangerous information. You should never assume that information found on the Internet is entirely trustworthy. Unless you are confident that the information obtained is from a reputable source (like the NHS), approach it with scepticism and caution. Ask yourself, is the author or sponsor of the website clearly identified? Is the author or source reputable? Does the information contradict what everyone else seems to be saying about the subject? Does the information make common sense? What is the purpose of the website? Is someone trying to sell you something or win you over to a point of view?

One way to determine the purpose of the website is to look at the URL (the address located at the top of the screen, starting with http://). For example, the URL for the Royal Osteoporosis Society is:

https://www.theros.org.uk/

At the end of the main part of a UK-based website's URL, you will most commonly see .edu, .ac, .org, .gov, or .com. For non-U.S. websites, the very last letters will represent the country of origin. Many websites end in .com, so you will have to investigate whether a site is affiliated with a school, not-for-profit organisation, government agency, or commercial enterprise. You may also see others, such as .biz or .info. This gives you a clue about the nature of the organisation that owns the website. College or university website addresses end in .edu or .ac. Not-for-profit organisation website addresses end in .org. UK government agency website addresses end in .gov. Commercial organisation website addresses end in .com.

As a rule of thumb, .edu, .org, .ac, and .gov are fairly trustworthy sites (although be aware that a not-for-profit organisation can be formed to promote just about anything). A website address with a URL that ends with .com is usually a commercial organisation trying to sell you a product or service. This doesn't mean that a commercial website can't be a good one. On the contrary, there are many outstanding commercial sites dedicated to providing high-quality,

trustworthy information. The BMJ (formerly known as The British Medical Journal) signalled by bmj.com is one such example. These sites are often able to cover the costs of providing this service only by selling advertising or by accepting grants from commercial firms.

In the case of the example we used earlier, www.theros.org.uk/, we know that www. stands for World Wide Web; theros stands for The Royal Osteoporosis Society; .org tell us it is a not-for-profit organisation, and .uk tells us it is a United Kingdom website. When you search for government websites in the UK, it is advisable to add .uk at the end of the address. Without this you may be referred to U.S. sites. Although these are likely to be reliable, they do not have information relating specifically to the UK situation.

A note of caution should be added about the use of the website Wikipedia. This is a free Internet encyclopaedia that is created by general users. These users are able to change or edit anything on the site, and although most of the information is accurate it is not always so. There are some editorial controls in place but care needs to be taken when using it.

The Internet and Social Networking Sites

Most people know about search engines such as Google. But many don't know about Google Scholar, which lists peer-reviewed science articles. Peer-reviewed articles are checked for accuracy and trustworthiness by panels of professionals in the field. You can use Google Scholar just like Google to find the scientific literature on almost any topic. In your search results, you can always see the short abstracts for the articles. Often you can see the entire articles as well.

Social networking sites and blogs are everywhere on the Internet. Sites such as Facebook, Twitter, and Instagram are currently very popular, but everything might change by the time this book is published! These sites enable the average person to communicate easily with others who want to listen (or read). Some sites, such as Facebook, require that users choose who will be allowed to read the thoughts they post. Others, such as Blogger, are more like personal journals that are open to anyone who finds them on the Internet.

You can find people living with long-term health conditions who are eager to share their experiences on these sites. Some have discussion forums where groups of people get together to share information and opinions. The information and support on these sites can be valuable but be cautious: some sites propose unproven and dangerous ideas.

Discussion Groups on the Internet

Yahoo, Google, and other websites offer discussion groups for just about anything you can imagine. Anyone can start a discussion group about any subject. The people who start the groups typically run these groups. For any single health condition, there may be dozens of discussion groups. You can join them and the discussions if you wish, or you can just 'surf' (read without interacting). For a person with Gaucher disease, for example, a discussion group may allow them to connect to people who share their experiences. This may be the only opportunity to talk with someone else with

their rare condition. For someone with bipolar disorder, it might be difficult to talk with someone face-to-face about their mental health concerns. To find discussion groups, go to the Google or Yahoo (or other) search engine home page and search for a link to 'groups'. Check to see that the group has a moderator who enforces the rules of the group. Some condition-specific charities also run discussion groups. For example, you can access the Diabetes Support Forum (an online community where you can exchange knowledge and experiences with other people with diabetes, family and carers) on the Diabetes UK website.

Please keep in mind that the Internet changes by the second. Our guidelines reflect conditions at the time this book was written.

Technology Enabled Care Services (TECS)

The term 'Technology Enabled Care Services' (TECS) refers to technologies that help people to manage and control long-term conditions and sustain independence. They enable the remote exchange of information, primarily between a patient and a healthcare professional, to assist in diagnosing or monitoring health status or promoting good health.

TECS aim to empower people and support them to take greater control of their own health and care, working in partnership with health and care professionals, families, carers, and the voluntary sector. Increasingly TECS are being seen by the NHS as convenient, accessible, and cost-effective ways of providing care for people with long-term conditions, as they have the potential to transform the way in which people can engage in and control their own healthcare, empowering them to manage their care in a way that is right for them.

TECS include:

- **Telehealth.** The remote monitoring of people in their own homes to anticipate an increase in severity of a condition or symptom and to help build their self-care skills

- **Telecare.** Technologies used in people's homes and communities to minimise risk and provide urgent notification of adverse events

- **Telemedicine and Teleconsultations.** Remote peer-to-peer support between clinicians and consultations between patients and clinicians

- **Telecoaching.** Telephone advice from a coach to support people in building their knowledge, skills, and confidence to change behaviours

- **Self-care apps.** Applications that raise awareness and help people self-manage

There are hundreds of thousands of health 'apps' (short for 'mobile application', designed for use on a mobile device, such as a mobile phone or tablet) available for download. The NHS Apps Library is therefore a good place to start your search for trusted health and well-being apps. The apps included in the NHS Apps Library have been assessed to be clinically safe and secure to use and can help people take an active role in managing their own physical and mental health.

Becoming an effective resource detective is one of the jobs of a good self-manager. We hope that this chapter has given you some ideas about how to determine what you need and how to find help in your community. Knowing how to search for resources will serve you better than simply being handed a list of resource agencies.

Useful Websites

advicelocal: https://advicelocal.uk/find-an-adviser

Age UK: http://ageuk.org.uk/

Blogger: https://www.blogger.com/

British Heart Foundation: http://bhf.org.uk/

Carers UK: https://www.carersuk.org/

Citizens Advice: https://citizensadvice.org.uk/

Diabetes UK (Diabetes Support Forum):
    https://www.diabetes.org.uk/how_we_help/community/diabetes-support-forum

Facebook: https://en-gb.facebook.com/

Gauchers Association: https://www.gaucher.org.uk/

Google Scholar: http://scholar.google.com/

GOV.UK: https://gov.uk/

Instagram: https://www.instagram.com/

Kent County Council: https://kent.gov.uk/social-care-and-health/

Macmillan Cancer Support: https://macmillan.org.uk/

NHS 111: https://111.nhs.uk/ or telephone 111

NHS Apps Library: https://nhs.uk/apps-library/

NHS England: https://nhs.uk/conditions/

NHS Northern Ireland: https://nidirect.gov.uk/services/health-conditions/

NHS Scotland: https://nhsinform.scot/illnesses-and-conditions/

NHS Wales: https://nhsdirect.wales.nhs.uk/

Reading Well: https://reading-well.org.uk/books/books-on-prescription/long-term-conditions/

Royal Osteoporosis Society: https://theros.org.uk/

Salvation Army: https://salvationarmy.org/

Stroke Association: https://www.stroke.org.uk/

The British Medical Journal (BMJ): https://www.bmj.com/

Twitter: http://twitter.com

Versus Arthritis: https://versusarthritis.org/

Wikipedia: https://wikipedia.org/

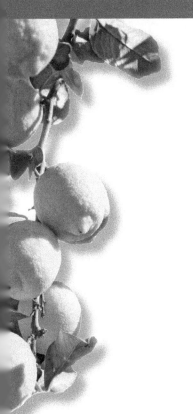

CHAPTER 4

Understanding and Managing Common Conditions

*I*N THIS CHAPTER WE DISCUSS SOME OF THE MOST COMMON long-term conditions, including heart disease, lung disease, and arthritis. Diabetes is discussed in a separate chapter (Chapter 14, *Managing Diabetes*) because there are many specific self-management issues involved in living with diabetes.

Even if we do not list and discuss your specific condition in detail, this book is still for you. Across long-term conditions, self-management skills are more common than different. A good way to learn more about your condition is to search the internet for the national organisation that supports your specific condition. For example, Parkinson's UK, Cancer Research UK, and the MS Society all have helpful resources for people who live with those conditions.

Heart Disease, High Blood Pressure, and Stroke*

The medical community knows a lot about the treatment of heart disease, high blood pressure, and stroke. There are many ways to prevent and treat these life-threatening conditions. Most people with heart conditions, and even many of those who have had strokes, can look forward to long, healthy, and enjoyable lives.

There are many forms of heart disease. Sometimes the problem is a physical block. For example, in atherosclerosis, the arteries that supply the heart muscle are clogged. Atherosclerosis causes coronary artery disease (CAD). Sometimes the problem is due to muscular damage. When a person has heart failure, the heart muscle is damaged and unable to push blood effectively to the lungs and the rest of the body. When the valves inside the heart are damaged, the result is valvular heart disease. Blood may not effectively reach the rest of the body. The electrical system that controls the beating of the heart can also be disrupted. This causes the heart to beat too fast, too slow, or abnormally. (When the heart beats irregularly, it is called arrhythmia.) In this section, we discuss all of these heart problems as well as other problems with the circulatory system, including strokes and high blood pressure.

Understanding Coronary Artery Disease

Coronary artery disease (CAD), which is caused by atherosclerosis, is the most common form of heart disease. CAD causes most heart attacks and heart failure. Coronary arteries are blood vessel 'pipelines' that wrap around the heart. (See Figure 4.1 on the next page.) The coronary arteries deliver oxygen and nutrients that the heart needs to perform its job. Healthy arteries are elastic, flexible, and strong. The inside lining of a healthy artery is smooth, so blood flows easily. When a person has atherosclerosis, their arteries narrow as they become clogged with cholesterol and other substances. The blocked or narrowed area is called a stenosis.

Atherosclerosis is a gradual process that occurs over many years. The first step is damage to the wall of the artery. High cholesterol, high triglycerides (the fats you use for energy which come from the fatty food you eat), diabetes, smoking, and high blood pressure can all cause damage. This damage allows the low-density lipoprotein cholesterol (LDL cholesterol, the 'bad' cholesterol) to enter the artery wall and cause inflammation. Some people have this damage as early as their teens.

---

*Special thanks to Eleanor Levin, MD, for contributions to this section. For the UK edition, special thanks to Northern Ireland Chest, Heart & Stroke (NICHS), Louise Heron RN DipHE, SCHN Bsc Hons, and Rachael Thornton BPharm(Hons), PGClinDip, MRPharmS, IP, MFRPSII, for their contributions to and review of this section.

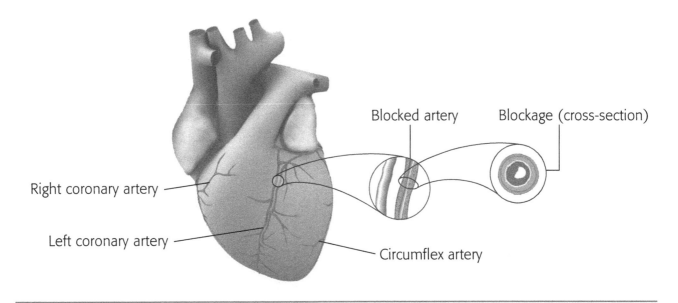

Figure 4.1 **The Arteries of the Heart**

Over time, more cholesterol is deposited in the arteries. Fatty areas called plaques grow larger and larger. Plaques can completely block off blood flow in an artery. Plaques can also crack open, causing blood clots. When blood flow to the heart is blocked, angina (temporary chest pain) or a heart attack can occur. A heart attack is also known as a myocardial infarction (MI). If a heart attack is not treated immediately, permanent damage to the heart muscle can result. When a part of the heart muscle has been damaged, that part can no longer effectively pump blood.

The pain of angina or a heart attack may be on the left side of the chest over the heart, but the pain may also spread to the shoulders, arms, neck, and jaw. Some people with angina or a heart attack also experience nausea, sweating, shortness of breath, and fatigue. These are the most common symptoms for men.

Symptoms of heart disease in women may be different to men's symptoms. Women may feel a subtler pressure, squeezing, fullness, or pain in the centre of the chest. They may also feel burning or numbness that can spread to the back or shoulders. Or women with heart disease may be unusually tired and experience shortness of breath, nausea, cold sweats, dizziness, and anxiety. These symptoms are subtler than the crushing chest pain often associated with men's heart attacks. This may be because women tend to have blockages not only in their main arteries but also in the smaller arteries that supply blood to the heart. This condition is called small vessel heart disease.

Many women show up in A&E after heart damage has already occurred. This is because their symptoms are not the ones that most people think of as heart attack warnings. Be familiar with all the symptoms of heart attack and stroke and seek help. It is important to get treatment as soon as possible to dissolve blood clots and prevent heart or brain damage. Minutes matter! (See 'Seek Emergency Care Immediately' on page 50.)

Seek Emergency Care Immediately

When you have heart attack or stroke symptoms, *you must seek medical help immediately.* New treatments are available that can dissolve or remove blood clots in the blood vessels of the heart and brain. These restore blood flow and prevent heart or brain damage. However, these treatments *must be given within hours of the heart attack or stroke* – the sooner, the better. Call 999 if you have any of the following symptoms. *Do not wait!*

Heart Attack Warning Signs:

- Severe, crushing, or squeezing chest pain

- Pain or discomfort in one or both arms, the back, neck, jaw, or stomach

- Chest pain lasting longer than 5 minutes when there is no apparent cause and pain is not relieved by rest or heart medications (like glyceryl trinitrate or GTN)

- Chest pain occurring with any of the following: rapid or irregular heartbeat, sweating, nausea or vomiting, shortness of breath, light-headedness or passing out, or unusual weakness. For women, chest pain may not be present with these symptoms.

If you think you are having a heart attack:

1. Stop what you are doing.
2. Sit down.
3. Call 999. *(Do not try to drive yourself to the hospital or home.)*
4. The NHS advises that while waiting for an ambulance, it may help to chew and then swallow a tablet of aspirin (ideally 300mg), as long as the person having a heart attack is not allergic to aspirin.

Minutes matter! Fast action can save a life – maybe your own. Don't wait more than 5 minutes to call 999.

Understanding Arrhythmias

People with heart disease may notice irregular heartbeats (palpitations). This is caused by irregularities in the conduction system (the electrical wiring) of the heart. Damage to this system can result in irregular heartbeats, skipped beats, or slow or racing beats. Doctors refer to these irregularities as arrhythmias or dysrhythmias.

Most irregular heartbeats are minor and not dangerous. However, there are some types of arrhythmias that cause problems. Dangerous arrhythmias are sometimes accompanied by episodes of fainting, dizziness, shortness of breath, or irregular heartbeats lasting minutes.

These arrhythmias may be more dangerous for people with severely weakened hearts and those with heart failure.

Sometimes the heart can beat irregularly, and you may not notice the difference. If you notice irregular heartbeats, take note of how frequently they occur, how long they last, how fast your heart is beating (check your pulse or fitness monitor), and how you feel during the episode. This information will help your doctor decide if your arrhythmias are dangerous. Remember that infrequent, short bouts of irregular beats are common for people both with and without heart disease. They are generally not cause for concern and should not require any change in activity or treatment.

Understanding Peripheral Vascular Disease

Peripheral vascular disease (PVD) occurs when the arteries in the legs stiffen and narrow, which blocks blood flow to the legs. PVD is also called peripheral arterial disease (PAD) or peripheral artery occlusive disease (PAOD). Atherosclerosis in the legs is usually the result of a similar disease process that happens with atherosclerosis in coronary artery disease (CAD).

The main symptom of PVD is leg pain when walking (claudication). Some people with PVD may also experience leg sores that don't heal or heal slowly. Some of the treatments for PVD are the same as those for heart disease, and they include stopping smoking (most important), exercise, medications, and sometimes surgery to help restore blood flow to the legs.

Understanding Heart Failure

'Heart failure' does not mean that your heart has stopped working or is going to stop. It means that your heart's ability to pump blood is reduced. Sometimes this is due to weakness or damage to the muscular wall of the heart. Or the walls of the heart chambers may become stiff and restrict the amount of blood available to pump out to your body. The weakness or stiffness of the heart muscle can be due to coronary artery disease, a heart attack, high blood pressure, heart valve problems, arrhythmias, diabetes, aging, or abnormalities to the heart walls or tissue around the heart (pericardial sac). The condition is sometimes called congestive heart failure because fluid tends to collect in the lungs and legs. Heart failure can be treated and its symptoms managed, even when the heart cannot be returned to normal.

What are the signs and symptoms of heart failure?

- **Excessive tiredness, fatigue, and weakness.** When your heart is not pumping with enough force, your muscles do not get enough oxygen. You may be more tired than usual and not have enough energy for normal activities.

- **Shortness of breath.** Sometimes breathing becomes more difficult due to excess fluid in your lungs. You may have trouble catching your breath, a frequent or hacking cough, or difficulty breathing when lying flat. You may wake up at night due to difficulty breathing. If you need to prop yourself up with many pillows or sleep in a recliner, this may be a sign of heart failure.

- **Weight gain and swelling.** These are common signs of heart failure. The weight gain is due to fluid retention. When your body is holding on to extra fluid, your weight goes up. Sometimes weight gain happens rapidly (in days), and sometimes it happens more slowly. You may have swelling (oedema) in your feet and ankles, your shoes and socks may be too tight, rings on your fingers may become too tight, your stomach may feel bloated, and there may be a tightness at your waistline.

- **Frequent urination.** When you urinate (pass water), your kidneys are helping your body get rid of extra fluid. You may need to urinate more often at night (nocturia) or at other times.

Self-management skills for heart failure: tracking your weight and eating a low-sodium diet

Although heart failure is a serious condition, keeping daily track of your weight, eating a low-sodium diet, and taking medications as prescribed can relieve symptoms and prevent unnecessary trips to the hospital.

It is important that you weigh yourself properly and frequently if you are to recognise signs of heart failure. Here's how to do it:

■ Weigh yourself at about the same time every day. For example, weigh yourself every morning, just after waking up (after urinating and before eating).

■ Weigh yourself each time wearing the same amount of clothing or without clothing.

■ Use the same scales. Check to be sure the scales are set to zero before weighing yourself. Make sure the scales are on a hard, even surface.

■ Write your weight in a daily weight chart or other record (a calendar works well).

■ Weigh yourself again if you have doubts about the scales or your weight.

■ Bring your daily weight chart to all your medical appointments.

■ Speak to your GP if you have a weight gain of 2 to 3 pounds (0.91 to 1.4 kilograms) or more in a day, a gain of 5 pounds (2.3 kilograms) or more in 5 days, shortness of breath, or increased swelling of feet or ankles.

In addition to weighing yourself, eat a low-sodium diet. Sodium is an important mineral that helps regulate fluid levels in your body. Too much sodium, however, makes your body hold on to too much fluid. Salt is one of our major sources of sodium. People with heart failure need to eat less sodium to avoid retaining excess fluid that can back up in their lungs and cause shortness of breath. To learn more about healthy eating and how to keep your sodium level low, see pages 245–256.

Understanding Stroke

Strokes happen when a blood vessel in the brain is blocked or bursts. When a blood vessel is not able to deliver blood to your brain, problems occur. Without blood and the oxygen blood carries, part of the brain starts to die. The part of the body or function controlled by the damaged area of the brain can't work properly.

There are two types of stroke:

■ An ischemic stroke (the most common stroke) happens when a blood clot blocks a blood vessel in the brain. The clot may form in the blood vessel in the brain or travel from somewhere else, such as the heart valves or arteries in the neck.

■ A haemorrhagic stroke happens when an artery in the brain leaks or bursts. This causes bleeding inside the brain.

Brain damage from a stroke can begin within minutes. It is important to know the symptoms of stroke and act fast (see 'Stroke Warning Signs: Seek Emergency Care Immediately' on page 53). Quick treatment to dissolve the clot within the first 4 hours (earlier is better!) can help limit

Stroke Warning Signs: Seek Emergency Care Immediately

Stroke Warning Signs: Act FAST

Use the letters in "F.A.S.T." to spot stroke signs and know when to call 999.

F	A	S	T
Face Drooping	Arm Weakness	Speech	Time to Call 999
Does one side of the face droop or is it numb? Ask the person to smile. Is the person's smile uneven or lopsided?	Is one arm weak or numb? Ask the person to raise both arms. Does one arm drift downward?	Is speech slurred? Is the person unable to speak or hard to understand? Ask the person to repeat a simple sentence.	If the person shows any of these symptoms, even if the symptoms go away, call 999 and get them to the hospital immediately.

Additional Symptoms of Stroke

If someone shows any of these symptoms, call 999 immediately.

Sudden Numbness	Sudden NUMBNESS or weakness of face, arm, or leg, especially on one side of the body
Sudden Confusion	Sudden CONFUSION, trouble speaking or understanding speech
Sudden Trouble Seeing	Sudden TROUBLE SEEING in one or both eyes
Sudden Trouble Walking	Sudden TROUBLE WALKING, dizziness, loss of balance or coordination
Sudden Severe Headache	Sudden SEVERE HEADACHE with no known cause
BE PREPARED	Learn more about the stroke warning signs and symptoms.

https://www.stroke.org.uk/what-is-stroke/what-are-the-symptoms-of-stroke

Minutes matter! FAST action can save a life – maybe your own. Don't wait more than 5 minutes to call 999.

damage to the brain. This increases the chance of a full recovery. If you are with someone who has these symptoms, call 999 even if the person says no. You may prevent brain damage and save a life.

Sometimes the symptoms of a stroke develop and then go away within minutes. This is called a transient ischemic attack (TIA) or 'mini-stroke'. Do not ignore these symptoms. These symptoms may be a warning sign that a stroke may soon happen. See your doctor if you have symptoms that seem like a stroke, even if the symptoms go away quickly. Getting early treatment for a TIA can help prevent a stroke.

If you have had a stroke and are recovering, you may notice improvements for several months or more. Stroke rehabilitation ('rehab') programmes can be especially helpful in recovery as well as in preventing future strokes. Rehabilitation programmes are most helpful if started as soon after a stroke as your doctor says is safe. This is usually days, not weeks, after your stroke. If you have had a stroke or are at risk of a stroke, keeping your blood pressure under control is very important. Other ways of self-managing to prevent strokes or recover from strokes include not smoking, getting regular exercise, keeping cholesterol, blood pressure (and diabetes if you have it) under control, and taking certain medications.

Understanding High Blood Pressure

High blood pressure (hypertension) increases your risk of heart disease, stroke, and kidney and eye damage. Blood pressure is a measurement of the amount of pressure in an artery. Blood pressure is expressed as two numbers. The *systolic* pressure (the higher first number) is the pressure in the artery when the heart contracts and pushes out a wave of blood. The *diastolic* pressure (the lower second number) is the pressure when the heart relaxes between contractions.

The two pressures are recorded in millimetres of mercury (mm Hg). Therefore, a blood pressure of 120/80 ('120 over 80') means that the systolic pressure is 120 mm Hg and the diastolic pressure is 80 mm Hg. Both numbers are important because a high reading for either type of pressure can cause damage.

High blood pressure is often called the 'silent disease'. Most people who have it have no symptoms and cannot really tell if their blood pressure is high without measuring it. The only way to know if your blood pressure is within normal range is to measure it. Unfortunately, because people with high blood pressure often feel perfectly well, they find it hard to believe that anything is wrong. As a result, they may not want treatment.

But the silent disease may not stay silent. Over years, untreated high blood pressure can damage blood vessels throughout the body. In some people this damage to blood vessels can cause strokes, heart attacks, heart failure, or damage to the eyes or kidneys. The reason for treating high blood pressure is to prevent these serious complications. That's why it is extremely important to treat hypertension even if you feel perfectly well.

Why do you have hypertension?

Although a family history of high blood pressure, eating too much salt, being very overweight, and drinking too much alcohol may all contribute, in most cases the exact cause is unknown. Over 90% of hypertension is called 'primary' or 'essential', which means that the cause is not known.

What is normal blood pressure?

Current NHS blood pressure guidelines are as follows, but be aware that guidelines change:

Ideal	Top number (systolic) between 90 and 120 and bottom number (diastolic) between 60 and 80
At risk	Top number (systolic) between 120 and 140, and bottom number (diastolic) between 80 and 90
High	Top number (systolic) 140 or higher, and bottom number (diastolic) 90 or higher
High (for people over 80)	Top number (systolic) 150 or higher, and bottom number (diastolic) 90 or higher

Everyone's blood pressure will be slightly different. What's considered low or high for you may be normal for someone else.

For most people, lower blood pressure usually means less risk of health complications. And for some people – for example, those with diabetes or long-term kidney conditions – it may be important to keep their blood pressure in a lower range. Note that guidelines change, and it is best to discuss appropriate targets for your situation with your doctor.

Your blood pressure varies from minute to minute. Hypertension is diagnosed when blood pressure measurements are high during two or more separate measurements. Except in severe cases, a hypertension diagnosis is never based on a single measurement. That's one reason why it is important to have repeated measurements of your blood pressure.

Self-management skills for high blood pressure: home blood pressure monitoring

Some people's blood pressure tends to go up only in the doctor's office. This is a stress reaction called 'white-coat hypertension'. It is very helpful to have additional measurements for both diagnosing hypertension and monitoring blood pressure treatment. There are many ways to get your blood pressure checked. Ask at the pharmacy, or talk to a health trainer or any healthcare professional.

You can also get a machine and take your blood pressure at home. Generally, blood pressure devices with an appropriately sized arm cuff are preferred over wrist or finger monitors. Check with your doctor or pharmacist before buying a home blood pressure device.

When using a home device, collect three or four blood pressure readings. See how these change depending on what you are doing. Follow the instructions carefully to get accurate results, including resting 5 minutes and keeping your feet flat on the floor. To help ensure accuracy take your blood pressure device and a record of your readings with you to the GP so that your machine and readings can be checked against your medical records. If your home measurements indicate that your pressure is rising over time, be sure to tell your doctor. Sometimes your GP can arrange for 24-hour ambulatory blood pressure monitoring. A blood pressure monitor is attached to your arm and records your blood pressure at regular intervals over the 24 hours. This gives the doctor more detailed information about your blood pressure.

Blood pressure can often be lowered by a combination of lifestyle changes (low-sodium diet, exercise, maintaining a healthy weight, limiting alcohol) and, when needed, medications. Understandably, some people are reluctant to use these medications due to fear of side effects. The surprising news is that many people with high blood pressure feel better with less fatigue and fewer headaches when they take the medications. If you are concerned or unsure about any of your medications you should arrange a medication review with your GP or pharmacist.

Treating Heart Disease, High Blood Pressure, and Stroke

There are many ways to prevent and treat heart disease, high blood pressure, and stroke. Patients with heart conditions, high blood pressure, and stroke often benefit from lifestyle changes (healthy diet, exercise, stress management, no smoking, limiting alcohol, etc.). Some patients may also benefit from medications, heart procedures, and surgery. In this section we discuss these options, beginning with medications.

Medications for a Healthy Heart*

People used to think that they should take heart medication only if lifestyle changes such as healthy eating and exercise failed to improve their condition. Newer research suggests that the way to get the greatest benefit is to combine certain medications with lifestyle changes.

A variety of medications are available to treat heart conditions and high blood pressure. Some of the medications may reduce symptoms such as chest pain, shortness of breath, fatigue, dizziness, or swelling. Some of these medications are also very useful in preventing future heart attacks, stroke, and kidney damage. Depending on the type of condition, your doctor may recommend one or more medications to:

- reduce cholesterol and lipids (such as statins)

- lower high blood pressure and improve heart function (such as angiotensin-converting enzyme inhibitors [ACE], angiotensin receptor blockers [ARBs], diuretics, beta-blockers, and calcium channel blockers)

- strengthen the pumping of the heart muscle (such as digoxin)

- dilate blood vessels to improve blood flow to the heart to relieve chest pain (such as nitrates)

---

*Because research on medications and treatments is rapidly progressing, medication names and options may differ from the information in this chapter. Consult your doctor, a pharmacist, a recent medications reference book, or an online medications reference for the latest information or if you have specific questions. But remember that the latest treatments are not always more effective. New treatments may not have as much information about safety and how they act with other medications that have been in use for many years.

- reduce the amount of excess fluids or swelling (such as diuretics or 'water pills')

- restore or control irregular heartbeats (such as antiarrhythmics)

- thin blood and prevent clots (such as anticoagulants)

If you have heart disease, diabetes, stroke, peripheral arterial disease, long-term kidney disease, or an abdominal aortic aneurysm, be sure to consult your GP to find out if any of these heart-protective medications are right for you. If one medication is not working for you or is causing side effects, discuss this with your doctor. Together you can usually find an alternative medication that will work. The side effects of most medications are manageable compared with the serious consequences of high blood pressure, heart attack, and stroke. Most heart medications are taken for a lifetime to reduce the risk of heart disease, heart failure, and stroke. They are not addictive and usually can be used safely over many years. Do not start or stop these medications without discussing it with your doctors.

Heart and Blood Vessel Procedures and Surgery

Sometimes medications alone are not sufficient. Several types of heart procedures and surgery may be helpful, including the following:

- **Coronary or 'balloon' angioplasty.** Coronary angioplasty opens blockages and relieves the symptoms of coronary artery disease by improving blood flow to the heart. A catheter (long, narrow tube) with a balloon at the tip is inserted into the artery and inflated to widen a narrow passage in the vessel. Your doctor may choose to insert a tiny mesh tube called a stent to help keep the narrowed vessel open. Many stents contain medications ('drug-eluting stents') that may help prevent the artery from clogging up again.

- **Coronary artery bypass surgery.** Bypass surgery creates a new route for blood flow to your heart. A surgeon uses a blood vessel from your leg or chest to create a detour around the blockage in the coronary artery. One or more blocked arteries may be bypassed. The surgery usually requires several days in the hospital, and the recovery time can be weeks to months.

- **Valve replacement.** Sometimes it is necessary to have heart surgery to repair or replace a damaged heart valve.

- **Procedures and devices for rhythm problems.** Devices such as pacemakers and implantable cardioverter defibrillators (ICDs) may be permanently attached to the heart to treat abnormal heart rhythms. Another option is a procedure called cardiac ablation, where surgeons deactivate tissue in your heart that triggers an abnormal heart rhythm.

- **Endarterectomy.** Sometimes surgery is done on the carotid arteries in the neck to remove plaque blockage and reduce the risk of stroke.

Self-Management Skills for Heart Disease, High Blood Pressure, and Stroke: Lifestyle Changes and Nonmedication Treatments

There are three general approaches to help prevent and treat heart conditions: lifestyle changes, medications, and procedures, such as surgery. Lifestyle changes are very important and should be combined with the medication or surgery options just discussed.

Heart attacks, strokes, and high blood pressure can often be prevented or controlled by making the following lifestyle changes:

- **Not smoking.** Smoking damages the inner lining of the blood vessels and raises blood pressure. Quitting is the best thing you can do for your health. For more information on smoking, see pages 109–113.

- **Exercising.** Exercise strengthens your heart. It can also lower your cholesterol and blood pressure and help you control your weight. Inactive people more than double their risk for heart disease. Even small amounts of daily physical activity can lower your risk of heart disease and help you feel better and have more energy. For more information, see 'Exercising with Heart Disease and Stroke' on pages 60–62 in this chapter, Chapter 7, *Being Physically Active*, and Chapter 8, *Exercising to Make Life Easier*.

- **Eating less 'bad' fat.** The type of fat you eat is important. Certain types of fats in the diet can raise cholesterol levels and cause fatty deposits called plaque to build up and narrow your blood vessels. The higher your LDL ('bad') cholesterol level, the greater your risk for heart disease. For information on good and bad fats and healthy eating, see Chapter 10, *Healthy Eating*. Unfortunately, not all cholesterol can be controlled by what you eat. The body also makes cholesterol, which means that some people have a genetic tendency to produce too much cholesterol and consequently medications may be necessary. No matter how it is done, through lifestyle changes or medications or both, lowering cholesterol considerably reduces the risk of heart attacks and strokes.

- **Eating less salt.** Salt contains sodium and too much sodium can cause high blood pressure. High blood pressure means your heart works harder to pump blood around your body. The NHS recommends that adults should eat no more than 6g of salt a day (2.4g of sodium), which is around 1 level teaspoon. This includes salt you add to your food and salt that is already in it. The American Heart Association recommends that people with high blood pressure or heart disease should eat no more no more than 3.75g of salt (1.5g of sodium) per day. Some food labels may only state the sodium content – don't confuse salt and sodium figures. To convert salt to sodium, you need to divide the salt amount by 2.5. For example, 2.5g of salt per 100g is 1g of sodium per 100g. Read labels and watch for hidden salt and sodium in foods, especially processed foods. See Chapter 10, *Healthy Eating*, for tips on reducing sodium. The British Heart Foundation has produced a short guide called *Taking Control of Salt* to explain how eating too much salt can cause high blood pressure, which can lead to a heart attack or stroke. It also provides practical tips on how to cut down on salt. You can download this guide at https://www.bhf.org.uk/informationsupport/publications/healthy-eating-and-drinking/taking-control-of-salt.

Some people with heart failure may also be advised by their doctor to limit their daily fluid intake.

- **Maintaining a healthy weight.** Being overweight makes your heart work harder and can raise your LDL ('bad') cholesterol and blood pressure and increase your chances of developing diabetes. Even losing a few excess pounds can often bring blood pressure down. The highest risk is excess weight around the midsection. Regular exercise and healthy eating are the most important steps to help prevent weight gain, maintain weight, or lose weight. See Chapter 7, *Being Physically Active*, Chapter 8, *Exercising to Make Life Easier,* and Chapter 10, *Healthy Eating.*

- **Managing emotional stress and social isolation.** Stress raises your blood pressure and heart rate, which can damage the lining of the blood vessels. This can lead to heart disease. See the section on stress in Chapter 5, *Understanding and Managing Common*

Symptoms and Emotions, and Chapter 6, *Using Your Mind to Manage Symptoms.*

- **Limiting alcohol.** If you drink alcohol, do so in moderation. The NHS advises men and women not to drink more than 14 units per week on a regular basis. This is equivalent to drinking no more than 6 pints of average-strength beer (4% ABV) or 7 medium-sized glasses of wine (175ml, 12% ABV) a week. To keep health risks from alcohol at a low level, spread your drinking over 3 or more days if you regularly drink as much as 14 units a week, and if you want to cut down try to have several drink-free days each week. Drinking more alcohol increases such dangers as alcoholism, high blood pressure, obesity, stroke, breast cancer, suicide, and accidents.

- **Limiting recreational drugs:** Recreational drug use such as marijuana (cannabis) may also increase your risk of stroke and heart disease.

- **Controlling diabetes.** If you have diabetes, your risk for heart disease more than doubles because high blood glucose damages the blood vessels and nerves. By controlling your blood glucose and taking certain heart-protective medications, you can greatly lower the risk of heart attack and stroke. See Chapter 14, *Managing Diabetes.*

- **Controlling high blood pressure.** Healthy blood pressure is critical to reducing the strain on your heart as well as preventing stroke.

The combination of a healthy lifestyle, selective use of medications, and heart procedures has dramatically lowered the risk of heart attack, stroke, and early death. People who have experienced heart disease and stroke can live long, full lives. It is up to you to eat well and exercise, manage stress, and take your medications as prescribed. If you do your part, your healthcare team will be much more effective. Part of good care and self-management for people with serious heart conditions involves planning for the future and making their wishes known regarding end-of-life issues and medical care (see Chapter 16, *Planning for the Future: Fears and Reality*).

Exercising with Heart Disease and Stroke*

Exercise can be both safe and helpful for many people with heart conditions, including those who have had bypass surgery. Work closely with your healthcare professionals to find the best exercise programme for your needs. Regular, well-chosen exercise is an important part of treatment and rehabilitation. Exercise can lower your risk for future problems, reduce the need for hospitalisation, and improve your quality of life. You can find more information about exercise in Chapter 7, *Being Physically Active*, and Chapter 8, *Exercising to Make Life Easier.*

When Not to Exercise with Heart Disease

With some heart conditions, you must limit the kinds and amount of exercise you do. Follow your doctor's advice about exercise and exertion if you have poor blood flow to the heart (ischemia), if you experience irregular heartbeats (arrhythmia), or if your heart is unable to pump enough blood to the rest of your body. Your doctor may want to change your treatment before giving you clearance to exercise. For example, if

you have an arrhythmia, your doctor may want to treat you with a medication that controls your heartbeat. Remember to always check with your doctor or cardiac nurse before starting a new exercise programme.

Exercising with Heart Disease

The British Heart Foundation has produced a booklet called *Keep Your Heart Healthy*, which advises people living with heart conditions to speak to their doctor, nurse, cardiac rehab team, physiotherapist or exercise specialist about the best way to increase their physical activity (see the 'Useful Websites' section at the end of this chapter for more information). This is especially important if you are not used to doing any physical activity. In addition, the target heart rate when exercising will be different for people living with a range of heart conditions. This is why it is necessary to speak with your healthcare professionals to take advice on your individual safe range.

There are many different ways to keep active and it's important to find activities that are safe

---

*For the UK edition, special thanks to Brid Cronin, Senior Physiotherapist Cardiac Rehabilitation, for contributions to this section.

and right for you. It is also important to gradually build up your activity levels. The following are exercise considerations for people with different kinds of heart conditions.

■ Make sure you warm up for 15 minutes and cool down for 10 minutes before and after doing any exercise.

■ Strengthening activities such as isometrics (which involves tightening muscles while not moving), weightlifting, or rowing can increase blood pressure and stress your heart. This can be dangerous if you have uncontrolled high blood pressure or your heart has trouble pumping. If you and your doctor think strengthening is important for you, pay special attention to not holding your breath while you exercise. Remember to breathe out as you exert. One way to be sure to breathe is to count out loud or breathe out through pursed lips.

■ If you have not exercised since your heart condition began, you and your doctor may decide that supervision by experienced professionals is a good way to start. Cardiac rehabilitation ('cardiac rehab') programmes usually provide a mix of exercise and education sessions tailored to each individual. They may take place in a hospital or community setting such as a leisure centre, or even at your home. A cardiac rehab programme offered by a hospital is free of charge. Exercise sessions which you might do as an ongoing programme may have a small cost attached, but you will continue to be monitored by specially trained exercise advisers. Some Heart Support Groups organise cheaper exercise classes. You can find out where your nearest cardiac rehabilitation programme is by visiting http://www.cardiac-rehabilitation.net or by calling the British Heart Foundation Heart Helpline (see the 'Useful Websites' section at the end of this chapter for more information.)

■ Once your doctor clears you for activity, keep the intensity well below the level that causes symptoms such as chest pain or severe shortness of breath. For maximum benefit your heart exercise should feel 'somewhat hard', which means you should feel slightly warm, have no angina or palpitations (though you feel your heart is beating harder or faster than when you are sitting), and can comfortably keep going for another 10 to 15 minutes. You should always be able to 'walk and talk'. If you become so breathless that you cannot talk, slow down or stop until you can breathe easily and then continue.

■ If your heart has decreased pumping strength, avoid activities that cause you to strain. Try conditioning activities such as light calisthenics (gymnastic-type exercises to achieve fitness), walking, swimming, and stationary cycling.

■ Exercising while lying down – such as swimming or pedalling a recumbent stationary bicycle (a bicycle that places the rider in a laid-back reclining position) – can help improve the efficiency of the heart's pumping action. This is less tiring than exercising while standing up.

■ Be especially cautious about outdoor exercise when it is very cold, hot, or humid. Stay hydrated, especially on hot days, unless you have been told to restrict fluids.

■ Always remember that if you develop new or different symptoms, such as chest pain, shortness of breath, dizziness, rapid or irregular heartbeat, excessive sweating, feelings of unusual and excessive tiredness or unusual pain (not associated with muscle soreness, which can be anywhere in your body) you should stop what you are doing and contact your doctor.

Exercising with Stroke

If you have had a stroke that affected your arm or leg, you may have had physical and occupational therapy. You may recognise many of the exercises in this book (Chapter 8, *Exercising to Make Life Easier*) as the ones you did in therapy. If you are still seeing a physiotherapist or doing a home exercise programme, talk with the therapist about adding new activities. If you are making your own exercise decisions now, you can use the exercises in this book to continue to improve flexibility, strength, endurance, and balance.

If you have weakness in your arm or leg or have trouble with balance, it is important that you think of safety when you choose which exercises to do. Some ideas for adapting exercises to meet your needs include having another person with you when you exercise, sitting instead of standing, and using a table, sturdy chair, or wall rail for support. You can also think of ways for your stronger side to help your weaker side. For example, a stationary bicycle with toe clips on the pedals allows your stronger leg to help

both legs exercise. Doing arm exercises holding a walking stick or towel in both hands allows both arms to move. Remember, even if your arm or leg weakness is permanent, you can still increase your physical activity and general health with exercise.

If you are nervous about falling when exercising at home, speak to your GP about a referral to an NHS Falls Prevention Programme or ask for a balance assessment, which will be carried out by a physiotherapist.

Exercising with Peripheral Vascular Disease (Claudication)

The leg pain (claudication) that develops during exercise generally limits exercise for people with peripheral vascular disease (PVD). The good news is that conditioning exercises can help improve endurance and reduce leg pain for most people. Start with short walks or by cycling short distances. Continue to the point when you start to have leg pain. Stop and rest or slow down until the discomfort eases and then start again. At the beginning, repeat this cycle for just 5 to 10 minutes, increasing the time gradually as you get more comfortable. Many people find that they can gradually increase the length of time they can walk comfortably or exercise with this method. A good goal is to be able to walk or cycle for at least 30 minutes. You can do this either all at one time or in three 10-minute sessions. This benefits both circulation and fitness levels. If leg pain continues to keep you from being physically active, talk to your doctor about your options. Remember, arm exercises won't usually cause leg pain, so be sure to include them as an important part of your overall conditioning programme.

Long-term Lung Disease*

Shortness of breath, tightness in the chest, wheezing, persistent coughing, and thick mucus: if you have long-term lung disease, these symptoms may be all too familiar. When your lungs aren't working well, you may have trouble getting enough oxygen to your organs. You also may not be able to get rid of unhealthy waste air containing carbon dioxide. There are many types of lung disease; the most common are asthma, chronic bronchitis, and emphysema. In each of these diseases, something gets in the way (an obstruction) of the airflow in and out of your lungs. We often refer to chronic bronchitis and emphysema as chronic obstructive pulmonary disease (COPD). Asthma, chronic bronchitis, and emphysema often overlap, so you may have one or more of them.

Because research on medications and treatments is rapidly progressing, medication names and options may differ from the information in this chapter. Consult your doctor, a pharmacist, a recent medications reference book, or an online medications reference for the latest information or if you have specific questions. But remember that the latest treatments are not always more effective. New treatments may not have as much information about safety and how they act with other medications that have been in use for many years.

Pulmonary function tests (PFTs or spirometry tests) are useful to evaluate your lung problem and the types of treatment that might help you. Although treatment varies somewhat depending on the specific symptoms and disease, many of the principles and strategies of long-term lung condition management are similar. Self-management involves taking appropriate medications, adjusting and managing your medications, self-monitoring symptoms and lung function, avoiding irritants and triggers, using breathing exercises, and adjusting physical activity and exercise. You will find information on all of these self-management tools in this section.

Understanding Asthma

With asthma, inflammation and swelling of the airways causes the muscle in the walls of the airways to tighten (bronchospasm) (see Figure 4.2). The airways (bronchioles) in the lungs are very sensitive. Irritants such as smoke, pollens, dust, or cold air make the lung muscles contract and the airways narrow (see Figure 4.3). As the airway narrows, the flow of air is obstructed or blocked. This causes an 'asthma attack', characterised by shortness of breath, coughing, chest tightness, and wheezing. (Wheezing is the high-pitched whistling sound you hear when air pushes through your narrowed airways.) Asthma attacks are also called flares or flare-ups. The goal of treatment for an attack is to relax the temporarily tightened airway muscles.

*Special thanks Roberto Benzo, MD, Mindful Breathing Lab, Mayo Clinic, for contributions to this section. For the UK edition, special thanks to the Enhanced Respiratory Service Team (Bury & Rochdale Care Organisation), Northern Ireland Chest, Heart & Stroke (NICHS), and Rachael Thornton BPharm(Hons), PGClinDip, MRPharmS, IP, MFRPSII for their contributions to and review of this section.

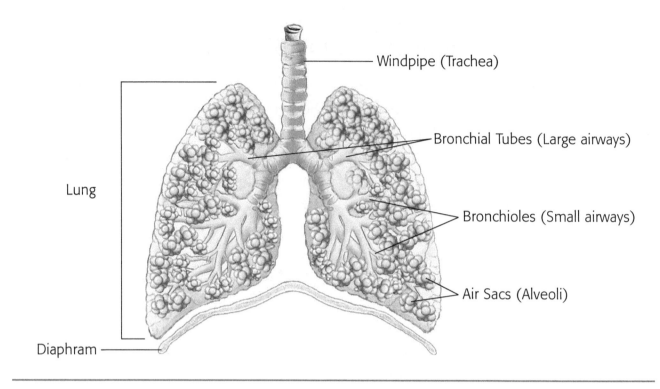

Figure 4.2 **Normal Lungs**

Irritants (sometimes called triggers) make the muscles contract and also cause inflammation of the airways (see pages 69–71 for more information about irritants and triggers). When this happens, the airways swell and produce mucus. To make things worse, the lining of the airways also releases chemicals that make them even more sensitive to irritants. This causes a vicious cycle leading to more bronchospasm and more inflammation.

Medications that relax the muscles in the airways (bronchodilators) can treat an acute flare-up of asthma, but that may not be enough. Effective treatment must include avoiding irritants and the use of anti-inflammatory medications such as corticosteroids. You may need to take anti-inflammatory medications *even when you have no symptoms.* These medications reduce the swelling, inflammation, and excessive sensitivity of the airways.

Asthma varies greatly from person to person. Symptoms may include mild wheezing or shortness of breath at night (asthma symptoms can be worse during sleep). Your attacks may be mild and infrequent or severe and life threatening. You can manage asthma, but you must be

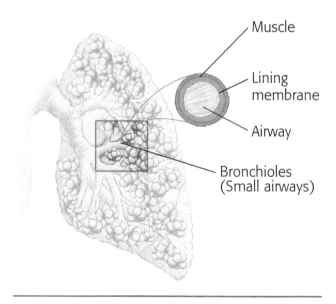

Figure 4.3 **The Bronchiole or Small Airway**

an active partner. Learn your triggers and avoid them. Take action to prevent symptoms and acute attacks. Your healthcare professional may also teach you to monitor your lung function. Your doctor or nurse will give you an asthma management plan, which will help you to manage your asthma. Learn how to breathe well, exercise properly, and use medications effectively. Although these measures cannot completely cure or reverse the condition, they can help you reduce symptoms and live a full, active life. Active self-management should allow you to participate fully in work and leisure activities, sleep through the night without coughing or wheezing, and avoid urgent visits to the GP or A&E department.

Understanding Long-Term Bronchitis

When you have long-term bronchitis, the walls inside your airways become swollen and thick. This inflammation narrows the airways and interferes with breathing. The inflammation also causes the glands that line the airways to produce large amounts of thick mucus. You may have a long-term cough that produces excessive amounts of mucus and shortness of breath.

Smoking is the primary cause of long-term bronchitis. Air pollutants, dust, and toxic fumes can also inflame and swell the airways. The keys to management are to stop smoking, use bronchodilator medications, take advantage of pulmonary rehabilitation services, and avoid being around second-hand smoke and other irritants. If you do these things, especially early in the disease, you can often prevent it from becoming worse. If you have long-term bronchitis, get an influenza (flu) vaccine injection once a year

and a one-time pneumococcal pneumonia vaccine. If you have a lung condition or are above age 65, you may need a second pneumonia vaccination. Try to avoid exposure to anyone who has a cold or flu. These infections can make bronchitis much worse. Your doctor may also recommend the use of medications to thin and liquefy mucus as well as occasional treatment with antibiotics and steroids if symptoms get worse. Symptoms may include increased cough with yellow-brown sputum, increased shortness of breath, or fever.

Understanding Emphysema

Emphysema damages the tiny air sacs (alveoli) at the very ends of the airways (see Figure 4.2). The air sacs lose their natural elasticity, become overstretched, and often break. When the air sacs are damaged, it is harder for your blood to get oxygen and to get rid of carbon dioxide. The tiniest airways also narrow, lose their elasticity, and tend to collapse when you breathe out. This traps the stale air in the air sacs and prevents fresh air from coming in.

Emphysema can destroy a large amount of your lung tissue before you have any symptoms. This is because most of us have more lung capacity than we need. However, eventually the lung capacity decreases to the point where you begin to notice shortness of breath with activity or exercise. As the condition progresses, shortness of breath is triggered by less and less activity. It may be present even at rest. You may also have a cough that produces mucus.

Smoking is the major cause of emphysema. Although cigarette smoking is by far the most common and most dangerous cause of emphysema, vaping and cigar and pipe smoking are also damaging. Even if you do not smoke or vape, daily exposure to second-hand smoke can damage your lungs. It is important that your home, car, and workplace be smoke-free. There is also a rare hereditary type of emphysema, called alpha-1 antitrypsin deficiency, that people get who do not have enough of the enzyme that protects the elastic tissue in the lungs.

Emphysema tends to get worse over time, especially if you continue smoking. The key to preventing emphysema from worsening is avoiding all smoking and vaping and becoming physically active. Although quitting smoking sooner rather than later is better, quitting at any stage of the disease can help preserve your remaining lung function. People with emphysema can benefit from a variety of self-management skills, from proper breathing to exercise. Self-management skills can help you lead an active life. Twenty minutes of daily physical activity, such as walking, is proven to slow the progress of both long-term bronchitis and emphysema. Medications and oxygen, which we discuss later in this section, can sometimes be helpful in emphysema management as well.

Treating Long-Term Lung Disease: Medications*

Medications cannot cure long-term lung disease, but they can help you breathe easier. Effective management of a lung condition often involves more than one medication. Do not worry if you are prescribed several medications. Depending upon the type of lung condition, you may be prescribed the following:

■ **Bronchodilator medications** relax and open airways in patients with asthma and COPD. Usually inhaled, these medications act quickly and are used as needed to treat suddenly worsening symptoms or before exercising. A commonly used bronchodilator is a salbutamol inhaler. Always carry these 'reliever' inhalers with you so you will have them at the first sign of increasing symptoms. Long-acting bronchodilator medications may be combined with a steroid medication to help people who have frequent flare-ups.

■ **Anti-inflammatory medications** are sometimes referred to as 'preventer' inhalers. These gradually reduce the inflammation and swelling of the airways and decrease

---

*For the UK edition, special thanks to the Enhanced Respiratory Service Team (Bury & Rochdale Care Organisation), Northern Ireland Chest, Heart & Stroke (NICHS), and Rachael Thornton BPharm(Hons), PGClinDip, MRPharmS, IP, MFRPSII, for their contributions to and review of this section.

Because research on medications and treatments is rapidly progressing, medication names and options may differ from the information in this chapter. Consult your doctor, a pharmacist, a recent medications reference book, or an online medications reference for the latest information or if you have specific questions. But remember that the latest treatments are not always more effective. New treatments may not have as much information about safety and how they act with other medications that have been in use for many years.

sensitivity to irritants and allergens. The most commonly prescribed anti-inflammatory medications are inhaler corticosteroids. Long-acting bronchodilators also have some anti-inflammatory properties and are not rapid acting. They are therefore not helpful for the immediate treatment of severe asthma attacks. Sometimes you may be prescribed a short course of oral corticosteroid medications to treat more severe COPD attacks. It is very important to take oral corticosteroid medications exactly as prescribed each day. Oral corticosteroid medications are generally safe in short courses.

■ **Mucolytics** may be prescribed to help make the mucus thinner and easier to cough up. However, there is limited evidence about how effective these medications are.

■ **Specific antibiotics** are also sometimes prescribed for a prolonged time for chronic lung conditions where you have had repeated infections.

Some medications relieve symptoms, whereas others prevent symptoms. Some medications are used to both treat and prevent symptoms. When the medications are being used to prevent symptoms, they must be taken regularly, *even when symptoms are not present.* Too often people stop taking their medications because they feel better. As your symptoms improve, discuss with your doctor which medications to continue and which may be reduced or stopped.

Some people worry that they will become addicted to their medications or that they may become 'immune' and no longer respond to the medication. None of the medications used to treat lung conditions are addictive. Nor do patients become 'immune' to the medications. If your medications are not controlling your symptoms, discuss this with your GP so that you can make adjustments. And stay tuned. New medications are being introduced that hold great promise for improving a long-term lung condition. If you are concerned or unsure about any of your medications, you should arrange a medication review with your GP or pharmacist.

Metered-Dose Inhalers

You can inhale some lung medications, including bronchodilators and corticosteroids. They come in a special canister called a metered-dose inhaler (MDI). When used properly, inhalers are a highly effective way to quickly deliver medication. By breathing the medication directly into the lungs it can act faster and more effectively. This can also reduce side effects. The key to using a metered-dose inhaler is to first exhale gently to empty your lungs and then inhale slowly through your mouth at the same time as you press down on the MDI canister to release the medication. Hold your breath for 10 seconds and then wait a minute before taking any additional puffs. This gives the previous puff time to work. Always read the instructions, and if you are not sure ask your pharmacist or nurse for advice.

There are many different devices to deliver medication. Some devices have a spacer or chamber into which you first spray the medication from the inhaler. You then inhale the medication from the spacer. The spacer makes it more likely that you can inhale the smaller, lighter droplets of medication further into your airways. The spacer also collects some of the larger, heavier droplets of medication that would otherwise settle in your mouth or throat. This can reduce side effects, such as oral yeast infections in the case of inhaled steroids.

Dry powder inhalers (DPIs) deliver medication in powder form. DPIs are used without a spacer. When using a dry powder inhaler, exhale first and then inhale *rapidly and deeply*. Note that in contrast to the *slow* inhalation for metered-dose inhalers, with dry powder inhalers the inhalation needs to be *rapid*. Many inhalers have counters built in so you can easily tell how many doses are left.

If you are prescribed an inhaler, be sure to get help in using it properly. Pharmacists or other healthcare professionals can help you learn the most effective and safe technique to use your inhaler. Using an inhaler properly is more difficult than swallowing a pill. It takes proper instruction and some practice. (See 'Tips for Correctly Using an Inhaler'. Asthma UK has also produced a series of short videos on how to use your inhaler properly – see the 'Useful Websites' section at the end of this chapter.) One study revealed that although 98% of patients said they knew how to use their inhalers properly, 94% made errors in using them. So even if you think you are an expert, have a health professional check out your technique every so often. Be sure to get clear instructions for your specific type of device. Improper use of inhalers is one of the primary reasons for difficulty in controlling symptoms. If you are using two types of inhalers, use the 'reliever' (bronchodilator) medication *first*. Wait several minutes for it to open up the breathing tubes so that the 'preventer' (inhaled anti-inflammatory) medication can get into your lungs better. After using

Tips for Correctly Using a Metered-Dose Inhaler

Be sure to:

- shake the canister
- hold the inhaler upside down (mouthpiece should be on the bottom)
- exhale before inhaling with the inhaler
- breathe through your nose
- inhale slowly
- hold your breath for 10 seconds
- never use an empty inhaler

an inhaler, rinse your mouth with water. This is especially important with inhaled anti-inflammatory medications. If you are unsure about using your inhalers, your pharmacist will be able to give you some advice.

Nebulisers

Nebulisers deliver 'quick relief' medication as a fine mist. These machines are used in the clinic or A&E to give a 5- to 10-minute 'breathing treatment'. Some people who cannot use an inhaler with a spacer may also use a nebuliser at home. Nebulisers can be a great help when you have a sudden flare-up of symptoms. However, when done correctly, taking four to six puffs of 'quick relief' medication from an inhaler works just as well as a breathing treatment with a nebuliser.

Oxygen Therapy

Some people with long-term lung conditions cannot get enough oxygen from ordinary air because their lungs are damaged. If you are tired and short of breath because there is too little oxygen in your blood, your doctor may order oxygen. Oxygen is helpful only if your oxygen level is low. It is not addictive. But some people try not to use it for fear of becoming dependent. Other people do not like to be seen with oxygen equipment. Supplemental oxygen can provide the extra boost your body needs to remain comfortable and enable you to do the things you want and need to do without extreme shortness of breath. Most important, oxygen therapy may slow down your condition and make your brain function better. Some people may require continuous oxygen, whereas others may need oxygen only to help them with certain activities, such as exercise or sleep.

Oxygen comes in large tanks of compressed gas or small portable tanks either as a gas or a liquid. If you are using oxygen, be sure to know the proper dose (flow rates, when to use it, and for how long), how to use the equipment, and when to order more. Do not worry: your oxygen tank will not explode or burn. However, oxygen can help other things burn, so keep the tank at least 10 feet away from any open flame, including cigarettes (which hopefully are not anywhere near you!). Oxygen concentrators are often used instead of cylinders, as they are safer and more convenient. There are also portable versions available.

Medications that Trigger Symptoms

Some medications, including anti-inflammatory medications such as aspirin, ibuprofen, naproxen, and beta-blockers (such as propranolol) can cause wheezing, shortness of breath, and coughing. ACE-inhibitor medications, such as ramipril and lisinopril, can also cause a dry, tickling long-term cough. If you suspect that you have symptoms related to a medication, do not stop your medication, but do talk to your doctor or pharmacist to get it reviewed.

Self-Management Skills for Long-Term Lung Disease*

In addition to taking appropriate medications, self-management of long-term lung conditions includes quitting smoking, being physically active, avoiding irritants and triggers and infections, and managing stress.

Quitting Smoking

Smoking is the main cause of long-term bronchitis and emphysema. Smoking is also a major trigger of asthma. Whether you smoke yourself or are around people who smoke, smoking irritates and damages the lungs. The poisonous gases in smoke paralyse the cilia, the tiny hair like 'sweepers' in your airways that help clean out dirt, mucus, and germs. The carbon monoxide in tobacco smoke robs your blood of oxygen and makes you feel tired and short of breath. The irritation from smoking makes infections more likely. This same irritation can permanently damage the air sacs in your lungs. Unfortunately, once your air sacs

*For the UK edition, special thanks to the Enhanced Respiratory Service Team (Bury & Rochdale Care Organisation), Northern Ireland Chest, Heart & Stroke (NICHS), and Rachael Thornton BPharm(Hons), PGClinDip, MRPharmS, IP, MFRPSII for their contributions to and review of this section.

are destroyed, they cannot be repaired. The good news is that most of these harmful effects can be eliminated by quitting smoking or vaping and avoiding second-hand smoke.

If you have tried to quit tobacco and failed, do not give up. This is a common experience. Get help. See the section on 'Smoking and Breathing Issues' on pages 109–113 for more information on how to quit smoking. You can search on the internet for the numbers of free NHS smoking cessation helplines in England, Scotland, and Wales. You can also search local Stop Smoking Services, which have trained advisers to support you either one-to-one or in a group. Your GP can refer you or you can phone your local stop smoking service to make an appointment with an adviser. This is not something you have to do on your own.

Physical Activity and Long-Term Lung Disease

An increase in physical activity greatly helps people with a long-term lung disease. Regular physical activity can increase the capacity of your heart and lungs. It can also improve your sense of well-being. You can choose your physical activities (see pages 170–177) and adjust your medications before exercising to prevent exercise-induced asthma. Always discuss with your GP or physiotherapist about how to include physical activity in your life. Do not miss out on this important part of managing your lung condition.

Air Pollution

Car exhaust, industrial wastes, household products, aerosol sprays, and wood smoke can irritate sensitive airways. On particularly smoggy days, check your radio or TV for air pollution alerts. Or check the Met Office website or a recommended app. If air quality is poor, stay indoors as much as possible.

Cold Weather or Steam

For some people, very cold air can irritate the airways. If you can't avoid the cold air, try breathing through a cold-weather mask (available at most pharmacists) or a scarf. For some people, steam, as from the shower, can also be a trigger.

Allergens

An allergen is anything that triggers an allergic reaction. If you have asthma, an attack may be triggered by almost anything you are allergic to (indoors and out). Avoiding your allergens completely can become a full-time job. Still, a few sensible measures significantly reduce exposure.

To avoid outdoor allergens, close the windows and use a portable air conditioner (if you have one) when pollen and mould spore counts are high. For some people, major allergic triggers are found indoors in the form of house dust mites, animal fur, and moulds. Often pets (dogs, cats, and birds) must be removed from the house or at least from bedrooms. Give dogs and cats a weekly bath to reduce allergens. House dust mites live in mattresses, pillows, carpets, upholstered furniture, and clothing. If dust mites are a trigger for you, vacuum your mattress and pillows and then cover them with an airtight cover. Wash bedding, including blankets and bedspreads, weekly in hot water. Avoid sleeping or lying on upholstered furniture. Remove carpets from the bedroom. If possible, avoid dusting and vacuuming and use a damp mop instead. All of this takes time, but in the long run the effort will pay off.

Perfumes, room deodorisers, fresh paint, and some cleaning products can trigger asthma symptoms. Sometimes indoor air cleaners can be helpful in reducing allergens in the air. Foods can be triggers for some people. The worst offenders are peanuts, beans, nuts, eggs, shellfish, and milk products. Food additives (such as preservatives in wine and dried apricots) can also sometimes trigger asthma symptoms.

If you cannot identify your triggers, allergy testing may be helpful. Immunotherapy ('allergy injections') help desensitise some people to certain allergens.

In addition to breathing problems, some people with long-term lung conditions also have gastric reflux. If you have gastric reflux, acid from your stomach backs up and irritates your oesophagus and airways. This may or may not cause heartburn symptoms. The irritation of the airways may cause coughing or trouble breathing. To treat reflux, keep your head and chest elevated when sleeping; avoid smoking, caffeine, and foods that irritate the stomach; and when necessary, take antacids and acid-blocking medications.

Infections

For individuals with lung problems, colds, flu, sinus infections, and infections of the airways and lungs can make breathing more difficult. Though you can't prevent all infections, you can reduce your risks. Get your flu and pneumonia vaccinations. Try to avoid people who have colds, wash your hands frequently, and don't rub your nose and eyes. Talk with your doctor about how to adjust your medications if you get an infection. Early treatment can often prevent serious illness and hospitalisation.

Emotional Stress

Stress does not cause long-term lung disease. However, it can make symptoms worse by causing your airways to tighten and your breathing to become rapid and shallow. Many of the breathing exercises, relaxation, and meditation exercises in this book (see Chapter 5, *Understanding and Managing Common Symptoms and Emotions*) can help prevent symptoms from getting worse. Learning how to manage your condition can also help you to feel more in control and less stressed.

Self-Monitoring Long-Term Lung Disease*

A lung condition changes over time. Sometimes it will be under better control than at other times. By monitoring your symptoms, you can often predict when a flare-up is coming and take action to keep it from getting worse.

There are two ways to self-monitor a lung condition. It is important to use at least one of them. For best results, use both symptom monitoring (for asthma, COPD, bronchitis, and emphysema) and peak flow monitoring (for asthma).

*For the UK edition, special thanks to the Enhanced Respiratory Service Team (Bury & Rochdale Care Organisation), Northern Ireland Chest, Heart & Stroke (NICHS), and Rachael Thornton BPharm(Hons), PGClinDip, MRPharmS, IP, MFRPSII, for their contributions to and review of this section.

Symptom Monitoring (for Asthma, COPD, Bronchitis, Emphysema)

Symptom monitoring requires that you pay attention to your symptoms and how they change. The following signs can tell you that a flare-up is coming:

- Symptoms (coughing, wheezing, shortness of breath, chest tightness, fatigue, increased or thickened sputum, or new fever) are worse, occur more often, or are greater in number than usual.

- More puffs than usual are needed of 'reliever' medication (such as a salbutamol inhaler), or the medication is required more often than twice a week (other than for physical activity).

- Symptoms cause you to wake up more frequently or interfere with work, school, or home activities.

If you have any of these symptoms, discuss them with your GP or other healthcare professional and develop a personal action plan (see page 73).

Peak Flow Monitoring (for Asthma)

This method of self-monitoring uses a tool called a peak flow meter. A peak flow meter measures whether your breathing tubes are open enough for normal breathing. Peak flow measurements can let you know when a flare-up is starting (*even before symptoms increase*). Peak flow measurements can also help you figure out how bad the flare-up will be.

If you have moderate or severe asthma, your peak flow meter can become your best friend.

Your peak flow meter can help you manage your asthma better. It can alert you to problems before they become severe. It can help you and your doctor know when to increase or safely reduce medications. It can help you distinguish between worsening asthma and breathlessness caused by anxiety or hyperventilation.

If you do not have a peak flow meter or are not sure how to use one, ask your healthcare professional. To use one, you need to measure your personal best peak flow when you are feeling well and in good control. This personal best measurement allows you to take quick action when your peak flow begins to drop. Because different meters can give different readings, use the same meter all the time.

When the peak flow reading is closer to your personal best measurement, your breathing tubes are more open and your asthma is under better control. When the peak flow reading is farther from your personal best, your breathing tubes are more closed. Even if you feel OK, a lower peak flow reading can warn you that a flare-up is starting. That means that you need to take action and adjust your medications.

Keep track of your symptoms and peak flow measurements by writing them in an asthma diary. (A healthcare professional can give you one, or you can make your own.) An asthma diary can help you understand what triggers your asthma, whether your medications are working, and when flare-ups are about to begin.

Work out an individual plan of action with your doctor as soon as you can. Asthma UK believes that everyone with asthma can benefit from using an asthma action plan.

A personal asthma action plan tells you, and anyone with you:

- which medication you take every day to prevent symptoms and cut your risk of an asthma attack

- what to do if your asthma symptoms are getting worse

- the emergency action to take if you're having an asthma attack and when to call 999.

You can download an asthma action plan template from the Asthma UK website (see the 'Useful Websites' section at the end of this chapter), which you can fill in with your GP or asthma nurse, so it's personal to you and your asthma. You can also do this by telephone or video call if your appointment isn't in the surgery. Ask them to save a copy onto your notes and send it to you by email, text message, or via WhatsApp.

If you wait until your symptoms get worse, they will be more difficult to treat. Early action and adjustment of your medications can make a critical difference.

Breathing Better

In addition to medications, there are other things you can do to improve your breathing. In this section we describe some self-management strategies to help you breathe better with a long-term lung condition.

Breathing exercises

A person breathes in and out nearly 18,000 times a day. It is not surprising that breathing is a central concern of people with lung conditions. Yet many people find it surprising that proper breathing is a skill that has to be learned. Breathing

properly is especially important for people with a lung condition. Breathing better will enhance the functioning of your respiratory system.

Pursed-lip breathing helps people living with asthma or COPD when they experience shortness of breath. This technique helps control shortness of breath, provides a quick and easy way to slow your pace of breathing, and makes each breath more effective. To use this simple technique, first breathe in naturally through your nose as if you are smelling a rose. Then breathe out slowly through tightly pressed (pursed) lips as if you are blowing out a candle (see page 107).

Diaphragmatic or *abdominal breathing* strengthens respiratory muscles (especially the diaphragm) and removes stale, trapped air from the lungs. One of the primary reasons why people with lung conditions feel short of breath and can't seem to get enough air in is that they don't get the old air out. Breathing exercises can help you empty your lungs more completely and take advantage of your full lung capacity. (See pages 106–107 for instructions on how to perform the diaphragmatic breathing technique.)

Good posture

If you are slouching or slumped over, it can be very difficult to breathe in and out. Certain positions make it easier to fill and empty your lungs. For example, if you are sitting, you may be able to breathe better if you lean forward from the hips with a straight back. It may also help to rest your forearms on your thighs or rest your head, shoulders, and arms on a pillow placed on a table. Or use several pillows at night to make breathing easier. See page 108 for more information.

Clearing your lungs

When excess mucus blocks your airways, it can be difficult to breathe. Your GP or asthma nurse may recommend certain exercises, positions, or devices to help you clear the mucus. Ask your doctor or asthma nurse if any techniques or devices might be helpful for you. Also remember that drinking at least six glasses of water a day (unless you have ankle swelling or are told to limit fluid intake by your doctor) may help liquefy and loosen mucus. See pages 105 and 108 for more information.

Exercising and Healthy Eating with Long-Term Lung Disease*

Eating well and exercising are two important self-management tools you can use to feel better and live a healthier life with long-term lung disease.

Exercising with a Long-Term Lung Disease

Exercise is among the simplest and best ways to improve your ability to live a full life with a long-term lung condition. Physical activity strengthens muscles, improves mood, increases energy level, and enhances efficiency of the heart and lungs. Although exercise does not reverse the damage disease causes to the lungs, it can improve your ability to function within whatever limits you have due to your lung condition.

When you start to exercise, it is very important to begin at a low intensity (for example, a slow rather than a brisk walk) and for short periods of time. You can gradually increase what you do as you find that you can do more with less shortness of breath. You will get the most benefit and enjoyment from an exercise programme if you communicate with your healthcare professionals to manage your symptoms and adjust medications.

Here are a few tips for exercising with long-term lung conditions:

- Some people with asthma may cough or wheeze when they exercise. If you do, discuss with your doctor if you can use two puffs of a fast-acting 'reliver' such as salbutamol 15 to 30 minutes before you start to exercise.

- Mild shortness of breath is normal during exercise, but if you become severely short of breath with only a little effort, your doctor may want to change your medications. It may take you some time to find the right combination of effort and medication to stay in your comfort zone.

- Take plenty of time to warm up (15 minutes) and cool down (10 minutes) during conditioning activities. Warming up and cooling down should include exercises

---

*For the UK edition, special thanks to the Enhanced Respiratory Service Team (Bury & Rochdale Care Organisation), Northern Ireland Chest, Heart & Stroke (NICHS), and Rachael Thornton BPharm(Hons), PGClinDip, MRPharmS, IP, MFRPSII, for their contributions to and review of this section.

such as pursed-lip breathing and diaphragmatic or abdominal breathing. (See pages 106–107.)

■ Exercise can be worrying if you are afraid of getting too short of breath. Everyone experiences a normal 'anticipatory' increase in heart rate and breathing rate even before exercise begins. Pursed-lip and diaphragmatic breathing can help you relax and stay calm.

■ Pay attention to your breathing. Make sure you breathe in deeply and slowly, and use pursed-lip breathing when you breathe out (see pages 107–108). Take two or three times longer when breathing out as you do breathing in. For example, if you are walking briskly and notice that you can take two steps while you're breathing in, breathe out through pursed lips over four to six steps. Breathing out slowly helps you exchange air better and may increase your endurance.

■ Remember that arm exercises may cause shortness of breath and a faster heart rate sooner than leg exercises.

■ Cold and dry air can make breathing and exercise more difficult. This is why swimming is an especially good activity for people with a long-term lung condition. Wearing a scarf or a mask over your face in cold weather may prevent the cold air from triggering asthma.

■ Strengthening exercises such as calisthenics, light weightlifting, and rowing may be helpful, particularly for people who have become weakened or deconditioned due to medications or other causes.

Choose any combination of physical activities you like (such as walking, gardening, and cycling) and can tolerate. The most important thing is to just do it.

Exercising with a Severe Lung Disease

If you can get out of bed, you can exercise 10 minutes a day. Every hour get up and walk slowly across the room or around a table for 1 minute. Doing this 10 times a day gives you 10 minutes of exercise. You can increase the time and distance of this daily exercise routine gradually as you feel stronger and more comfortable moving. Here are some things to remember as you start to get more active:

■ Don't hurry. Many people with lung conditions hurry to complete their exercise before their breath runs out. It is much better to slow down. Move slowly, breathing as you go. At first, this will take a real effort. With practice, you will find that you can go further more comfortably. If you are afraid to try this alone, have someone walk with you, carry a chair (a folding 'walking stick chair' might be useful), or use a walker with a seat so that you can sit down if necessary.

■ As you begin to feel stronger and more confident, walk 2 minutes every hour. You have just doubled your exercise and are now up to 20 minutes a day. When this feels comfortable, change your plan to walking 3 to 4 minutes every other hour. Do this for another week or two, and then try 5 minutes three or four times a day.

Next, try 6 to 7 minutes two or three times a day. Most people with a severe lung condition can build up to walking 10 to 20 minutes, once or twice a day, within a couple of months.

■ If being on your feet is a problem, try using a restorator (a portable exercise pedal bicycle for arms and legs). This is especially helpful if you have a low level of endurance, do not have standby help, or are afraid of exerting yourself too much. The restorator lets you sit where you are and use your legs to pedal. It's a good device to build confidence and get accustomed to physical activity in a secure atmosphere.

Healthy Eating with Lung Disease

Changing your eating habits will not cure long-term lung conditions, but it can help you feel better. Good nutrition makes being physically active easier, and it may help you to manage your emotions and fight infections. Most important, if you are obese, even a small weight loss through healthier eating (see page 253) can greatly improve breathing. If you are underweight or are losing weight and strength, talk to your GP for guidance.

Asthma, long-term bronchitis, and emphysema can be significantly improved. By working in partnership with your healthcare team, you can come up with a personal plan to reduce

Sleep Apnoea

If you snore and tend to feel sleepy during the day, you may have a type of breathing problem called sleep apnoea. If you have sleep apnoea, your throat blocks the flow of air during sleep. For short periods of time (10 seconds or more), you may stop breathing (this is called apnoea). If you have sleep apnoea, you probably don't know it until someone says something to you about your snoring. This condition is one of the most common undiagnosed serious health problems today.

Sleep apnoea may cause you to wake up feeling tired or with a headache, and it may make you feel sleepy or have trouble concentrating throughout the day. Sleep apnoea can also lead to more serious problems such as high blood pressure, heart disease, and stroke. It can even mimic the memory problems seen in dementia and Alzheimer's

disease. Sleep apnoea is diagnosed by doing a sleep test in a laboratory or wearing a small monitor at home.

You can treat sleep apnoea at home by making lifestyle changes. Losing weight if needed can be particularly important. Sleeping on your side, avoiding alcohol, not smoking, and using medication to relieve nasal congestion and allergies may also be helpful. After you have been tested, your doctor may recommend you use a breathing device. These continuous positive air pressure (CPAP) devices use gentle air pressure to keep tissues in the throat from blocking your airway. Sometimes this can make a big difference in quality of sleep and energy during the day. Your doctor may also recommend using a dental device (oral breathing device) or surgery to keep your airway open.

the symptoms and improve your ability to live a rich, rewarding life. The goal is to be confident that you can manage your condition and control your symptoms so that you can do daily activities, exercise, sleep comfortably, and avoid going to the hospital or A&E.

Long-Term Arthritis and Osteoporosis*

The word *arthritis* means 'inflammation of a joint'. However, as it has come to be used, the term now commonly refers to virtually any kind of inflammation or damage to a joint. Although most forms of arthritis cannot be cured, you can learn to reduce your pain, maintain your mobility, and use medications to manage symptoms, control the condition, and slow it down. The most common form of long-term arthritis is osteoarthritis. Osteoarthritis is the arthritis that generally affects people as they age. Symptoms include knobby fingers, painful hips, swollen knees, or back pain. Osteoarthritis is not caused by inflammation, although sometimes it may result in inflammation of a joint. It involves a wearing away of the cartilage that cushions the ends of bone and degeneration of the bones, ligaments, and tendons associated with the joint. The cause of osteoarthritis is not precisely known.

Many other kinds of long-term arthritis are due to inflammation. When the inflammation is caused by your own immune system attacking your joints, the most common forms are rheumatoid arthritis and psoriatic arthritis. In gout or pseudogout, crystals in your joints cause the inflammation. With these inflammatory diseases, the thin membrane lining the joint (synovium) becomes inflamed and swollen and makes extra fluid. As a result, the joint becomes swollen, warm, red, tender, and painful, and you may lose range of motion. If it continues, inflammatory arthritis can also result in destruction of cartilage and bone. If this destruction is not stopped, it can ultimately lead to deformity and loss of function.

Arthritic diseases do not affect joints only. Arthritis can result in cartilage loss and damage to nearby bone, ligaments, and tendons. Tendons attached to muscles move the joints, and ligaments stabilise the joints. When your joint lining is inflamed or the joint is swollen or deformed, those tendons, ligaments, and muscles can be affected. The tendons, ligaments, and muscles may become inflamed, swollen, stretched, displaced, thinned out, or even torn. There are also lubricated surfaces to make the movement easy in many places where tendons or muscles move over each other or over bones. These surfaces are called bursas. Bursas may also become inflamed or swollen, causing bursitis. In this way arthritis of any kind does not simply affect the joint.

---

*Special thanks to Stanford Shoor, MD, and Jeffrey Brown, MD, for contributions to this section. For the UK edition, special thanks to Versus Arthritis and Jean Thompson, MBE, for contributions to this section.

It can affect all the structures in the area around the joint.

Understanding Arthritis

There are different forms of arthritis. We describe each in more detail here.

1. **Osteoarthritis** is caused by the inability of cartilage to repair itself. The damage develops slowly, and inflammation can be present.

2. **Inflammatory arthritis** may be an 'auto-immune' disorder that is caused by your body's immune system inappropriately attacking and inflaming the joint lining. There are three general types of inflammatory arthritis: rheumatoid, spondyloarthritis, and psoriatic (which is actually a type of spondyloarthritis). Joint damage can occur quickly in inflammatory arthritis, so it is important to identify it and start treatment early. Some forms of inflammatory arthritis, such as Lyme disease or streptococcal and virus illnesses, may appear with infections. These types usually get better with antibiotic treatment or with time, but sometimes they become long-term. Rheumatoid arthritis is a disease in which the body's immune system appears to play a role in causing the disease. These types of illness are also called autoimmune diseases.

3. **Crystalline arthritis** results from crystals forming inside a joint and causing intense, acute inflammation. The common names for this kind of arthritis are gout and pseudogout.

Fibromyalgia is a condition that sometimes accompanies long-term arthritis, but it can also exist alone. Though not inflammatory, fibromyalgia causes painful tender points in muscles and soft tissue as well as joint pain. The cause of fibromyalgia is not yet known, but it may be due to how the nervous system handles pain signals. Anti-inflammatory medications do not usually help, although medications such as duloxetine (*Cymbalta, Yentreve*), gabapentin (*Neurontin*), or pregabalin (*Lyrica, Alzain, Lecaent, Rewisca*) may reduce pain. Self-management skills – especially exercise – that benefit patients with long-term arthritis are also beneficial for people with fibromyalgia.

Arthritis: More Than Pain

The irritation, inflammation, swelling, or joint deformity of arthritis can cause pain. The pain may be present all the time or only sometimes, as when moving the joint. Of all the symptoms of arthritis, pain is the most common. Arthritis can also limit movement. The limitation may be due to pain, swelling that prevents normal bending, deformity of the joint ligaments or tendons, or weakness in nearby muscles.

In addition, arthritis can cause problems in areas far away from the joint. For example, if arthritis affects the joints of one of your legs, you may favour that leg during walking or other motion. This changes your posture and places an extra burden on other muscles and joints. This can create pain on the other side of your body or in other areas in addition to the site of the arthritis.

Stiffness of joints and muscles may also occur, particularly after periods of rest such as sleeping and sitting. The stiffness makes it difficult to move. If you can get going, or if you can heat the affected joint and muscles (with a hot pad or hot shower), the stiffness may lessen or disappear. For most people with osteoarthritis, the stiffness after rest usually lasts only a short time (30 to 60 minutes). In contrast, stiffness due to inflammatory arthritis, such as rheumatoid or psoriatic arthritis, typically lasts more than 1 hour, or it can last all day.

Another common consequence of arthritis is fatigue. Inflammation itself causes fatigue. So does long-term pain, and so does the effort of movement when joints and muscles don't work right. In addition, fatigue can be caused by the worries and fears that often accompany arthritis. Whatever its cause or combination of causes, fatigue is an issue many arthritis patients must confront.

Depression may also accompany long-term arthritis. People with long-term arthritis often have trouble doing what they need or want to do. This can make you feel helpless, angry, and withdrawn, which may lead to depression. Depression can make other symptoms such as pain, fatigue, and disability seem worse. It can reduce your work or social functioning. It can damage family relationships, as well as your capacity for independent living. Usually the depression comes from the difficulties caused by the arthritis and is not a long-term mental illness. Often this type of depression improves when the arthritis improves. You can also address this depression with self-management practices (see Chapter 5, *Understanding and Managing Common Symptoms and Emotions*) and, if needed, by the use of antidepressant medication.

Arthritis: What Does Your Future Hold?

Proper self-management can greatly help reduce and prevent disability from arthritis. Successful self-management depends largely on the participation of the person with arthritis and sometimes the person's family. It is not possible to predict the future accurately for any individual. It depends partly on medical treatment, partly on the individual's own self-management efforts, and partly on chance.

If left untreated, osteoarthritis has different outcomes for different people. For some people, the condition progresses steadily, causing increasing disability. For others, the condition waxes and wanes over many years, possibly getting slowly worse but maybe not. With treatment, most patients can reduce the limitations from arthritis. For some people, treatment slows or stops arthritis symptoms. However, with long-term arthritis due to inflammation, such as rheumatoid or psoriatic arthritis, joint damage can occur early in the disease. There are effective treatments for inflammatory arthritis, so it is important to see your doctor as soon as possible if you have inflammatory arthritis (see the discussion on DMARDs, page 82). There is no real cure for any of the forms of long-term arthritis. Medications usually suppress inflammation and symptoms, but with inflammatory arthritis or gout, medication must often be continued for long time periods.

Most people with long-term arthritis can lead normal or nearly normal lives. Proper use of medications and self-management practices make this possible. Do not abandon major life plans. Adjust them to meet your treatment needs, and remember that you can change treatment plans to meet your particular needs or wishes. Although arthritis can have very damaging effects, much can be done to offset or eliminate these effects. The remainder of this chapter describes appropriate management techniques and points you to helpful self-management techniques described in detail elsewhere in this book.

Treating Osteoarthritis*

Osteoarthritis is a result of a wear-and-repair process in the cartilage and bones in your joints. The wearing of the tissues causes the body to try and repair itself, but the repair process isn't perfect and sometimes causes changes to the structure of the joint. Cartilage cushions the ends of your bones and allows them to move smoothly over one another. Because of this wear-and-repair process, the bone surfaces become rough and painful when in motion. The roughness may also irritate your joint lining (the synovium), causing it to produce more than normal amounts of joint fluid. The extra fluid results in swelling. Occasionally, small pieces of damaged cartilage break off, float in the fluid, catch on a moving surface, and increase pain. Also, bone ends may grow small spurs (called osteophytes). These spurs are most common on fingers, hips, knees, and the spine. They give the knobby appearance to fingers in osteoarthritis. Although osteoarthritis can affect any joint, it most commonly affects the hands, knees, hips, shoulders, and spine. In general, symptoms of osteoarthritis increase with age.

Osteoarthritis happens when your cartilage does not repair itself. There is no specific medical treatment to prevent or stop the cartilage changes, and currently there is no cure for any of the forms of long-term arthritis. The goal of treatment is to maintain joint function and reduce pain. Surprisingly, many patients may appear to have significant osteoarthritis on examination and X-rays, but they have few or no symptoms or limitations.

If you have osteoarthritis, the saying 'use it or lose it' is particularly true. If you don't use the affected joints, they will slowly lose mobility, and your surrounding muscles and tendons will weaken. Fortunately, exercise does not make osteoarthritis worse, and as movement improves with exercise and surrounding tissues strengthen, pain often declines. For this reason, exercise is the most important part of treatment. We describe exercise later in this chapter, in Chapter 7, *Being Physically Active*, and in Chapter 8, *Exercising to Make Life Easier*. Being overweight can increase pain in your weight-bearing joints such as hips

---

*Because research on medications and treatments is rapidly progressing, medication names and options may differ from the information in this chapter. Consult your doctor, a pharmacist, a recent medications reference book, or an online medication reference for the latest information or if you have specific questions. But remember that the latest treatments are not always more effective. New treatments may not have as much information about safety and how they act with other medications that have been in use for many years.

and knees. Weight loss – even just losing a modest amount – can reduce pain in the joints commonly affected with osteoarthritis.

Cartilage needs joint motion and some weight bearing to stay healthy. Because osteoarthritis damages joint cartilage, an exercise programme also protects cartilage. In much the same way that a sponge soaks up and squeezes out water, joint cartilage soaks up nutrients and fluid and gets rid of waste products by being squeezed when you move the joint. If you don't move your joints regularly, cartilage deteriorates.

For osteoarthritic pain, the most readily available medications are acetaminophen (*Paracetamol*) and aspirin. Other medications can also be effective such as ibuprofen (*Nurofen*) and naproxen which are available on prescription (as tablets or as liquid that you drink). You can also obtain pain relief without a prescription (such as period pain medication. Brands include *Feminax Ultra, Period Pain Reliever, and Boots Period Pain Relief*). Aspirin, ibuprofen, and naproxen are nonsteroidal anti-inflammatory drugs, or NSAIDs. You can take NSAIDs in pill form, or as patches, or apply them in gel form or as cream directly to the skin. When there is no inflammation involved in the arthritis, as is commonly the case with osteoarthritis, the anti-inflammatory activity of NSAIDS is not important. The benefit from these medications, like the benefit from acetaminophen (which is not an anti-inflammatory drug), is their pain-reducing effect.

Heat and pain-controlling measures such as relaxation and cognitive distraction can be very helpful (see Chapter 5, *Understanding and Managing Common Symptoms and Emotions*, and Chapter 6, *Using Your Mind to Manage Symptoms*). Applying heat before exercise often makes exercise easier. For pain at night in hands, feet, or knees, wearing gloves, socks, and a sleeve over the knees can often improve sleep. If you sleep on your side, placing a pillow between your knees can also be helpful. Braces or other assistive devices, such as walking sticks for knee or hip osteoarthritis or knee braces for certain types of knee arthritis, may reduce pain and increase mobility.

When swelling from irritation or mild inflammation is present, the problem can often be corrected by draining the joint and injecting it with a corticosteroid medication. This sometimes has a long-term benefit.

If osteoarthritis progresses to deformity, discomfort, and weakness that make normal living impossible, surgical intervention, such as joint replacement or joint modification, may be an option. Joint replacement, such as knee or hip replacement, can reduce pain and increase function. Although joint surgery to treat osteoarthritis can be effective, you should consider surgery only if other treatments are not satisfactory.

Two additional therapies for osteoarthritis have become available. Both are thought to have the potential to improve or substitute damaged cartilage. They are glucosamine, which is taken daily in pill form, and hyaluronan, which is injected into the joint as a lubricant. Studies suggest that glucosamine provides short-term relief of symptoms in some people, similar to low doses of aspirin. However, these studies are not clear, and long-term benefits have not been established. Fortunately, glucosamine appears to have no significant adverse effects. Hyaluronan use is more complicated because it requires injections into the joint. As of the time of writing this book, neither glucosamine nor hyaluronan appear to benefit most people with osteoarthritis or other types of arthritis. If you want to consider either of these medications, you should discuss their use and appropriateness for you with your GP or consultant.

Treating Inflammatory and Crystalline Arthritis

The most common medications for long-term inflammatory and crystalline arthritis fall into the following categories:*

- **Nonsteroidal anti-inflammatory drugs (NSAIDs).** These medications have both pain-reducing and, in high enough doses, anti-inflammatory effects. They are usually the first medications used to treat inflammatory arthritis because, although they do not treat the underlying condition, they are often helpful and tend to have the least severe side effects. NSAIDs include aspirin, ibuprofen, naproxen, meloxicam, celecoxib, sulindac, and diclofenac. Acetaminophen (Paracetamol) is not an NSAID, but it is also used to reduce pain. It has no anti-inflammatory effect. Most of the NSAIDs can cause nausea or stomach upset, but this can be minimised by taking the medications with a meal or by taking medication such as omeprazole (*Losec* and *Losec MUPS*).

- **'Disease-modifying' antirheumatic drugs (DMARDs).** The term *disease-modifying* implies slower progression or reversal of inflammatory arthritis. Some of the newer medications target the substances produced by the body that cause inflammation and can be very helpful when other treatments fail. Some DMARDs are given intravenously, while others are injected subcutaneously (under the skin) or taken by mouth. They are occasionally associated with serious infections or toxic side effects. Sometimes an initially effective DMARD will lose its effectiveness and another medication will need to be used. DMARDs are not prescribed for osteoarthritis.

  In recent years, evidence has shown that earlier use of DMARDs slows the progression of disease. Because NSAIDs do not achieve such slowing, most patients with rheumatoid arthritis now receive treatment with disease-modifying agents early in the

---

*Because research on medications and treatments is rapidly progressing, medication names and options may differ from the information in this chapter. Consult your doctor, a pharmacist, a recent medications reference book, or an online medication reference for the latest information or if you have specific questions. But remember that the latest treatments are not always more effective. New treatments may not have as much information about safety and how they act with other medications that have been in use for many years.

course of their condition. This early benefit from DMARDs may also apply to other forms of long-term inflammatory arthritis. Use of these medications should be discussed with a rheumatologist (a physician with special training in treating arthritis and associated conditions).

■ **Corticosteroids.** Corticosteroids are powerful anti-inflammatory medications that also suppress the body's immune system. Both effects are helpful with inflammatory arthritis, especially for rheumatic autoimmune diseases in which the body's immune system appears to play a role. Most corticosteroids are synthetic versions of a normal human hormone called cortisol, which is present in our bodies. Corticosteroids are the most rapid acting and effective of the anti-arthritic medications. However, they may cause serious adverse effects when used for long periods of time. Prednisone is the most common corticosteroid. Prednisone is often given with another anti-inflammatory medication for a faster response. Corticosteroids can be taken in pill form or injected into a joint or muscle.

■ **Medications to treat gout.** Acute gout, which causes severe inflammation in one or a few joints, is treated with anti-inflammatory medications such as NSAIDs, corticosteroids (either in pill form or by joint or muscle injection), or colchicine. Once the inflammation is treated, the anti-inflammatory medication is slowly decreased and stopped. If flares of acute gout reoccur frequently, you may be given medications to lower uric acid blood levels and prevent flare-ups. Allopurinol (*Zyloric* and *Urictoand*) and febuxostat (*Uloric*) lower uric acid blood levels in people with long-term or recurrent gout. Once started, these medications must be taken regularly to prevent attacks.

For inflammatory arthritis, medications taken in pill form, such as methotrexate, hydroxycholorquine (*Plaquenil*) or leflunomide (*Arava*) are frequently used in combination with self-injected medications such as etanercept (*Enbrel*) or adalimumab (*Humira*). Healthcare teams determine the best combinations based on your individual response. Recent evidence shows that no one combination is clearly better than the others.

Today, many of the medications we discuss here are used for any type of inflammatory arthritis. The choice of medications depends on the person's condition and responses. Commonly, milder medications are used first, and more powerful ones are used when milder ones fail. As mentioned earlier, stronger medications are now often used earlier in rheumatoid or psoriatic arthritis to try to prevent joint destruction.

It is almost impossible to predict whether any medication will be helpful. Therefore, the treatment of long-term arthritis with medications is a trial-and-error process. For long-term inflammatory arthritis, medications other than corticosteroids only occasionally provide an immediate benefit. Corticosteroids work quickly; DMARDs usually take weeks to months before the full effects of the medications are felt.

All medications can harm as well as help. Sometimes a medication can be very helpful for your arthritis but cause so many side effects that you cannot use it. It is impossible to predict which medications will cause side effects for which patients. With some medications, patients may not recognise bad side effects. In these cases, the healthcare team must monitor patient response with liver or kidney tests, blood or urine tests, or other tests. If you are starting on any medication treatment for long-term arthritis, make sure you understand the signs and symptoms of potential harm, including rash or upset stomach. Notify your GP if these symptoms appear. Also, ask your doctor if you need regular blood or urine tests to monitor for effects of your medications.

Sometimes, despite medication treatment, joints are damaged to the point where they no longer work effectively. Fortunately, many types of joints can be replaced with modern surgical techniques. This can often significantly relieve pain and improve function, especially for hips and knees.

Self-Management Skills for Long-term Arthritis*

People with long-term arthritis can often lead productive, satisfying, and independent lives. The most important step in achieving this is to take an active part in managing your own arthritis. In addition to medications or surgery, self-management skills can help you live a healthy and active life with long-term arthritis. The goal of proper management is not only to avoid pain and reduce inflammation; it is to maintain the maximum possible use of affected joints. This involves maintaining the greatest motion of the joint and the greatest strength in muscles, tendons, and ligaments surrounding the joint. The key to this is exercise – an essential part of any good self-management programme. Exercise should be regular, consistent, and as much as you can safely tolerate. Exercise will not make your arthritis worse. In fact, failing to exercise can increase arthritis symptoms because of loss of joint mobility and physical deconditioning. Regular joint motion can decrease joint pain and swelling.

Sitting or lying down for long periods can worsen your posture, reduce your joint flexibility, and cause weakness even in your joints that are not affected by arthritis. After a period of inactivity, stiffness is common. This is especially true after sleeping. You can reduce stiffness by

---

*Because research on medications and treatments is rapidly progressing, medication names and options may differ from the information in this chapter. Consult your doctor, a pharmacist, a recent medications reference book, or an online medication reference for the latest information or if you have specific questions. But remember that the latest treatments are not always more effective. New treatments may not have as much information about safety and how they act with other medications that have been in use for many years.

doing mild exercise in bed before you get up or by taking a hot bath or shower. For some people, mild exercise before going to bed can also reduce stiffness the next morning.

You can find specific exercise information for people with arthritis later in this section. We also describe appropriate exercise programmes in detail in Chapter 7, *Being Physically Active*, and Chapter 8, *Exercising to Make Life Easier*. To maintain general physical condition, you need to exercise as many joints as possible, including your joints without arthritis. However, long-term arthritis can affect the bones of the neck. Therefore, it is best to avoid extreme neck movements or positions that can place strain on the back of the neck or head. It's also worth noting that extreme movements for any joint affected by arthritis should probably be avoided. Any form of exercise should build up in intensity only gradually.

Because heat makes exercise easier, exercise when you are warm. For example, exercise during or after a bath. Or for hands and wrists, exercise after you wash dishes. In addition to improving mobility, heat is also useful to reduce pain in joints and muscles, at least temporarily. When combined with rest, it can be very soothing. Some people find it helpful to apply ice to a warm joint.

It is important to control fatigue. Rest periods between activities and restful sleep at night are essential. (Learn more about sleeping better in Chapter 5, *Understanding and Managing Common Symptoms and Emotions*.) When pain disturbs sleep at night, different types of beds (firm beds, foam beds, air beds) can be of significant help. For some people with arthritis, low doses of antidepressant medication at bedtime will effectively control night pain and improve sleep.

When joint function remains limited, assistive devices can be helpful. Many types of devices are available, including braces, walking sticks, special shoes, grippers, reachers (used for reaching items placed overhead or on the floor), and walkers. (See Chapter 9, *Organising Your Life for Freedom and Safety* for information about assistive devices.)

If you are overweight, losing weight (even a small amount) can greatly reduce the pain and extra burden on joints. This is especially true for joints that bear weight, such as the hips, knees, and feet. There is some evidence that eating oils from certain types of fish can help people with rheumatoid arthritis; however, the benefit is probably small. What you eat has little effect on most types of long-term arthritis, particularly osteoarthritis and rheumatoid arthritis. What you eat, however, is important for gout. Alcohol and certain meats can increase the risk of gout attacks. People with gout should discuss their diet with their GP.

Sometimes in the struggle against arthritis, people become depressed. Usually this depression is related directly to the consequences of long-term arthritis and is not a sign of mental illness. It is important to recognise the depression and to seek advice from healthcare professionals. There are many ways to combat depression. You can read more about depression in Chapter 5, *Understanding and Managing Common Symptoms and Emotions*.

Understanding and Treating Osteoporosis*

Osteoporosis is not arthritis. It is a condition that affects the bones and is usually a result of ageing. If you have osteoporosis, your bones lose calcium and become more brittle. Then they are more susceptible to fracture than normal. Normal bone structure is maintained primarily by calcium and vitamin D intake and physical activity. In women, the hormone oestrogen also affects bone structure. After menopause, when oestrogen production declines, osteoporosis risk increases for women. As people age and are less physically active, bone weakening becomes more likely. Other factors increase the risk of osteoporosis, including smoking and heavy drinking, some endocrine diseases, and long-term use of corticosteroids.

Although osteoporosis can cause bone pain, it usually does not cause specific symptoms. A diagnosis of osteoporosis is made by a DXA scan (bone density test). Most doctors use the DXA scan for people who are at risk of osteoporosis. DXA scan results establish the diagnosis, determine its severity, and guide treatment. How often should you have DXA scans? Because bone density changes very slowly, the interval between DXA scans should be at least two years in order to detect changes in bone density.

The prevention and treatment of osteoporosis may involve taking dietary supplements and taking the steps listed in 'To Prevent or Slow Osteoporosis' on pages 88-89. It is particularly important to get an appropriate amount of calcium and vitamin D. If your osteoporosis does not respond to these steps or is severe, there are medications that can strengthen bones. Bisphosphonates, such as alendronate (*Fosamax* and *Bonosto*), ibandronate (*Boniva*), risedronate (*Actonel*), etidronate (*Didronel*), and zoledronic acid (*Zometa* and *Aclasta*), can treat osteoporosis. These medications are taken in pill form once per week (alendronate and risedronate), once per month (ibandronate), or by IV infusion (zoledronic acid) once per year. If you cannot tolerate bisphosphonates or can't take them for another medical reason, your doctor may prescribe other classes of osteoporosis medications, depending on the severity of the osteoporosis and your other medical conditions. Discuss treatments with your doctor.

Osteopenia is calcium loss from bone that has not reached the level of calcium loss seen in osteoporosis. Osteopenia can also be diagnosed by DXA scan. You can usually manage osteopenia by taking supplements and following the advice in the box on pages 88–89. Medications are unnecessary unless osteopenia is progressing.

---

*Because research on medications and treatments is rapidly progressing, medication names and options may differ from the information in this chapter. Consult your doctor, a pharmacist, a recent medications reference book, or an online medication reference for the latest information or if you have specific questions. But remember that the latest treatments are not always more effective. New treatments may not have as much information about safety and how they act with other medications that have been in use for many years.

Exercising with Long-term Arthritis or Osteoporosis

Regular exercise is crucial to the management of all types of long-term arthritis and osteoporosis.

Exercising with Long-term Inflammatory Arthritis

Exercise is important for all types of long-term inflammatory arthritis. Exercise maintains joint mobility, and it strengthens ligaments and tendons around the joint. It also maintains or increases the strength of muscles that move your joints. Gentle flexibility exercises can also help with morning stiffness. When a joint is inflamed, mild exercise is good. Appropriate exercise will not damage joints in people with long-term arthritis. Exercise should not be painful. Medication can reduce inflammation so you can exercise more easily. Try some of the exercises in Chapter 8. Exercise each affected joint. As your joints become more flexible and less painful, add strengthening exercises. Gradually increase resistance with weights, elastic bands, compressible balls, and spring structures. The goal is to achieve maximum comfortable function for the affected joints.

Exercising with Osteoporosis

Osteoporosis begins primarily as a problem with joint cartilage, so your exercise programme should include taking care of cartilage. Cartilage needs joint motion and some weight bearing to stay healthy. As we noted earlier, in much the same way that a sponge soaks up and squeezes out water, joint cartilage soaks up nutrients and fluid and gets rid of waste products by being squeezed when you move your joints. If your joints are not moved regularly, cartilage deteriorates. Good posture, strong muscles, and good endurance, as well as shoes that absorb the shocks of walking, are important ways to protect cartilage and reduce joint pain.

Move all joints with osteoporosis through their full range of motion several times daily to maintain flexibility and cartilage health. Judge your activity level so that exercises do not increase your pain. After you spend time on your feet, spend at least an hour off your feet. This gives your cartilage time to decompress. If one knee or leg is worse than the other, use a walking stick on the opposite side of a painful knee to reduce joint stress. Make sure the walking stick is the proper height for you. When you use stairs, lead with your good leg when going up and lead with your bad leg when coming down. Certain types of knee braces can also help. Performing knee-strengthening exercises (Exercises 21 and 22 on page 195 in Chapter 8) daily can help reduce your knee pain and protect the joint. If you have a painful hip, experiment with a walking stick on the same or opposite side. Explore which works better for you.

Regular weight-bearing exercise plays an important part in preventing osteoporosis and strengthening bones. Endurance and strengthening exercises are the most effective for strengthening bone that show signs of osteoporosis. Weight-bearing exercise (such as walking and lifting light weights) puts stress on bones and helps maintain and promote calcium in bone.

To Prevent or Slow Osteoporosis

- **Get enough calcium.** The NHS recommends that adults aged 19 to 64 need 700mg of calcium a day, all of which you should be able to get from your daily diet. The best sources are milk and foods made from milk. If you avoid milk products because you don't like them, do not eat animal products, or have problems digesting milk sugar (lactose intolerance), you can still get enough calcium from your diet. Try milk products in small amounts, or eat other foods at the same time, like cereal with milk. If you are lactose intolerant, use lactase tablets to help digest the lactose, or try eating foods that are lower in lactose, such as kefir or yogurt. Some fruits and vegetables are high in calcium, including kale, greens, bok choy, broccoli, calcium-treated tofu, and cooked dried beans. There are also foods available with added calcium, such as soy milk, juices, cereals, and pasta. Most experts agree that the best and safest way to get calcium is through your diet, not by taking supplements. If you think you may not be getting enough calcium, talk to your GP or a registered dietitian about your diet. They will tell you if you need to take calcium supplements.

- **Get enough vitamin D.** Although you can get vitamin D in some foods and from the sun, you may need to take a vitamin D supplement. Public Health England recommends taking a 10mcg supplement during autumn and winter. But people in certain groups at risk of not having enough exposure to sunlight, or whose skin is not able to absorb enough vitamin D from the level of sunshine in the UK, are encouraged to take a daily supplement of 10mcg all year round. Check with your GP before taking a supplement, as recommendations may change.

- **Be physically active.** Walk, bicycle, or dance. It is also very important to do strengthening exercises for the shoulders, arms, and upper back.

That is why swimming, which is an excellent form of exercise but is not weight bearing, may not be as helpful for people with osteoporosis.

Flexibility and exercises that strengthen your back and abdomen are important for maintaining good posture. Look for the 'VIP' exercises in Chapter 8 to choose strengthening exercises. Start and maintain a regular exercise programme that includes some walking and general flexibility and strengthening of your shoulders, hips, back, and stomach muscles.

■ ■ ■

Although long-term conditions such as heart disease, lung disease, and arthritis are not curable, the self-management skills in this chapter can lessen symptoms, prevent complications, and help you work in partnership with your healthcare team.

- You may want to avoid lifting heavy objects and high-impact exercise, especially if you have osteoporosis.

- Sit up straight and don't slouch. Good sitting posture puts less pressure on the back.

- Don't bend down to touch your toes when standing. This puts unnecessary pressure on your back. If you want to stretch your legs or back, lie on your back and bring your knees up toward your chest.

- Limit alcohol to no more than the recommended number of 14 units per week for men and women (see page 59).

- Don't smoke or vape. If you do, stop or reduce your smoking.

- Prevent falls to protect yourself from injury in the following ways:
  - Remove throw rugs, electrical cords, and items left on the stairs that may cause you to trip and fall.

- Make sure that your home is well lit, including staircases and hallways.

- Do not walk on ice, polished floors, or other slippery surfaces.

- Avoid walking in unfamiliar places.

- Use a walking stick or walker if your balance is poor.

- Install grab bars, especially in the bathroom, to keep you safe at home.

- Wear low-heeled shoes with good arch supports and rubber soles.

- Check your vision and get new glasses if you do not see well.

- Regain and maintain your balance. Check out the balance exercises in Chapter 8, *Exercising to Make Life Easier*.

- Discuss with your GP if medications might strengthen your weakened bones.

In this chapter we discussed some common long-term conditions, including heart disease, lung disease, and arthritis. Across long-term conditions, self-management skills are more common than different. You can use the information and self-management tools in this chapter to successfully manage your long-term conditions.

Useful Websites

Asthma UK (How to use your inhaler correctly): https://www.asthma.org.uk/advice/inhaler-videos/

Asthma UK (Your asthma action plan): https://www.asthma.org.uk/advice/manage-your-asthma/action-plan/

British Heart Foundation (Cardiac rehab): https://www.bhf.org.uk/informationsupport/support
/practical-support/cardiac-rehabilitation/

British Heart Foundation (Find your nearest cardiac rehab programme): http://www.cardiac
-rehabilitation.net/

British Heart Foundation (Heart Support Groups): https://www.bhf.org.uk/informationsupport
/heart-matters-magazine/wellbeing/cardiac-rehab/heart-support-groups

British Heart Foundation (Heart Helpline): https://www.bhf.org.uk/informationsupport/heart
-helpline or telephone 0300 330 3311

British Lung Foundation: https://www.blf.org.uk/

Cancer Research UK: https://www.cancerresearchuk.org/

Met Office (Weather forecasts): https://www.metoffice.gov.uk/weather/forecast/

Multiple Sclerosis Society of Great Britain: https://www.mssociety.org.uk/

NHS (Alcohol facts): https://www.nhs.uk/live-well/alcohol-support/calculating-alcohol-units/

NHS (Calcium guidelines): https://www.nhs.uk/conditions/vitamins-and-minerals/calcium/

NHS (Heart attack): https://www.nhs.uk/conditions/heart-attack/

NHS (High blood pressure): https://www.nhs.uk/conditions/high-blood-pressure-hypertension/

NHS (Salt the facts): https://www.nhs.uk/live-well/eat-well/salt-nutrition/

NHS (Stop smoking services): https://www.nhs.uk/live-well/quit-smoking/nhs-stop-smoking
-services-help-you-quit/

NHS (Stop smoking services – local): https://www.nhs.uk/smokefree/help-and-advice/local
-support-services-helplines#bt4Q3X2d7CKUh5Ml.97

NICHS (Northern Ireland Chest Heart & Stroke): https://nichs.org.uk/

Parkinsons UK: https://www.parkinsons.org.uk/

Public Health England: https://www.gov.uk/government/news/phe-publishes-new-advice-on
-vitamin-d

Versus Arthritis: https://www.versusarthritis.org/

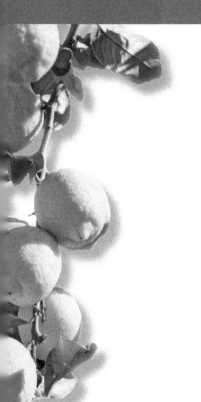

Understanding and Managing Common Symptoms and Emotions

IF YOU HAVE A LONG-TERM CONDITION, you usually experience symptoms. Symptoms are signals from your body that something unusual is happening. They can include physical sensations like fatigue, shortness of breath, pain and itching, or emotions like anger, fear, and low mood. They can also be combinations of both, such as sleep problems and stress. Often other people cannot see your symptoms, and sometimes they are very difficult to describe. Some symptoms are common and most people with the same conditions as you will have them. When they intrude in your life they can feel unpredictable, and the ways they affect you are very personal. One thing that's really important is that your symptoms can affect each other, making it difficult to manage, and this can also cause new

For the UK edition special thanks to Dr Patrick Hill, Clinical Psychologist, for contributions to this chapter.

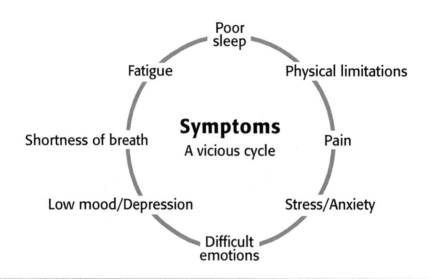

Figure 5.1 **The Vicious Cycle of Symptoms**

symptoms. You might find yourself in a vicious circle, or cycle of symptoms (see Figure 5.1).

You can find ways to break the vicious cycle of symptoms. Whatever causes your symptoms, the ways to manage many of them are often similar. The tools you need to manage them are in the self-management toolbox we discussed in Chapter 2, *Becoming an Active Self-Manager*. This chapter discusses some common symptoms, their causes, and the tools you can use to manage them. Additional thinking tools – ways you can use your mind to help deal with many of these symptoms – are discussed in Chapter 6, *Using Your Mind to Manage Symptoms*.

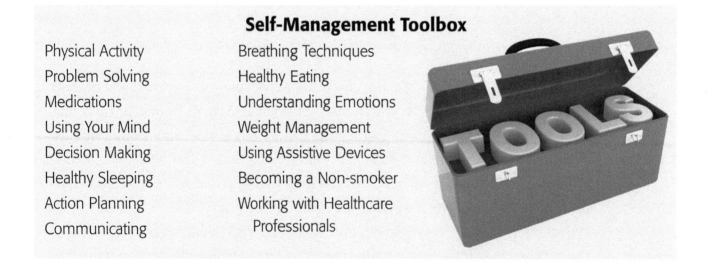

Self-Management Toolbox

Physical Activity	Breathing Techniques
Problem Solving	Healthy Eating
Medications	Understanding Emotions
Using Your Mind	Weight Management
Decision Making	Using Assistive Devices
Healthy Sleeping	Becoming a Non-smoker
Action Planning	Working with Healthcare
Communicating	Professionals

Dealing with Common Symptoms

Learning to manage symptoms is a lot like problem solving, discussed in Chapter 2, *Becoming an Active Self-Manager*. First, you name the symptom you are experiencing. Next, you figure out why you might be experiencing the symptom now. This might sound simple, but it is not always easy. You may have many different symptoms. Each symptom can have various causes and interact with other symptoms. The ways these symptoms affect your life also varies. All of these can become very tangled, like a knot that is hard to untie.

Keeping a Symptom Diary

To manage symptoms, it is helpful to figure out how you can untangle the threads that make up the knot. One way you can do this is to keep a daily diary, like the example below. The easiest way to begin doing this is to write down your symptoms on your calendar each day and add some notes. It is important to write notes about what you were doing before the symptom started or got worse. After a week or two, you may see a pattern. For example, you go out to dinner every Saturday evening and wake up in the night with stomach pain. After a few weekends, you realise that when you go out, you eat

too much and that is what causes the pain. Once you know this, you can try to eat less next time. Or you may notice that every time you go dancing, your feet hurt. And this does not happen when you walk to the park. Is it because you wear different shoes to walk and to dance? For many people, seeing patterns is the first step in successful symptom self-management.

As you read through this chapter, you will notice that different problems can cause similar symptoms, and many symptoms have the same causes. You may also notice that one symptom may cause other symptoms. For example, pain may change the way you walk. You may avoid putting your weight on a sore hip or knee. This new way of walking may change your balance and cause new pain or cause you to fall. As you recognise your symptoms and understand the possible causes of your symptoms, you will be able to find better ways to deal with them. You may also find ways to prevent or lessen some symptoms.

Sample Symptom Diary

Mon.	Tue.	Wed.	Thur.	Fri.	Sat.	Sun.
Supermarket shop	Babysat grandkids Pain later	Tired	Water exercise Felt great	Little stiff Cleaned house	Dinner out Felt bad	Tired
Mon.	**Tue.**	**Wed.**	**Thur.**	**Fri.**	**Sat.**	**Sun.**
Supermarket shop	Babysat grandkids Pain later	Tired	Water exercise Felt great	Cleaned house	Felt great	Felt great Dinner out Felt bad Disrupted sleep

A Word About Coronavirus (COVID-19)

At the time of writing we find ourselves in the middle of a global coronavirus pandemic. Coronavirus (COVID-19) can make anyone seriously ill. But for some people, especially people living with long-term conditions, the risk is higher.

The following advice comes from the NHS website and is specific to England (correct as of July 2020). There is separate guidance for Scotland, Wales, and Northern Ireland, which you can download at

https://www.gov.uk/coronavirus

People who are considered *clinically extremely vulnerable* include people living with long-term conditions such as cancer, severe lung conditions, and serious heart conditions. Also, people with a condition that means they have a very high risk of getting infections, people who are taking medicine that makes them much more likely to get infections, and pregnant women.

If you're at high risk from coronavirus, you're advised to take extra steps to protect yourself. This is called *shielding.* At the end of this chapter you will find a link to the NHS website which provides advice for people who are shielding.

People at moderate risk from coronavirus are considered to be *clinically vulnerable.* This includes people who are aged over 70, people who live with long-term lung conditions, heart conditions, diabetes, long-term kidney conditions, and liver conditions. Also, people who have a condition affecting the brain or nerves (such as Parkinson's disease, motor neurone disease, multiple sclerosis, and cerebral palsy), people who have a condition that means they have a high risk of getting infections or are taking medicine that can affect the immune system (such as low doses of steroids), people who are very obese (a BMI of 40 or above), and pregnant women.

Using Different Symptom-Management Tools

Review the tools in the box on page 35 and start using them. Be sure to keep the following tips in mind:

- Choose a tool to try. Be sure to give this tool a fair trial. We recommend that you practice a tool for at least two weeks before deciding if it is going to be helpful.

- Try other tools, giving each a trial period. It is important to try more than one tool because some tools may be more useful for certain symptoms. You might also find that you simply like some tools more than others.

- Think about how and when you will use each tool. For example, some of these tools may need more lifestyle changes than others. The best symptom managers learn to use a variety of tools. These depend on your condition and what you want and need to do each day.

A report by Public Health England found that other things might also mean you are more likely to get seriously ill from coronavirus. These include your age (your risk increases as you get older), being a man, where in the country you live (the risk is higher in poorer areas), being from a Black, Asian, or minority ethnic background, being born outside the UK or Ireland, living in a care home, and having certain jobs, such as nurse, taxi driver, and security guard.

NHS England has a service for people with ongoing health issues after having coronavirus. The 'Your COVID Recovery' online portal provides information and advice, access to healthcare professionals and a tailored rehabilitation programme for those who qualify. For more information, visit

https://www.yourcovidrecovery.nhs.uk

In addition, a number of charities have worked with the NHS to produce advice about coronavirus and certain health conditions. These can be downloaded at

https://www.nhs.uk/conditions/coronavirus-covid-19/people-at-higher-risk/other-conditions-and-coronavirus

Nobody knows exactly what the long-term effects of coronavirus will be, especially for people living with long-term conditions. So as a good self-manager, it's your job to make sure you are up to date with the latest guidance.

So as a good self-manager, it's your job to make sure you are up to date with the latest guidance. You can do this by searching the Internet for

https://www.gov.uk/coronavirus

■ Place some reminders in your home and workplace to remind you to practice your self-management tools. Both practice and regular use are important for mastering new skills. For example, place stickers or notes where you'll see them, such as on your mirror, near the phone, in your office, on your computer, or on the car's dashboard. Change the notes from time to time so that you'll continue to notice them.

■ Try linking the practice of each new tool with something you already do. For example, practice relaxation breathing techniques as part of your cool-down from exercise. Or ask a friend or family member to remind you to practice each day. You may end up having a partner practicing with you!

Common Symptoms

These are the common symptoms we discuss in this chapter and page references so you can find them quickly.

- Fatigue (page 96)
- Pain (page 98)
- Shortness of Breath (page 104)
- Disrupted sleep (page 113)
- Low mood/Depression (page 117)

- Anger (page 122)
- Stress (page 124)
- Memory problems (page 129)
- Itching (page 130)
- Urinary Incontinence (page 132)

Fatigue

Fatigue is extreme tiredness following mental or physical exertion or illness. It is more than just feeling tired and is not, as some might say, 'all in your mind'. Fatigue is probably the most common symptom people with long-term conditions face, and is a very real problem for many people. Those with long-term conditions can often experience fatigue when they feel as though they haven't done very much.

Like other symptoms, you cannot see fatigue, and people who do not have a long-term condition cannot usually understand how you feel. Partners, family members, friends, and colleagues do not always understand how fatigue from your long-term condition can affect you. They might think that you are just not interested in certain activities or that you want to be alone. Sometimes you may not even know when fatigue is making you feel bad or unhappy or choose to avoid others.

To manage fatigue, it is important to understand that several things can cause your fatigue:

- **The condition itself.** No matter what condition or conditions you have, you use more energy to complete your activities of daily living. When you have a long-term condition, your body does not use energy well. This is because your body needs the energy that could be going to your everyday activities to deal with your condition. One cause of fatigue is that your body might be releasing chemical signals to save energy and make you rest more. Some long-term conditions also cause anaemia (low blood haemoglobin in your red blood cells). Anaemia can cause fatigue. We discuss disease management in Chapter 4, *Understanding and Managing Common Conditions*.

- **Inactivity.** Muscles that you don't use regularly become deconditioned and don't work as well. Deconditioned muscles tire more easily than muscles in good condition. Your heart, which is a muscle, can also become deconditioned. When this happens, your heart does not pump blood well. Blood carries necessary nutrients and oxygen to other parts of the body. When your muscles do not receive these necessary nutrients and oxygen, they cannot work properly and you get fatigued. We discuss activity and exercise in Chapter 7, *Being Physically Active,* and Chapter 8, *Exercising to Make Life Easier.*

■ **Poor nutrition.** Food is our basic source of energy. If your fuel is of poor quality, is not enough, or is not digested well, fatigue can result. It is rare that vitamin deficiencies cause fatigue. For some people, excess weight results in fatigue. If you have extra weight, it can cause an increase in how much energy you need. Being underweight can also cause fatigue. This is especially true for people with COPD (chronic obstructive pulmonary disease – emphysema or chronic bronchitis). Many people with COPD lose weight because of changes in their eating habits. They feel fatigued because their bodies have less oxygen and also because they are taking in less fuel to keep their bodies going. We discuss nutrition in Chapter 10, *Healthy Eating.*

■ **Disrupted sleep.** For a variety of reasons, there are times when you do not sleep well, or your sleep pattern is disrupted. This can cause fatigue. We discuss how to manage disrupted sleep later in this chapter on page 113–116.

■ **Emotions.** Stress, anxiety, fear, worry, and low mood can also cause fatigue. You probably know that stress and feeling tired often go together, but do you know that fatigue is a major symptom of low mood? We discuss emotions in this chapter and stress management and relaxation techniques in Chapter 6, *Using Your Mind to Manage Symptoms.*

■ **Medications.** Some medications can cause fatigue. If you think one of your medications can be causing your fatigue, talk to your GP. Sometimes doctors can change your medication, the time of day you take it, or the dose. This may help your fatigue.

■ **An oversensitive nervous system.** One of the roles of your nervous system, which includes your brain and all the nerves in the body, is to protect you from things it thinks are harmful. When you have a long-term condition, your nervous system has a lot to deal with and can sometimes become oversensitive and create symptoms such as pain and fatigue much more than it needs to. It is only trying to protect itself, but it can end up stopping you doing the things you want to do, and this starts another vicious cycle of symptoms.

If fatigue is a problem, start by looking for the cause. A symptom diary or journal, which we discussed earlier in this chapter, is a good place to start. Begin with the easiest things that you can do to control or improve your fatigue. Are you eating healthily? Are you exercising? Are you getting enough good-quality sleep? Are you managing your stress? If you answer "no" to any of these questions, you are on your way to finding one or more of the reasons for your fatigue.

The most important thing to remember about fatigue is that *it may be caused by something other than your condition, such as an oversensitive nervous system or a cold virus. Or it may be that your condition is causing only part of your fatigue.* Managing fatigue means doing something about its possible causes and usually means using several self-management tools, such as relaxation, managing activity, sleep management, and communicating with others.

For example, it's quite common that people with long-term conditions get frustrated when they are not able to do their normal activities and try to get everything done when they feel better. However, they then do too much, and this can cause an increase in symptoms such as pain, breathlessness, and fatigue. They then find they have to rest for a few days to recover, which causes more frustration and low mood. Often they have to take more medication and as a result can't sleep well, and the whole vicious cycle starts again.

Take another example. People often say that they can't exercise because they are too fatigued. This is probably true. If you haven't been able to exercise for a while, your body will have become deconditioned or weaker. When you try to exercise you won't be able to do what you used to, which can start a vicious cycle. You are fatigued because of a lack of exercise, and you don't exercise because of the fatigue. Getting yourself to do a little exercise is the answer. When you start, it will probably need to be a lot less than you think. You don't have to run a marathon or take a daily weightlifting class. The important thing is to make a plan to get moving and stick to it. It's really important not to overdo it when you start, or this will cause more fatigue. Think about what you can manage on a not-so-good day and make a plan to just do that, even if you feel like doing more. This may feel like you are not doing anything very much, but you can build it up slowly if you do it regularly. Try going outdoors and taking a short walk. If this is not possible, walk around your house or try some gentle chair exercises. See Chapter 7, *Being Physically Active*, and Chapter 8, *Exercising to Make Life Easier*, for more information on getting started with an exercise programme. Even moving just a minute during each hour you are awake can make a difference.

If emotions are causing fatigue, rest will probably not help. In fact, it may make you feel worse. This can be true especially if your fatigue is a sign of low mood or even depression. We talk about depression a little later in this chapter. If you feel that your fatigue may be from stress, read the sections 'Dealing with Stress' in this chapter and 'Positive Thinking and Self-Talk' on page 151 in Chapter 6, *Using Your Mind to Manage Symptoms*.

Pain

Pain is another common symptom for people who are managing long-term conditions. Pain is created by your nervous system to protect you. This may sound odd if you experience constant pain, but this can happen when your system has become oversensitive. One of the roles of your nervous system, which includes your brain and all the nerves in the body, is to protect you from things it has learned are harmful. It does this by monitoring what is happening both inside and outside your body through messages it receives via all the nerves in the body and 'sounding the alarm' if it thinks there is a threat of harm. It does this by creating sensations or symptoms to get your attention. For example, if you put your hand too near a dangerous heat source, such as a fire, it will create pain in your hand to make you remove it from the danger before any damage occurs.

The most important thing to understand is that pain is created by complex processes in your brain and nervous system, not by your body where you feel the pain. Because it is complex and the whole brain gets involved in creating pain, many other factors, such as mood, stress, attention, time, and place, all play a part in how much pain you experience.

When you have long-term conditions, your nervous system has a lot to deal with and can sometimes become oversensitive and create symptoms such as pain much more than it needs to. It is only trying to protect itself, but it can end up stopping you doing the things you want to do, and this starts another vicious cycle of symptoms.

It is very important to note that we are *not* saying that pain is all in your head. This is not true. All pain is real, but it is created by your nervous system according to what it thinks is going on, and sometimes it makes mistakes.

As with most symptoms of long-term conditions, pain has many causes, which we discuss in the following list. You might notice that these are similar to the causes for fatigue. These two symptoms – pain and fatigue – often strike together.

▪ **The condition itself.** In the beginning pain can come from inflammation, damage in joints and tissues, a lack of sufficient blood flow to muscles or organs, or irritated nerves. There can be other causes, depend-

ing on your condition. However, it is almost impossible to predict how much pain someone will have by just looking at the body structures, because the pain process is so complicated and involves psychological, emotional, and social factors.

▪ **Tense muscles.** When the nervous system creates pain anywhere in your body, the muscles in that area become tense in order to protect the area. This is a natural reaction to pain. You tense up to try to protect the painful area. When you have a long-term condition, you may experience pain for months or years and the muscles can become almost permanently tense. A problem with this is that tense muscles can feel normal after a while. We know that muscle tension always makes pain worse. We often have double trouble as people with long-term conditions often have tense, weak muscles, which can lead to muscle spasm.

▪ **Muscle deconditioning.** When you have a long-term condition, you might become less active. This lack of activity can lead to weak muscles. If a muscle is weak, it may complain anytime you use it. That is why even a tiny bit of activity can sometimes cause pain and stiffness. And this is why it is important to get your body used to being used and to *keep* it used to being used.

▪ **Disrupted sleep pattern.** Pain can make it difficult to get enough good-quality sleep, as it's often difficult to get comfortable in bed. People with long-term conditions often don't get enough deep sleep, which means that they don't feel restored in the morning even if they have slept for a long time. Disrupted sleep affects the way the body self-manages and can make dealing with pain and fatigue even more difficult.

■ **Stress, anxiety, low mood, and difficult emotions such as anger, fear, and frustration.** It is normal for people living with a long-term condition to have difficult feelings and emotions. How you feel emotionally will affect symptoms like pain and fatigue. When you are stressed, angry, afraid, or low, everything, including your pain, seems worse. Often these feelings make people 'think the worst' about everything around them. For example, when you are sad, you may think your pain, which is already bad, is never going to improve.

■ **Medications.** Medicines all have side effects. Medication for pain can cause problems elsewhere in your body, such as your gut, or tiredness or changes in your thinking. If you think that medications are causing your pain, talk with your GP.

Long-Term Pain and the Mind-Body Connection

If you are reading this section carefully, you probably have chronic or long-term pain. This is defined as any pain that goes on beyond 3 months. Many people have pain that lasts for months or years. Long-term pain is not well understood, and it is therefore difficult for many non-specialist doctors to explain. We now know that it is a complex sensation that is produced by multiple parts of the whole nervous system working together (modern MRI scanners have helped us to see this). So long-

term pain is not something you are imagining. By managing things like activity, mood, stress, sleep, diet, and exercise you can have an effect on it. People who are good at self-managing their long-term pain tell us that they still experience it, but they are able to get on with their lives and they control it rather than have the pain control them.

Low mood and feelings of anxiety, anger, frustration, and loss of control can make your experience of pain much worse. Don't forget that your pain is *not* 'all in your head'. However, as many people know from experience, emotions, mood, stress, and paying attention to pain are all important influences on how they feel pain. Quite often people find themselves in conflict, with their mind wanting to do things that their body won't let them. Philosophers used to think of the mind and body as separate things, but that's not a helpful model to use.

Here are four examples of ways in which the mind and body interact:

■ **Inactivity.** As we mentioned earlier, pain can cause you to avoid physical activity. Inactivity causes you to lose strength and flexibility. The weaker and more out of condition you become, the more frustrated and low you feel. This will make your pain more difficult to manage and create one of the vicious cycles we mentioned before.

■ **Overdoing.** Because of the frustration of not being able to do things, on your better days you might be determined to prove that you can still be active, so you do too much. This can trigger your nervous system to produce more pain to try and stop you and can cause more inactivity, more difficult emotions (such as frustration and anger), and more consequently pain.

■ **Misunderstanding.** Your friends, family, manager, and work colleagues might not understand that you have long-term pain. They might dismiss your pain as 'not real'. Or they might expect you to be 'better' after a while, especially if you have had to take time off work. For most people, others not understanding is a huge cause of frustration.

■ **Overprotection and Under-protection.** Friends, family, managers, and work colleagues might stop you doing things which they think 'will make you worse' or make excuses for not participating in social activities. This can make you feel and act more dependent and disabled. Equally, some people close to you can start to ignore the fact that you have pain and expect you to be 'back to normal'. This is just as frustrating.

Fortunately, you can interrupt this vicious cycle. Pain doesn't have to be a life sentence. It can be a new beginning. You can develop tools to keep in your self-management toolbox, including the following:

■ redirecting your mind's attention

■ challenging negative thoughts

■ working on having more positive emotions

■ slowly increasing your activity and reconditioning yourself

To help you understand how your moods, activities, and conditions affect your pain, keep a diary. Start with something like the symptom dairy we discussed earlier in this chapter (see

page 93). Begin by making entries in the diary three times a day.

1. Record the date and time.

2. Describe the situation or activity (watching TV, doing housework, working at the computer, arguing, or whatever you happen to be doing).

3. Describe what you did, if anything (took medication, had a massage, did a relaxation exercise, went for a walk, etc.). Note if this helped, did not help, or made no difference.

After you have kept the diary for a week, look for patterns in what you wrote in it. For example, is your pain worse after sitting for a long time? Did you notice it less when you were engaged in a favourite hobby? Do you tend to have a pain flare-up after you have had an argument with a family member? Or when you are stressed, such as when paying your bills?

Once you have learned from your diary, it's time to look at the tools in your self-management toolbox.

Tools for Managing Pain

You cannot build a house with just a screwdriver. You also need a hammer and a saw. In the same way, you often need several tools to manage pain. Luckily, there are many tools for managing pain available to you.

Exercise

Exercise and physical activity are important. We discuss the benefits of exercise and tips for starting an exercise programme in Chapter 7, *Being Physically Active*, and Chapter 8, *Exercising to Make Life Easier*. If you are not able to do the things you want and need to do because of physical limitations, advice from a physiotherapist may be helpful. Remember, for many people the most risky thing relating to exercise is *not* doing it or doing too much and creating more pain.

Mind-made medicine

You can also use your mind through relaxation, imagery, visualisation, and distraction (see Chapter 6, *Using Your Mind to Manage Symptoms*). Positive thinking is another powerful way to stop the vicious cycle. Learn how to monitor and challenge negative thinking, worst-case thinking, and self-talk. Do you think your most negative thoughts when your pain is at its worst? Try to change that. Do you wake up in pain and say to yourself, 'I'm going to be miserable all day. I won't get anything done'? Instead, try telling yourself, 'I've got some pain this morning, so I'll start with some relaxation and stretching exercises. Then I'll do some of the easier things I want to get done this week.'

Staying social

People with long-term pain often become isolated. Sometimes you can feel alone even when you are in the middle of a group of friends. You may think that even people who are very helping and caring sometimes 'just don't understand' what you are going through. If you feel this way, these feelings may be causing you more pain. Research shows that emotions can make pain feel worse. Isolation can bring on depression, frustration, and anger. Keep in touch and active with other people even if you hurt. Connecting with other people who live with pain can help a

lot too. They do understand. Maybe you know someone else dealing with a long-term condition. Perhaps they can give you some support and tips on how to cope. Maybe you can help them. Subscribe to a pain newsletter or join a pain support group. Participate in an online discussion group. Don't try to handle your pain all by yourself.

Medications

All medications have side effects and your body also habituates or gets used to them over time. Most people find that a medicine that worked well at first stopped being so helpful after a few weeks and they needed more of it, but over time they got less pain relief and had more side effects. Does this sound familiar?

All medications that we have for pain are designed for short-term or acute pain, such as after surgery or an injury. They are not designed for long-term pain. You may be aware that stronger opioid medications which were once thought safe for long-term pain are now known not to be so. The general advice is to first build up your self-management toolbox and then get some advice from your doctor or pharmacist about how to reduce your pain medication. Don't start by reducing your medication, as your body may be used to it and it's likely that you will get withdrawal symptoms if you just start reducing the medication straightaway. Even if you reduce slowly, most people get some withdrawal symptoms and a temporary increase in pain. This will settle and most people tell us that after they stop taking pain medication their pain is actually no different.

The overprescribing of strong prescription pain medication is a significant problem in the

A Note for Long-Term Users of Prescription Opioids

Gradually reducing opioids can be scary and there may be some withdrawal symptoms and temporary increase in pain, but this will settle. So do not taper off opioids by yourself. Work with your doctor.

Problems with Opioids

There are at least three problems related to opioid use:

1. Opioids are being prescribed too freely because the risks are sometimes not well understood by either the patient or the prescriber. In addition, self-management of pain has not often been considered as a first-line option. Beyond short-term pain, opioids are not very effective and may cause many side effects. Many people are not taught the tools for dealing with long-term pain without opioids and are just told to reduce them, which can be quite frightening.

2. Because of government policy, there is now a movement to review all long-term prescription opioid use with the aim of either reducing or stopping use of these medications (deprescribing). Sometimes deprescribing leaves people fearful, and healthcare professionals often don't know

what else to suggest. There are strategies to get people off opioids and still address their pain: medically supervised slow tapering of their medication (taking less and less opioids over time) and helping people learn new ways to deal with pain. Helping people learn self-management tools for dealing with pain is one reason why we wrote this book.

3. Use of street (illegal) opioids is never a good idea. People who buy illegal opioids do not know the quality of the medications or even what medication they are taking. Using street medications or medication bought over the internet is very dangerous. People taking strong opioids need to be medically supervised. Talk to your doctor or pharmacist if you are worried about your medication.

For the UK edition, special thanks to Rachael Thornton, BPharm(Hons), PGClinDip, MRPharmS, IP, MFRPSII, for contributions to this section.

United States and a growing problem in the UK. At the time of writing this book the UK government has announced that all opioid medications (such as Morphine, Oxycodone, Fentanyl, Buprenorphine, and Tramadol) are to carry prominent warnings to inform people about their potentially addictive properties. It is important to discuss the use of these and all other powerful addictive medications with your doctor.

Marijuana (cannabis) and marijuana products

The use of cannabis products to treat pain is another complicated topic. As we write, the police can issue a warning or an on-the-spot fine of £90 if you're found in possession of cannabis.

Despite what you may read or what people may tell you, there isn't any good scientific evidence for the effectiveness of marijuana (cannabis) use. The studies that do exist are very flawed. We know that the self-management tools we describe here can be effective, so we strongly advise concentrating on building up your toolkit rather than relying on cannabis or other substances (either complementary or prescribed) to manage your long-term pain.

Three Final Notes About Pain Management

- If you have pain medication in your house, keep it where young people or visitors cannot get it. The most common source of abused prescription medication is the family medicine cabinet.

- Do not share prescription medication. You do not know how your medication may affect someone else. There may be a good reason for them not to use it, such as their having ulcers or a bleeding problem. Don't be responsible for someone having a severe reaction, or worse.

- If you, or someone you care for, are nearing the end of life (they are estimated to have 6 months or less to live) and pain is a problem, consider palliative or hospice care. Hospices are staffed by special teams of healthcare professionals who are experts in relieving end-of-life pain while enabling people to remain alert. At this point comfort is most important and medication has a very useful part to play, but this is different to managing a long-term condition.

Pain can be self-managed. There are many tools available, both non-medication and medication. You and your healthcare professionals can find the right tools for you. If you have long-term pain it will really help to become an active pain self-manager. If pain continues to be a major influence in your life, discuss your options with your doctor. You might also ask for a referral to a pain management clinic.

Shortness of Breath

When your lungs do not work well, your body does not get the oxygen it needs. Shortness of breath happens when the body is trying to get more oxygen. Like other symptoms, shortness of breath can have several causes, such as lung or heart disease, and stress. Where people have long-term lung conditions such as emphysema or bronchitis, it is often referred to as COPD (chronic obstructive pulmonary disease). People with heart conditions such as heart failure, or other conditions such as asthma, commonly

experience shortness of breath, which can be very frightening at times. Other issues can result in shortness of breath, such as excess weight. Added weight increases the amount of energy you use and how much oxygen you need. Weight also increases the workload for your heart.

Muscle deconditioning can also cause shortness of breath. Even your breathing muscles can become deconditioned. When muscles become deconditioned, they cannot do what they are supposed to do. They need more energy (and oxygen). In the case of deconditioned breathing muscles, the problem is even more complicated. If your breathing muscles are not strong, it is harder to cough and clear mucus from the lungs. When there is mucus in the lungs, there is less space for fresh air.

Just as there are different causes of shortness of breath, there are many things you can do to manage it.

- When you feel short of breath, don't stop what you are doing or hurry up to finish. Slow down. If shortness of breath continues, stop for a few minutes. If you are still short of breath, take medication if prescribed by your healthcare professional. Shortness of breath can be frightening. The fear you feel can cause two additional problems. First, when you are afraid, you release hormones such as adrenaline. This can cause more shortness of breath as it makes your breathing become fast and shallow. Second, you may stop activity for fear that this will hurt you. If you stop being active every time this happens, you will not be able to build up the endurance necessary to breath more easily. Take things slowly and in small steps, but don't stop unless you have to.

- Increase your activity gradually, usually by not more than 25% each week. If you are able to garden comfortably for 20 minutes now, next week increase your gardening time by just 5 minutes. Once you can garden comfortably for 25 minutes, again add a few more minutes. If you can ride a stationary bike for 4 minutes, great! Next week add a minute. Slow and steady wins the race.

- Don't smoke or vape, and – equally important – stay away from smokers. This might be difficult. Smoking friends or relatives might not realise how they are complicating your life. Your job is to tell them. Explain that their smoke is causing breathing problems for you and that you would appreciate it if they would not smoke around you. Also, make your house and especially your car 'no smoking' zones. Ask people to smoke outside. (For tips on stopping smoking, see pages 109–113.)

- If mucus and secretions are a problem, drink plenty of fluids (unless your doctor has told you to limit liquids). Fluids help thin the mucus and make it easier to cough up. Using a humidifier may also be helpful. Ask your doctor if these simple self-management steps can help you.

- Use medications and oxygen as prescribed. Make sure you are using your inhaler correctly. Many people think they are, but often they are not. (See 'Tips for Correctly Using a Metered-Dose Inhaler', page 68.) We sometimes hear that medications are harmful and overused. However, when you have a long-term condition, medications are often very helpful, even lifesaving. Don't skimp, cut down, or go without. Likewise, more is never better, so don't take more than your doctor tells you. If you think you need to adjust your medications, ask your doctor to make that decision. See Chapter 13, *Managing Your Treatment Decisions and Medications*.

A Word About Outdoor Air Pollution

Like everyone, you are exposed to outdoor air pollution every time you leave your home. This pollution comes from a mixture of particles and gases from car, bus, and lorry exhaust, power stations, factories, smog, forest fires, chemical reactions, and more. Pollution can cause problems for everyone, but especially for people who have breathing problems. The Daily Air Quality Index (DAQI) tells you about levels of air pollution and provides recommended actions and health advice (see the 'Useful Websites' section at the end of this chapter for more information about the DAQI).

What can you do to avoid air pollution risks?

■ Stay indoors on days when air pollution risks are high.

■ Keep windows closed and use air conditioning (if you have it) on hot days.

■ Avoid exercising near busy roads or sources of pollution such as factories and power stations.

■ Avoid woodburners, fireplaces, and people who are smoking.

■ Use your medications as directed by your healthcare professionals.

To help yourself and others, do your part to reduce pollution: if possible, use just a little less energy, drive a little less, buy a fuel-efficient vehicle, and use public transport. And do not smoke or vape.

Breathing Self-Management Tools

In this section, we discuss several tools that can help you breathe easier. You will find more tools in Chapter 15, *Working and Living with Long-Term (Chronic) Conditions*. If you aren't sure how to do these breathing techniques, ask a healthcare professional to show you how to do them the right way. You can also search the Internet for videos demonstrating better breathing techniques made by organisations like the British Lung Foundation. Also see Figure 5.2, Positions That Will Help if You Are Breathless or Short of Breath.

Diaphragmatic breathing ('belly breathing')

Diaphragmatic breathing is also called belly breathing. When you do it correctly, your stomach or abdomen (belly) expands with each breath. Your diaphragm is a big dome of muscle that moves up and down under your lungs to help them expand and contract when you breathe. Most people use the upper lungs and chest for breathing. Because diaphragmatic or belly breathing goes deeper, you need a little practice to learn how to do this and fully expand the lungs. Deep breathing strengthens the breathing muscles and makes them work better, so breathing is easier. One of the problems that causes shortness of breath, especially for people with emphysema, chronic bronchitis, or asthma, is deconditioning of the diaphragm and breathing muscles in the chest. When your muscles get weak, your lungs are not able to work the way they are supposed to. They do not fill well, and they don't get rid of old air.

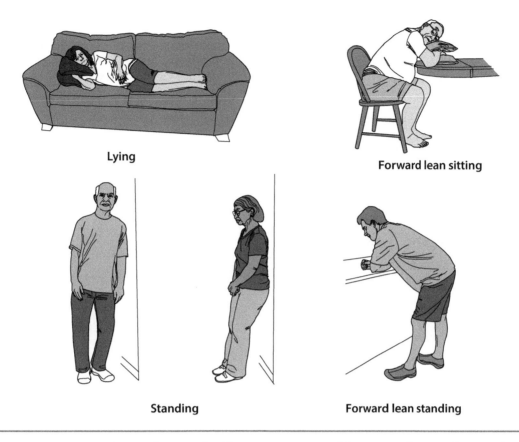

Lying

Forward lean sitting

Standing

Forward lean standing

Figure 5.2 **Positions That Help if You Are Breathless or Short of Breath**

To see a good example of diaphragmatic breathing, watch a sleeping baby breathe. You will notice (or perhaps you can remember) that all the movement of their breathing is in their stomach, not their chest. Somewhere along the line, most adults forgot how to do this. Follow these steps to belly-breathe correctly:

1. Lie on your back with pillows under your head and knees.

2. Place one hand on your stomach (at the base of your breastbone) and the other hand on your upper chest.

3. Breathe in slowly through your nose, allowing your stomach to expand outward. Imagine that your lungs are filling from the bottom up with fresh air. The hand on your stomach should move up, and the hand on your chest should not move or should move only slightly.

4. Breathe out slowly, through pursed lips (see the next section about pursed-lip breathing). At the same time, use your hand to gently push inward and upward on your abdomen.

5. Practice for 10 to 15 minutes, three or four times a day, until it becomes automatic. If you begin to feel a little dizzy, breathe out slower or rest.

You can also practice diaphragmatic breathing while sitting in a chair:

1. Relax your shoulders, arms, hands, and chest. Do not grip your knees or the arms of the chair.

2. Put one hand on your stomach and the other on your chest.

3. Breathe in through your nose, filling the area around your waist with air. Your chest hand should remain still and the hand on your stomach should move.

4. Breathe out without force or effort.

Once you are comfortable with this, you can practice belly breathing almost anytime or anywhere. Do it while you are lying down, sitting, standing, or walking. Diaphragmatic breathing can help strengthen and improve the coordination and efficiency of your breathing muscles, as well as decrease the amount of energy needed to breathe. What you will notice when you do this is that if you take a deep diaphragmatic breath, your whole upper body tenses up. It's like blowing air into a balloon. When you breathe out (like letting the air out of a balloon) your upper body will relax. So, once you have learned how to do this it can quickly relieve stress. You can use the breathing at any time and it can also be used with any of the relaxation techniques that use the power of your mind to manage your symptoms (described in Chapter 6, *Using Your Mind to Manage Symptoms*).

Pursed-lip breathing

Pursed-lip breathing usually happens naturally for people who have problems emptying their lungs. You can also use this tool if you are short of breath or breathless. Follow these steps to pursed-lip breathe:

1. Breathe in. Then purse your lips as if to blow out a candle or to whistle.

2. Using diaphragmatic breathing, breathe out through pursed lips without any force.

3. Remember to relax the upper chest, shoulders, arms, and hands while breathing out. Check for tension. Breathing out should take longer than breathing in.

By mastering pursed-lip breathing and doing it while doing other activities, you will be better able to manage your shortness of breath.

Huffing

The next two techniques, huffing and controlled coughing, can be helpful for removing secretions (mucus, phlegm). Huffing combines one or two forced huffs (puffs of breath) with diaphragmatic breathing. It is useful for removing secretions from small airways. Follow these steps to learn huffing:

1. Take in a breath as you would for diaphragmatic breathing.

2. Hold your breath for a moment.

3. Huff – keep your mouth open while squeezing your chest and abdominal muscles to force out the air (this is a little like panting).

4. If possible, do another huff before taking in another breath.

5. Take two or three diaphragmatic breaths.

6. Huff once or twice.

Controlled cough

A controlled cough can help remove secretions (phlegm) from larger airways. Follow these steps to use this tool:

1. Take in a full, slow diaphragmatic breath.

2. Keep shoulders and hands relaxed.

To prevent or stop uncontrolled coughing, these strategies may help

■ Avoid very dry air or steam.

■ Swallow as soon as you begin to cough.

■ Sip water.

■ Suck lozenges or boiled sweets.

■ Try diaphragmatic breathing, being sure to breathe in through your nose.

3. Hold the breath for a moment.

4. Cough (tighten the stomach muscles to force the air out).

Smoking and Breathing Issues*

If you smoke or use alternative tobacco products such as chewing tobacco, e-cigarettes, a hookah (shisha) pipe, or cigars, this section is for you. Our intention is not to tell you off – we just want to give you some tools to add to your self-management toolbox. Consider the following facts about tobacco use:

■ Smokers are at greater risk of developing long-term conditions, including cancer, heart disease, stroke, diabetes, and COPD (chronic obstructive pulmonary disease, which includes emphysema and chronic bronchitis).

■ Smokers with long-term conditions have more risk of getting complications than non-smokers.

■ There is no risk-free level of exposure to secondhand smoke. Simply being in a room with someone who smokes, or has recently smoked, puts people at greater risk of developing long-term conditions and can cause complications in pregnant women and children with asthma.

■ Smoking makes almost all long-term physical and mental health conditions worse.

*Tips for becoming a non-smoker***

Smoking and being around smokers is not good for your health or that of your children, grandchildren, colleagues, and friends. Although everyone knows that using tobacco is not good for you, quitting completely can be hard. Nicotine, one of the main ingredients in tobacco, is as addictive as heroin. The good news is that you *can* quit, and many people have. And you can quit even if you have not been successful at quitting in the past. In fact, every time you *try* to quit tobacco, your chance of success increases as you learn how to manage the pitfalls with each attempt!

Before we advise you about the tools to help you quit smoking, this is what we know about quitting:

■ The most successful way for most people to quit is to combine support like counselling

---

*For the UK edition, special thanks to Solutions4Health for their contributions to this section.

**With acknowledgment and thanks to the U.S. Department of Veterans Affairs. Much of the material in this section was adapted from its excellent publication, *HIV Provider Smoking Cessation Handbook*.

or quitting classes with medication. The most successful types of medications are a long-acting product like nicotine patches along with a short-acting product like gum, mouth spray, or an inhalator. Oral tablets like varenicline (*Champix*) are also very effective. They work differently to Nicotine Replacement Therapy (NRT) and take away most of the pleasurable effects of smoking. The tablets are only available on prescription from your GP. To find more resources, search the Internet for NHS Stop Smoking Services (see the 'Useful Websites' section at the end of this chapter).

■ Although many people try to quit 'cold turkey', fewer than 5 in 100 make it. Most people need medication and support; it is normal to need help.

■ E-cigarettes are the most popular aid to stop smoking in the UK, and one study has shown them to be nearly twice as effective as regular NRT. It's important to note that e-cigarettes haven't been through the same rigorous testing as Nicotine Replacement Therapy (NRT) and that not enough studies have looked at their long-term effects. However, from the research available to date, e-cigarette use is far less harmful than smoking when tobacco is stopped completely.

■ If alcohol has been a problem in your life and you are no longer drinking, stopping smoking does not need to affect your sobriety.

Taking the following active self-management steps can set you up for success when you make the decision to quit using tobacco:

■ Set a start date within the next 2 to 3 weeks. Give yourself enough time to prepare and plan.

■ Make an action plan. Review Chapter 2, *Becoming an Active Self-Manager*.

■ Tell your friends and family what you plan to do and ask for their support.

■ Ask any smokers you live with if they could smoke away from you.

■ Remove all tobacco products and smoking paraphernalia from your life, including your home, car, and place of work.

■ Making your house and car a smoke-free zone can help reinforce your non-smoking frame of mind.

■ Sign up for help – apps, websites, telephone support, one-to-one support, or group sessions can improve your chances of stopping and staying stopped.

■ Expect some challenges in the first tobacco-free weeks, especially nicotine withdrawal. Symptoms of withdrawal may include a desperate desire to smoke, irritability, anxiety, restlessness, hunger, depression, food cravings, headache, and trouble sleeping. Not everyone gets all these symptoms, and using medication with support will help take the edge off cravings.

■ Talk to your GP and ask about Nicotine Replacement Therapy (NRT), varenicline (*Champix*) or other medications that can help you quit smoking. (See the next section for more on NRT.)

■ Most importantly, remain a non-smoker through the first few weeks of the quitting process. Just having one puff of a cigarette can take you back to day one. Once you get past the first month, your chances of long-term success increase dramatically!

Nicotine-replacement medications

Medications such as Nicotine Replacement Therapy (NRT) can help you quit smoking and remain a non-smoker. The most common medications replace the nicotine you no longer get from tobacco once you quit smoking. You might wonder why medications containing nicotine are better than cigarettes. Cigarettes have lots of dangerous chemicals in them in addition to nicotine. By not smoking, you are not putting all these harmful chemicals through your body, only a reduced dose of nicotine from the NRT. And NRT can be tapered, which means you take less medicine gradually over time. This tapering process ensures that you get less and less nicotine as your body adjusts to being nicotine-free.

E-cigarettes, also known as 'vaping', are usually available to buy from vape shops. It is recommended you get advice from a reputable vape shop if you decide to go down this route. As with licensed NRT it is usually recommended to 'titrate' (adjust) down on the nicotine strength over time and stop its use as early as possible after 8 to 12 weeks. It's important not to smoke whilst vaping, as the harm caused by smoking will still be present.

Nicotine-replacement medications come in many forms: patches, lozenges, gum, nose and mouth spray, and inhalators. Not all of these are exactly the same. Consider the following information when you choose a product:

▪ Patches take 3 to 12 hours to reach their highest dose. Once they reach their peak, patches deliver a steady dose of nicotine for as long as they are on the skin.

▪ Nicotine gum takes about 30 minutes to reach peak nicotine level, and then levels drop slowly over 2 to 3 hours. It is advisable not to eat or drink 15 minutes before using the gum, or while you are using it. There is a special technique to chewing the gum: you chew for a few moments, then rest it between your gum and your cheek. Once the strong taste fades, you can chew again for a few moments before resting it again.

▪ Nicotine lozenges work in a similar way to gum. Suck a lozenge for a few moments before resting it between your gum and cheek until it dissolves.

▪ Nasal and mouth sprays work faster than gum. They are a good option for those who like to get nicotine into their system rapidly. The inhalators are shaped like cigarettes, so they provide a familiar hand-to-mouth substitute for smokers trying to quit.

Although you can buy Nicotine Replacement Therapy without a prescription, we strongly recommend that you talk to your GP before choosing and using these products. There are two reasons for doing this:

▪ It is often better to use more than one NRT method. Some medications that can help you quit smoking can only be obtained by prescription, and they can be helpful. Only you and your doctor can make the best decision about what is right for you.

▪ One of the main reasons people go back to smoking is because they do not use their

NRT products properly (poor technique), or are underdosing on treatment (using one product instead of two) and then terminating the treatment too early. It's recommended that you use the NRT for a minimum of 8 weeks.

Dealing with withdrawal and preventing relapse

If you are a former smoker, there will be times when you want to smoke. This is true whether you smoked for 6 hours or 6 years. These urges decrease over time, but there is no denying that they do occur. When this happens, think DEADS (delay, escape, avoid, distract, substitute):

- **Delay.** The urge will usually go away in 5 to 10 minutes if you wait. Tell yourself, 'This urge *will* go away, and I am not going to have a cigarette because I don't want to be a smoker.' See Chapter 6, *Using Your Mind to Manage Symptoms*.

- **Escape.** Sometimes urges hit during times of stress or if someone else is smoking around you. In either case, leave the environment that is triggering your craving. Go outside and take a short walk, or just leave the room. You will probably soon feel ready to go back to the situation.

- **Avoid.** Avoid places and situations where you are tempted to smoke. If you always smoke when you take a coffee break, take your break somewhere that is smoke-free. This is especially true in the first couple of days. You may find it easier to quit when you are away from your regular routine.

- **Distract.** If an urge hits, find something else to do right away. Choose an activity to do in a place where you cannot smoke, such as taking a shower or reading a book in a place where smoking is not allowed.

- **Substitute.** Chew on a toothpick, eat a piece of fruit, or chew sugarless gum. Use something to substitute for the cigarette. But be careful not to replace tobacco with empty calories such as sweets or crisps.

Chewing tobacco

Some people think that chewing tobacco is not as bad for your health as smoking is. Unfortunately, this is not true. Chewing tobacco causes

Smoking and Coronavirus (COVID-19)

Public Health England guidance (based on available evidence as of 29 May 2020) advises that people who smoke generally have an increased risk of contracting respiratory infections and of developing more severe symptoms once infected. COVID-19 symptoms may, therefore, be more severe if you smoke. Stopping smoking will bring immediate benefits to your health, even if you have an existing smoking-related disease. Smokers are at increased risk of viral and bacterial infections, including pneumonia. These risks can be immediately reduced by stopping smoking. There is also some evidence that current smoking compared with never smoking is associated with greater disease severity in those hospitalised for COVID-19.

the same problems that smoked tobacco causes. In addition, it can cause mouth and throat cancer. The good news is that you can use the same advice in this section to stop using chewing tobacco.

Disrupted Sleep

Not getting good-quality sleep on a regular basis causes all kinds of problems, some of which we have only learned about recently. Some of the well-known consequences of not getting enough sleep are fatigue, problems concentrating, irritability, pain, and weight gain. Improving the quality of your sleep can help you manage many symptoms, regardless of the cause.

How Much Sleep Do You Need?

Different people need different amounts of sleep. Most adults do best with about 7 to 9 hours. If you are alert, feel rested, and function well during the day, chances are you're getting enough sleep.

Sleep is a very basic need, like food and water. All living things seem to do it. Getting less sleep one night is not a big problem. But if you don't get enough sleep night after night, your quality of life and mood may suffer.

As people age, they tend to have a harder time falling asleep and more trouble staying asleep. A common myth is that people need less sleep as they age. Not true. Many older adults report being less satisfied with their quality of sleep and more tired during the day.

Getting a Good Night's Sleep

The self-management techniques for getting better sleep that we offer here are scientifically proven. They help most people sleep better. They are not 'quick fixes' like sleep medications, but in the long run they give you better (and safer) results. Allow yourself at least 2 to 4 weeks to see some improvement and 10 to 12 weeks for long-term improvement.

Things to do before you get into bed

■ **Get a comfortable bed.** This usually means a good-quality, firm mattress that supports the spine and does not allow your body to roll to the middle of the bed. Airbeds or foam mattresses are helpful for some people with long-term pain because they support weight evenly by conforming to your body's shape. An electric blanket or mattress pad, set on low heat, is good at providing heat while you sleep, especially on cool or damp nights. A wool mattress pad that does not use electricity is another option to keep you warm. If you decide to use electric bedding, be sure to follow the instructions carefully to prevent getting burned.

■ **Warm your hands and feet** with gloves or socks. For painful knees, cut the toes off warm socks and use the cut socks as sleeves over your knees.

■ **Find a comfortable sleeping position.** The best position depends on you and your condition. Sometimes small pillows in the right places can relieve pain and discomfort.

Experiment with different positions and pillows. Also check with your healthcare professional for specific recommendations given your condition.

- **Raise your head off the bed** 4 to 6 inches to make breathing easier. This is especially helpful if you have heartburn or gastric reflux. There are blocks for this purpose, and they often have adjustable heights. You place the blocks under the bed's legs at the head of the bed. A pile of pillows under your head and shoulders can also work for some people.

- **Keep the room at a comfortable temperature.** The Sleep Council recommends that a cool 16–18°C (60–65°F) is thought to be an ideal temperature in a bedroom.

- **Use a humidifier** if you live where the air is dry. Warm, moist air can make breathing and sleeping easier.

- **Make your bedroom safe and comfortable.** Keep a lamp and telephone by your bed. If you use a walking stick or walking frame, keep it by the bed so you can use it when you get up during the night. Make sure to put it where you will not trip over it.

- **Keep your glasses by the bed.** If you need to get up in the middle of the night, you can easily put on your glasses and see where you are going!

Things to avoid before bedtime

- **Avoid eating** just before bedtime. If going to sleep on an empty stomach keeps you awake and hungry, try drinking a glass of warm milk at bedtime.

- **Avoid alcohol.** You may think that alcohol helps you sleep better because it makes you feel relaxed and sleepy, but it does not. Alcohol is a sedative and in fact alcohol disturbs your sleep cycle. Alcohol before bedtime will disrupt your natural sleep cycle and is not recommended.

- **Avoid caffeine late in the day.** Caffeine is a stimulant and stays active in your body for about 8 hours. Caffeine interferes with the chemistry in your brain that helps regulate your sleep. Coffee, tea, fizzy drinks, and chocolate all contain caffeine. Be careful with these items as evening approaches or stop them earlier in the day. Some people are quite sensitive to caffeine and remember that decaffeinated does not mean no caffeine, it means reduced caffeine.

- **Avoid smoking or vaping.** The nicotine in cigarettes and e-cigarettes is also a stimulant. So don't smoke before bedtime and particularly not if you wake up in the night and can't get back to sleep. Falling asleep with a lit cigarette can be a fire hazard.

- **Avoid diet pills.** Diet pills often contain stimulants, which could cause problems with falling asleep and staying asleep.

- **Avoid sleeping pills.** Although 'sleeping pills' sound like the perfect solution for disrupted sleep, they become less effective over time. They also disrupt your natural sleep cycle. Many sleeping pills have a rebound effect – that is, if you stop taking them, it is even harder to get to sleep. Some people get a 'hangover' effect from sleep medication – they feel 'groggy' all morning. You may have more problems after trying sleeping pills than you had when you first started taking them. Use nondrug sleep tools and avoid sleeping pills.

- **Avoid using a computer, tablet, or mobile phone and avoid watching TV** for about an hour before you go to bed. The kind of light that comes from computers and TV screens can disrupt natural sleep rhythms. Don't do these things in bed.

- **Avoid diuretics (water pills) before bedtime.** It may be a better option to take diuretics in the morning so that your sleep is not interrupted by frequent trips to the toilet. Unless your doctor has recommended otherwise, don't reduce the amount of fluids you drink. Fluids are important for your health.

How to develop a routine

- **Maintain a regular rest and sleep schedule.** Try to go to bed at the same time every night and get up at the same time every morning. If you want to take a short nap during the day, take it in the afternoon. But remember that any sleep counts, so your will need less sleep at night. In hot countries where people take a siesta they tend to go to bed later. Do not take a nap after your evening meal. Stay awake until you are ready to go to bed.

- **Reset your sleep clock when necessary.** If your sleep schedule gets off track (for example, you go to bed at 4:00 A.M. and sleep until noon), you need to reset your body's sleep clock. Try going to bed an hour earlier or later each day until you reach the hour you want to be your bedtime. This

may sound strange, but it seems to be the best way to reset your sleep clock.

- **Exercise at regular times each day.** Exercise helps you get better-quality sleep. It also helps set a regular pattern for your day. However, don't exercise right before bedtime.

- **Get out in the sun every morning,** even if it is only for 15 or 20 minutes. This helps your body clock to become synched back in with daylight and rhythms become regular.

- **Have a bedtime routine every night before going to bed.** This can be anything from listening to the news on the radio to reading a chapter of a book to taking a warm bath. By making and sticking to a 'get ready for bed' routine, you tell your body that it's time to wind down and relax.

- **If possible, use your bedroom only for sleeping and sex.** If you find that you get into bed and you can't fall asleep, get out of bed. Go into another room and have some things to do that make you feel sleepy again. Keep the lights low when you wake up in the night.

What to do when you can't get back to sleep

Many people get to sleep without a problem but wake up with the 'middle of the night worries'. They can't stop their racing minds. Then they get more worried because they cannot get back to sleep. If you do wake up, keep your mind busy with pleasurable or interesting thoughts. This will chase off the worries and help you get back to sleep. Try a distraction tool to quiet your mind, such as counting backward from 100 by threes or naming a flower for every letter of the alphabet. The relaxation tools in Chapter 6, *Using Your Mind to Manage Symptoms*, may also help. If you really can't get back to sleep after a short time, get up and do something. Read a book, take a warm bath, or play a game of solitaire (not on your phone or tablet). After 15 or 20 minutes, go back to bed.

Some people find it helps to set a 'worry time'. (See 'Worry Time' on page 157 in Chapter 6, *Using Your Mind to Manage Symptoms*.) If a racing mind keeps you awake, schedule a 'worry time' each day well before bedtime. Write down your problems and worries and make a to-do list to get them off your mind. You can relax and sleep well that night, knowing that you don't have to think about it until tomorrow's worry time.

The most important thing to do is not worry about not sleeping. Quite often people start to worry that they are not getting enough good-quality sleep. Such worries will make it worse! If you have a few disrupted nights your body will take the sleep it needs and restore a natural pattern. Use the different techniques to manage your worries and your sleep will sort itself out.

You can find lots of information, advice, and tools to support you to get a better night's sleep on The Sleep Council's website at

https://sleepcouncil.org.uk

Getting Professional Help with Disrupted Sleep

You can solve most disrupted sleep issues with the tools and techniques we have discussed in this section, but there are times when you need professional assistance. When should you get help?

- If your insomnia doesn't go away after 6 months, and self-help tools don't help.

- If your lack of sleep is causing serious problems in your daytime activities (such as at work or in your social relationships).

- If you have problems staying awake during the day. This is especially important if your daytime sleepiness causes or comes close to causing an accident.

- If your sleep is disrupted by breathing difficulties, including loud snoring with long pauses, chest pain, heartburn, leg twitching, excessive pain, or other physical conditions. (Ask your sleep partner about this, or if you live alone, look online for sleep monitors or apps for your smartphone.)

- If you have difficulty sleeping when you are feeling low.

- If your sleep is disrupted when you use alcohol, sleeping medications, or opioids.

If sleep is a real problem for you, ask your GP for a referral to a sleep clinic for expert help. Don't put off asking for help. Most disrupted sleep issues can be solved. Once they're gone, you'll enjoy a better night's sleep and better health.

Low Mood and Depression

Most people who have long-term conditions often experience episodes of low mood. There are different degrees of low mood, from feeling occasionally sad or blue to depression. Sometimes people do not know they are depressed. More often they may not want to admit it. How you manage your mood makes the difference.

What Are Low Mood and Depression?

Feeling sad sometimes is natural. 'Normal' sadness is a temporary feeling. It often happens after a specific event or loss. People sometimes use the word *depressed* to describe feeling low, sad, or disappointed: 'I'm really depressed about missing out visiting with my friends.' You can feel low or sad but still be involved with others and find joy in other areas of your life. Sometimes a low mood lasts longer, such as when you lose a loved one or are diagnosed with a serious illness.

For some people, unhappy and sad feelings or low mood are another symptom of their long-term condition, and like pain or fatigue they need to be managed. For others, depression can itself be a long-term condition.

If your sad feelings are severe, long-lasting, or happen often, you might be dealing with depression. Serious depression takes the pleasure out of life. It leaves you feeling hopeless, helpless, and worthless. With severe depression, you may become emotionally numb, and even crying doesn't help. Depression affects everything: the way you think, the way you act, the way you interact with others, and even the way your body functions.

Sometimes unrealistic cheeriness covers up what the person is really feeling. The wise observer will recognise that the mood is fake or fragile. Refusal to accept offers of help, even if there is an obvious need for it, is a frequent symptom of unrecognised depression.

Long-term or clinical forms of depression may involve the use of self-management tools, but they also require professional help, which often includes counselling and medication. Therefore if you feel unhappy for more than a few weeks, or think about harming yourself it is very important to talk to your GP, so that together you can discuss the different options to help treat and manage your depression. Clinical depression is a biological illness and can be treated. Also, if you are taking medication for depression and are thinking about stopping, talk to your GP first. Many medications should not be stopped suddenly and need to be reduced slowly.

What Causes Low Mood and Depression?

Depression is not caused by personal weakness, laziness, or lack of willpower. Genetics, your long-term condition, and medications can all play a role in depression. Negative thoughts can also cause a low mood and keep it going. You can get stuck in a loop with negative thoughts, and they can become automatic and occur over and over. The following feelings and emotions can also cause low mood or depression:

■ **Fear, anxiety, or uncertainty about the future.** Worries about finances, your condition or treatment, or concerns about your family can cause low mood or make it worse. It is often best to face these issues as soon as possible. If you do, you and your family may spend less time worrying and have more time to enjoy life. Facing issues that you are worried about can have a healing effect. We talk more about these issues and how to deal with them in Chapter 16, *Planning for the Future: Fears and Reality*.

■ **Frustration.** Frustration can have many causes. You might think, 'I just can't do what I want', 'I feel so helpless', 'I used to be able to do this myself', or 'Why doesn't anyone understand me?' The longer you focus on these feelings, the more alone and isolated you are likely to feel.

■ **Thinking the worst.** We all think about the worst thing that can happen sometimes. For example, if your pain hasn't improved, you may think you will end up in a wheelchair or confined to your home. You keep thinking about it until you believe the worst will happen. Doctors call this 'catastrophising', and we discuss this in Chapter 6, *Using Your Mind to Manage Symptoms*. Jumping to the worst conclusions and focusing on them can cause or add to many symptoms. Emotions are powerful and negative emotions can make symptoms worse.

■ **Loss of control over your life.** Many things can make you feel as if you are losing control. You may have to rely on medications, see a doctor on a regular basis, and change your eating habits. You might have to count on others to help you do things such as

preparing meals, bathing, dressing, shopping, and going to appointments. This feeling of loss of control can make you lose faith in yourself and your abilities. However, you can be a self-manager and the 'coach' for your team of family, friends, and healthcare professionals. Even if you are not able to do everything yourself, you can still be in charge.

Depressed feelings can lead to withdrawal, isolation, and lack of physical activity. These behaviours can come back to create more depressed feelings. The more you behave this way, the more likely you are to drive away the people who can support and comfort you. Friends and family want to help, but often they don't really know what to do to help. As their efforts to comfort and reassure are rejected, they might give up and quit trying. Then you wind up saying, 'See, nobody cares.' This again reinforces the feelings of loss and loneliness.

All these factors, along with others, can contribute to an imbalance in the chemicals in your brain that are called neurotransmitters. This imbalance can have a negative effect on the way you think, feel, and act. But actively changing the way you think and behave can be a powerful and effective way to change your brain chemistry for the better and lighten low mood and depression. (See 'Managing Low Mood and Depression on pages 119–122.)

Am I Depressed?

Here is a quick test for depression: Ask yourself what you do to have fun. If you do not have a quick answer, consider the other symptoms of depression listed here.

Think about your mood over the past 2 weeks. Which of the following have you experienced?

- **Little interest or pleasure in doing things.** Not enjoying life or other people may be a sign of depression. Symptoms include not wanting to talk to anyone, to go out, or to answer the phone, e-mail, or doorbell.

- **Feeling down, depressed, or hopeless.** Feeling down for a long time can be a symptom of depression.

- **Trouble falling or staying asleep or sleeping too much.** Waking up and being unable to get to sleep or sleeping too much and not wanting to get out of bed can signal a problem.

- **Feeling tired or having little energy.** Fatigue – feeling tired all the time – is often a clear-cut symptom of depression.

- **Poor appetite or overeating.** This change may range from a loss of interest in food to unusually irregular or excessive eating.

- **Feeling bad about yourself.** Have you felt that you are a failure or have let yourself or your family down? Have you had a feeling of worthlessness, a negative image of your body, or doubts about your own self-worth? If so, it could be a sign of depression.

- **Trouble concentrating.** This includes finding it hard to do such things as reading a book or watching a film.

- **Lethargy or restlessness.** Have you been moving or speaking so slowly that other people have noticed? Or is the opposite true – have you been more fidgety or restless than usual? Either can be a sign of depression.

- **Wishing yourself harm or worse.** Thoughts that you would be better off dead or thoughts about hurting yourself are often a big sign of severe depression.

- **Crying for no obvious reason.** Do you find yourself frequently crying for no apparent reason?

Depressed people may also experience weight gain or loss, loss of interest in sex or intimacy, loss of interest in personal care and grooming, inability to make decisions, and more frequent accidents.

If several of these symptoms seem to apply to you, please seek help from your GP, a family member, good friends, a psychologist, or a social worker. Do not wait for these feelings to pass. If you are thinking about harming yourself or others, get help now. Don't let a tragedy happen to you and your loved ones. Help and support are available. You do not have to struggle with difficult feelings alone. Go to https://www.nhs.uk/conditions/suicide/ for details of free telephone helplines and tips on how to cope in the moment.

Fortunately, the treatments for depression are highly effective and can decrease the frequency, length, and severity of depression. You *can* manage your depression, just like you manage your other symptoms.

Managing Low Mood and Depression

The most effective treatments for low mood and depression are combinations of medications, counselling, and self-help. In this section we discuss these management tools.

Medications

Antidepressant medications can be highly effective. These medicines work by helping to balance brain chemistry. Most antidepressant medications take from several days to several weeks before they begin to work. Then they usually bring significant relief. Don't be discouraged if your doctor prescribes antidepressants and you don't feel better immediately. Stick with it.

Side effects of antidepressants are usually most noticeable in the first few weeks, and then they lessen or go away. If the side effects are not especially severe, keep taking your medication. As your body gets used to the medication, you will begin to feel better. It is important to remember to take antidepressant medications regularly as prescribed. If you stop taking your medication because you're feeling better (or worse), your depression can come back. Talk with your doctor before stopping or changing the dose. Taking these medications is not anything to be ashamed of. You would be surprised to learn how many people take them, including people you know.

Counselling and psychotherapy

The best scientific evidence for treating low mood and depression is for cognitive behavioural talking therapy. This can take several forms but, as with medications, talking therapy rarely has an immediate effect. It may be weeks (or longer) before you see improvement. Therapy typically involves regular sessions over some weeks and as you learn new ways to think and relate, counselling or psychotherapy may also help reduce the risk of your depression returning.

Self-management

Self-management can also be surprisingly effective. You can learn many successful psychotherapy techniques on your own.

The following skills and strategies can be used alone or in addition to medications and counselling:

- **Eliminate the negative.** Being alone and isolating yourself, crying a lot, getting angry and yelling, blaming your failure or bad mood on others, or using alcohol or other drugs usually leave you feeling worse.

  Some medications can make low mood worse or a side effect of mediation can be low mood. Talk to your doctor or pharmacist if you are concerned about this. They may be able to suggest an alternative with fewer side effects.

  Do you drink alcohol to feel better? Alcohol also amplifies low mood. To alleviate low mood and depression, it is important to avoid negative substances and influences.

- **Plan for pleasure.** When you are feeling low, the tendency is to withdraw, isolate yourself, and restrict activities. That is the opposite of what you should be doing. Maintaining or increasing activities is one of the best remedies for low mood. Go for a walk, look at a sunset, watch a funny film, get a massage, learn another language, take a cooking class, or join a social club. These activities can all help get you out of situations where you can get depressed.

  But sometimes having fun isn't such an easy prescription. You may have to make a deliberate effort to plan pleasurable activities. Even if you don't feel like doing it, try to stick to the schedule. You may find that a nature walk, cup of tea, or half-hour of listening to music improves your mood even if you didn't think it would. Don't leave good things to chance. Make up a schedule of your free time during the week and plan positive things to do during it that you like such as reading, gardening, cooking or listening to music, watching comedy or a film, take a long bath.

Make plans and carry them out. Look to the future. If you know that one time of the year is especially difficult, such as anniversaries or Christmas or a birthday, make specific plans for that period. Don't wait to see what happens. Be prepared.

■ **Take action.** Continue your daily activities. Get dressed every day, make your bed, get out of the house, go shopping, walk your dog. Plan and cook meals. Make a plan to do these things and share it with someone if you can – it will help you do them even when you don't feel like it. Taking action to solve problems right away gives the best relief from a low mood. The confidence-building feelings that come from successfully changing something – anything! – is more important than what or how much you change. Taking action is the important thing. Doing even a simple thing can boost your mood. Decide to reorganise a wardrobe, for instance, or call a friend for a chat.

Be careful not to set difficult goals or take on a lot of responsibility. Break large tasks into small ones, set some priorities, and do what you can as best you can.

Review the proven steps for taking successful action in Chapter 2, *Becoming an Active Self-Manager*.

It is best not to make big decisions when you are depressed. For example, don't move to a new area without first visiting for a few weeks. Moving can be a sign of withdrawal, and depression often intensifies when you are away from friends and loved ones. Besides, your troubles can move with you. At the same time, the support you may need to deal with your troubles may have been left behind.

■ **Socialise.** Don't isolate yourself. Seek out positive, optimistic people who can lighten your heavy feelings. Get involved in a community group, a book club, an adult education class, a self-help class, or an exercise or cooking class. If you can't get out, consider joining an online group. If you do this, be sure that the virtual group is moderated. Someone needs to be in charge to keep it safe and positive.

■ **Move your mood.** Physical activity lifts negative moods. When people have low mood they often complain that they feel too tired to exercise. But the feelings of fatigue you feel when you are depressed are not due to physical exhaustion. Try to exercise at least 20 to 30 minutes a day. Any sort of activity can lift your mood – from chair dancing to walking to a water exercise class. If you get yourself moving, you may find that you have more energy (see Chapter 7, *Being Physically Active*).

■ **Think positively.** Many people can be too critical of themselves, especially when they're depressed. You may find yourself thinking groundless, negative, untrue things about yourself. Do you think your health, for example, will never get better? Do you think you will never be able to do the things you used to? Thinking the worst makes negative or sad feelings worse.

As you challenge your automatic negative thoughts, begin to "rewrite" the negative stories you tell yourself (see 'Positive Thinking and Self-Talk' on page 150 in Chapter 6, *Using Your Mind to Manage Symptoms*). For example, one of your beliefs may be, 'Unless I do everything perfectly, I'm a failure.' Revise this belief to, 'Success is doing the best that I can in any situation.' Also, when you are depressed, it's easy to forget that anything nice has happened at all. Make a list of some of the good or positive events in your life.

■ **Do something for someone else.** Lending a helping hand is one of the best ways to change a low mood. But it is one of the least commonly used tools to fight a low mood. Babysit for a friend or relative, walk someone's dog, read a story to a person who is ill, or volunteer at a food bank. Helping others can help you appreciate your own situation. Your problems might not appear so overwhelming. Helping others is the best way to help yourself. See 'Practice Acts of Kindness' on page 159 in Chapter 6, *Using Your Mind to Manage Symptoms*.

Don't be discouraged if it takes some time to feel better. If these self-help tools alone are not enough, get help from your GP, a mental health professional, or contact one of the many organisations, such as Mind, that are there to help people who are struggling with their mental health. Talk therapy or antidepressant medications (or both) can go a long way toward relieving depression. Seeking professional help and taking medications are not signs of weakness. They are signs of strength.

Anger

Anger is a common response to having a long-term condition. The unpredictability of living with a long-term condition can initially challenge your independence and control. People who learn how to self-manage effectively do find that living with one or more long-term conditions becomes less random and unpredictable over time, as they begin to understand how various factors interact and patterns form. But it's also common at the beginning to feel angry about having to deal with your condition and

you may find yourself asking, 'Why me?' This is a normal response to a long-term condition. Some people express their frustration, low mood, or anxiety through anger.

You may be angry with yourself, family, friends, healthcare professionals, or the world in general. For example, you may be angry with yourself for not taking better care of yourself. You may be irritable around your family and friends because they don't do things the way you want. Or you might be angry with your doctors because they cannot fix your problems. Sometimes your anger may shift to another target, as when you find yourself yelling at the dog.

Sometimes the health condition itself plays a part in mood changes or anger. For example, when people are very anxious or stressed or have had a stroke or are living with dementia these things can have a direct effect on the emotions, causing a person to cry for no reason or have temper flare-ups.

There are some important steps to learning how to manage your anger. You may need to talk to someone to do this as it's often hard to do it on your own. The first step is to recognise or admit that you are angry. You also need to figure out why you are angry. And finally, you need to know who or what is the object of your anger. Finally, you need to find more positive ways to express your emotions and defuse your anger.

Defusing Anger

Research tells us that people who vent their anger get angrier. But suppressing anger isn't the answer either. Suppressed angry feelings often smoulder and flare up later. There are two basic strategies you can use to reduce hostile feelings:

■ You can raise your anger threshold – that is, allow fewer things to trigger your anger in the first place.

■ You can choose how to react when you get angry – without either denying your feelings or giving in to the situation.

This sounds simple enough, but what gets in the way is the human tendency to see anger as coming from outside yourself – something over which you have little control. You may see yourself as a helpless victim. You may blame others and say, 'You make me so angry!' You may explode and then say, 'I couldn't help it.' You may see friends as selfish and insensitive, work colleagues as snobs or bullies, friends as unappreciative. So it can seem that your only choice is an outburst of anger. But with a little practice, anyone can master a new set of healthy and more effective responses.

There are several strategies you can use to help manage your anger. In this section we discuss each one.

Reason with yourself

How you interpret and explain a situation determines whether you will feel angry or not. You can learn to defuse anger by pausing and questioning your anger-producing thoughts. If you change your thoughts, you can change your response. You can decide whether to get angry and then decide whether or not to act.

At the first sign of anger, slowly count to three and ask yourself the following three questions:

■ **Is this important enough to get angry about?** Maybe whatever is making you angry isn't serious enough to spend the time and energy.

■ **Am I justified in getting angry?** Are you sure you know what is happening? You may need to gather more information and understand the situation better before jumping to conclusions or misinterpreting the intentions or actions of others.

■ **Will getting angry make a difference?** Often, getting angry and losing your cool does not work and may even have bad results. Exploding or venting increases your angry feelings, puts a strain on your relationships, and potentially damages your health.

Cool off

Any technique that relaxes or distracts you – such as meditating or taking a long walk – can help calm you down. Slow, deep breathing is one of the quickest and simplest ways to cool off (see page 107). When you notice anger building, take three slow, relaxed breaths before responding. Sometimes withdrawing and being alone for a little while can defuse the situation. Also, exercise is a good outlet for stress and anger.

Verbalise without blame

One important thing to do is to learn how to communicate about your anger, preferably without blaming or offending others. This can be done by using 'I' (rather than 'you') messages to express your feelings. (See the discussion of 'I' messages in Chapter 11, *Communicating with Family, Friends, and Healthcare Professionals*).

If you choose to express your anger with words, know that many people will not be able to help you. Many people are not very good at dealing with angry people. This is true even if the anger is justified or if you use 'I' messages.

Therefore, you might also find it useful to seek counselling or join a support group.

Modify your expectations

You might benefit from changing what you expect out of life. Changing your expectations can lessen your anger. You have done this throughout your life. For example, as a child you thought you could become anything – a fire fighter, a ballet dancer, or a doctor. As you grew older, however, you re-evaluated these expectations, along with your capabilities, talents, and interests. Based on this re-evaluation, you modified your plans.

You can deal with how long-term conditions affect your life in a similar way. For example, it may be unrealistic to expect that you will get 'all better'. However, it is realistic to expect to still do many pleasurable things. You can affect the progress of your condition. You can use management tools to slow your decline or prevent your symptoms or your condition from becoming worse. Changing your expectations can change your perspective too. Instead of dwelling on the 10% of things you can no longer do, think about the 90% of things you can still do.

Anger is a normal response to having a long-term condition. Part of learning to manage your condition involves acknowledging your anger and finding constructive ways to deal with it.

Stress

Stress is a common concern, whether or not you have a long-term condition. But what is stress? You might feel stress after negative events, such as the death of a loved one. But you might also feel stress with good events, such as the marriage of a child.

How Does Your Body Respond to Stress?

We all have a system in the body which comes into play when we feel stressed. It is activated by hormones, the one most widely known is adrenaline. When adrenaline is released into the bloodstream it causes physical changes in the body which help us to respond to events, most commonly when we have to deal with something that is potentially dangerous or harmful. Your son or daughter's wedding is clearly not dangerous, but you would be concerned as their parent that it all goes well.

When adrenaline is released your body gets organised very quickly to deal with whatever is happening. It reacts by preparing to take some action: your heart rate increases, your blood pressure rises, your muscles tense, your breathing becomes more rapid, your digestion slows, your mouth becomes dry, and you may begin sweating. Altogether we call this the 'stress response', or sometimes it is called the 'fight-or-flight response', which is a good name for it as at its most basic it is your body organising itself to fight or run away from a threat. When this response is switched on your muscles need to be supplied with oxygen and energy. Your breathing increases to take in as much oxygen as possible and to get rid of as much carbon dioxide as possible. Your heart rate increases to deliver the oxygen and nutrients to the muscles. Body functions that are not immediately necessary, such as the digestion of food and the body's natural immune responses, are slowed down.

How long do these responses last? In general, they only last until the stressful event passes.

Your body then returns to normal. Sometimes, though, your body does not return to normal. If your stress stays with you for any length of time, your body starts adapting to it. Sometimes people end up in fight-or-flight mode almost all the time and it starts to feel like a normal way of being. People who have long-term conditions which are difficult to manage often feel like this. Ongoing tension in the body of this kind will make your symptoms like pain and fatigue much harder to manage.

Although feeling stressed for long periods of time can be harmful, in other situations stress can be helpful. Stress can help you prepare to take on both mental and physical challenges (like taking exams or making necessary lifestyle changes) and help you to build resilience. The most important thing is to understand what happens to you physically and mentally when you are stressed and to learn how to manage your stress so that it doesn't overwhelm you. Learning how to relax properly and then to use this learning to stay relaxed as you go through your day is an important part of self-management.

Common Stressors

Stressors are the things that trigger the stress response or fight-or-flight response. Stressors don't often appear alone. Several stressors can occur at the same time. One stressor can lead to other stressors or even make the effects of existing ones worse. For instance, shortness of breath can cause anxiety, frustration, inactivity, and loss of physical endurance. In this section, we examine some of the most common sources of stress.

Physical stressors

Physical stressors can range from something as pleasant as lifting up your new-born niece to something as normal as everyday food shopping. The symptoms of your long-term condition, such as pain or fatigue, can also be physical stressors. It is very common for people to experience vicious cycles where more symptoms cause more stress, which in turn cause more symptoms and so on.

Mental and emotional stressors

Mental and emotional stressors can also be either pleasant or uncomfortable. The pleasure you feel from thinking about going out to see your friends might cause a similar stress response as feelings of frustration or worries about your condition.

Environmental stressors

Stress from what is around you also can be both good and bad. Environmental stressors may be as varied as a very hot or cold day, crowded shops, an uneven pavement, or loud traffic noise.

Chemical stressors

Certain chemicals can also increase stress. These include nicotine, alcohol, and caffeine. Some people smoke a cigarette, drink a glass of wine or beer, eat chocolate, or drink a cup of coffee to soothe their tension. What actually happens when you take things that contain nicotine or caffeine is that the relaxation you feel is because you are stopping mild feelings of withdrawal from these addictive substances – another vicious cycle. Generally eliminating or cutting down on things that contain these substances can help.

Recognising Stress

Living without stress isn't possible. We live in cultures and societies that create many stressors. Sometimes it is hard to recognise when we are stressed all the time as it starts to feel normal. Human beings are very adaptable, but this is not always a good thing. The following are some of the habits we get into when we are stressed all the time:

- biting your nails, 'twiddling' your hair, tapping your foot, or other repetitive habits
- clenching your jaw and sometimes grinding your teeth at night
- tension in your muscles such as neck and shoulders
- feeling anxious or irritable all the time
- forgetting things you usually don't forget
- difficulty concentrating
- not sleeping or waking up still feeling tired

By doing a regular relaxation exercise most people find they get better at spotting these habits or when they are beginning to get tense. Using regular deep breathing a number of times throughout the day can really help to change these habits. Take one or two deep breaths and try to relax. Also, a quick body scan (described in Chapter 6, *Using Your Mind to Manage Symptoms*) can help you recognise stress in your body. You will find many additional good ideas for coping with stress in Chapter 6.

In the next section we share some tools for dealing with stress.

Dealing with the Causes of Stress

Dealing well with the causes of stress doesn't have to be complicated. It can start with three simple steps:

1. **Name your stressors and make a list.** Consider every area of your life: family, relationships, health, job, finances, living environment, and so on.

2. **Sort your stressors.** For each stressor on your list, ask yourself: Is it important or unimportant? Is it changeable or unchangeable? Place each stressor in one of four categories (see the examples in Figure 5.3):

   ■ important and changeable

   ■ important and unchangeable

   ■ unimportant and changeable

   ■ unimportant and unchangeable

   For example, needing to quit smoking is changeable and, for most people, important. Loss of a loved one or a job is important and unchangeable. Things such as your favourite sports team losing, a traffic jam, or bad weather are unchangeable and may or may not be important. What really counts is what you think about each stressor.

3. **Match your strategy to each stressor.** Different strategies work for different stressors. Here are some ways to be more effective in managing each type of problem.

Important and changeable stressors.
You can best manage these types of stressors by taking action to change the situation. Helpful problem-solving skills include planning and goal setting (see Chapter 2, *Becoming an Active Self-Manager*), imagery (see page 145), Positive Thinking and Self-Talk (see page 151), and effective communication and asking for support from others (see Chapter 11, *Communicating with Family, Friends, and Healthcare Professionals*).

Important and unchangeable stressors.
These stressors are the most difficult to manage. They can make you feel helpless and hopeless. No matter what you do, you cannot make another person change, bring someone back from the dead, or delete traumatic experiences from your life. You cannot change the situation, but you can try one or more of the following strategies:

■ Change the way you think about the problem. For example, think how much worse it could be, focus on the positive and practice gratitude (see page 158), deny or ignore the problem, distract yourself (see page 150), or accept what you can't change.

■ Find some part of the problem that you can move to changeable on your list. For example, you can't stop a storm, but you can take steps to rebuild any damage it causes.

■ Reassess how important the problem is in light of your overall life and priorities (for example, maybe your neighbour's criticism isn't so important after all).

■ Change your emotional reactions to the situation to reduce your stress. You can't change what happened, but you can help yourself feel less distressed about it. Try writing down your deepest thoughts and feelings (see page 159), seeking support from others, helping others, enjoying your

Sorting your life problems

Important and Changeable	Unimportant and Changeable
▸ Argument with partner	▸ Irritating phone calls
▸ Trouble with boss	▸ Errands
▸ Meeting job deadlines	▸ Chores
▸ Quitting smoking	▸ Unnecessary meetings
Important and Unchangeable	**Unimportant and Unchangeable**
▸ Death of a loved one	▸ Bad weather
▸ Loss of job	▸ Spilled food on clothes
▸ Serious illness	▸ Traffic jams
▸ Natural disaster	▸ Neighbour's opinion

You can use this space to jot down your problems.

Important and Changeable	Unimportant and Changeable
▸ _____	▸ _____
▸ _____	▸ _____
▸ _____	▸ _____
▸ _____	▸ _____
Important and Unchangeable	**Unimportant and Unchangeable**
▸ _____	▸ _____
▸ _____	▸ _____
▸ _____	▸ _____
▸ _____	▸ _____

Figure 5.3 **Sorting Your Stressors**

senses, relaxing, using imagery, enjoying humour, or exercising.

- Seek professional help. Sometimes people need help from a psychologist or a counsellor. Trained mental healthcare professionals can help you to live with important unchangeable stressors.

Unimportant and changeable stressors.

If a stressor is unimportant, first try just letting it go or putting it off until later. Or if you can control it with relatively little effort, go ahead and deal with it. Solving small problems builds your skills and confidence to tackle bigger ones. The same strategies that work for important and changeable stressors work for unimportant and changeable stressors.

Unimportant and unchangeable stressors.
The best solution for unimportant and unchangeable problems is to ignore them. Starting now, you have permission to let go of unimportant concerns. These are common hassles, and everybody has their share of them. Don't let them bother you. Distract yourself from these problems with humour, relaxation, or imagery or by focusing on more pleasurable things.

Using Problem Solving to Deal with Stress

You can successfully manage some types of stress by modifying the situation. But others seem to sneak up on you when you don't expect them. If you know that certain situations will be stressful, develop ways to deal with them before they happen. Try to rehearse, in your mind, what you will do when this happens so that you will be ready.

You can prepare for some future stressful situations such as being stuck in traffic, going on a trip, or preparing a meal. First, look at what about it is stressful. Is it that you hate to be late? Are trips stressful because you are not sure about your destination? Does making a meal involve too many steps and demand too much energy?

Once you have determined the problem, begin looking for possible ways to reduce the stress. Can you leave earlier? Can you let someone else drive? Can you call someone at your destination to ask about wheelchair access, local public transport, and other concerns? Can you prepare food in the morning? Can you take a short nap in the early afternoon?

After you have identified some possible solutions, select one to try the next time you are in the situation. Then evaluate the results. (This is the problem-solving approach we discussed in Chapter 2, *Becoming an Active Self-Manager*.)

We have also discussed tools for dealing with stress. They include getting enough sleep, exercising, eating well, and thinking techniques. Many of the tools for difficult emotions also work for stress. But sometimes stress is so overwhelming that these tools are not enough. These are times when good self-managers need consultants such as counsellors, social workers, psychologists, or psychiatrists.

Stress, like every other symptom, has many causes and can therefore be managed in many ways. It is up to you to examine the problem and try to find solutions that meet your needs and suit your lifestyle. And remember, stress can help you focus, grow, and deal with challenges.

Memory and Concentration

Many people worry about changes in their memory, particularly as they age. We know that many people with long-term conditions notice that they have 'cognitive' difficulties.

This means difficulties that relate to the normal processes of thoughts and thinking. In practice this can mean trouble remembering or problems concentrating on things they didn't used to find difficult, such as reading or following a story on a TV programme. There can be a number of things that can contribute to this:

- **Stress and low mood** have an effect on thinking processes, making it harder to see positive aspects of situations and more difficult to recall positive experiences.

- **Disrupted sleep** will interfere with your brain's ability to process and store memories.

- **Medication side effects** – some medications like pregabalin, gabapentin, and amitriptyline can have an effect on your ability to concentrate and remember things.

- **Pain** is a well-known 'interrupter' of normal thinking, making it hard to lay down memories.

So there are a number of common factors which affect these cognitive areas, and developing your self-management skills to manage stress, low mood, sleep disruption, and reduce your medication will usually help with these cognitive difficulties.

There are also conditions that cause serious and dramatic memory loss. These include Alzheimer's and other types of dementia. This is not a normal part of ageing. Symptoms for Alzheimer's and dementia vary widely. If you suspect that you or someone you know has symptoms of Alzheimer's and similar conditions, it is important to get these problems as assessed soon as possible. The treatments available may relieve some symptoms and help you maintain your independence longer. Knowing what you are dealing with allows you to take part in decisions about care, living options, and financial and legal matters. You can also start building a social network sooner and increase your chances of participating in clinical drug trials that help advance research.

If you are concerned about Alzheimer's or a similar condition, contact the Alzheimer's Society or Dementia UK for advice on a range of topics and to find support near you (contact details for both organisations are listed under the 'Useful Websites' section at the end of this chapter).

Itching

Itching is one of the hardest symptoms to deal with. It is any sensation that causes an urge to scratch. Like other symptoms, itching can have many different causes. Some of these causes are understood. When you get an insect bite or have contact with plants such as stinging nettles, your body releases chemicals called histamines. Histamines irritate nerve endings and cause itching. In some conditions, such as when someone's liver is damaged, it cannot remove bile products which are deposited in the skin, causing itching. Other causes of itching are not well understood. In kidney disease, itching may be severe. However, the exact cause is not clear. There are also other conditions, such as psoriasis, where the causes of itching are not easily explained. No matter what causes your itching, things such as warmth, wool clothing, and stress can make it worse. The next section discusses some ways to relieve itching.

Moisture

Dry skin tends to be itchy. Keep your skin moist by applying moisturising lotions or creams several times a day. When you choose a moisturiser, be careful. Be sure to read the list of ingredients. Avoid products that contain alcohol or other ingredients with names that end in *-ol*, as they tend to dry the skin. In general, the greasier the product, the better it works as a moisturiser. Creams or ointments are better moisturisers than lotions. Products such as Vaseline, olive oil, and vegetable shortening (such as Trex, Flora White, and Cookeen) are also very helpful.

When taking a bath or shower, use warm water and soak between 10 or 20 minutes. You can add bath oil, baking soda, or homemade bath oil to the water. To make your own bath oil, stir 2 teaspoons of olive oil into a large glass of milk and add it to the bath. When you get out of the water, pat yourself dry immediately and apply your cream.

If your itching is caused by the release of histamines during an allergic reaction or from having had contact with an irritating substance, wash off the oils or offending agent and apply cold compresses. Take an antihistamine to stop the reaction.

During cold weather it can be especially difficult to deal with itching because indoor heating tends to dry the skin. If this is a problem for you, a humidifier might help. Also try to keep your home and office as cool as you can without being uncomfortable.

Clothing

Your clothing can add to your itching sensations. The best rule of thumb is to wear what is comfortable. This is usually clothing made from material that is not scratchy. Most people find that soft natural fibres such as cotton allow the skin to 'breathe' better and are the least irritating to the skin.

Medications for Itching*

Antihistamines help if itching is caused by the release of histamines. You can buy antihistamines over the counter. There are two cheap antihistamines: Loratadine and Cetirizine, both of which are available in pharmacies and supermarkets. They are very similar, but ask a pharmacist if you are not sure which one to take as some can make people drowsy. Antihistamines with brand names such as *Benadryl, Piriton,* and *Clarityn* are the same as the generic versions but are much more expensive.

You can also buy medicated creams for itchy skin such as *Eurax* but most are not very effective. Steroid creams that contain cortisone can help itchy skin rashes associated with allergies. It is always sensible to ask the pharmacist about these over-the-counter products to ensure they are appropriate and will not cause problems with your prescribed medications.

Except for moisturising creams, no cream should be used on a long-term basis without talking to your doctor. If your itching continues, talk to your GP to have a review of your skin condition.

---

*For the UK edition, special thanks to Rachael Thornton, BPharm(Hons), PGClinDip, MRPharmS, IP, MFRPSII, for contributions to this section.

Stress and Itching

Anything that you can do to reduce stress will also help reduce itching. We have already discussed some of the ways to deal with stress earlier in this chapter. Chapter 6, *Using Your Mind to Manage Symptoms*, contains some additional stress reduction techniques.

Scratching

You probably want to scratch what itches, but this really does not help, especially for long-term itching, as it can lead to a vicious cycle where the more you scratch, the more you itch.

Unfortunately, it is hard to resist scratching. When you feel the need to scratch, try pressing or patting the skin. If you are not able to break this cycle yourself, ask your GP for a referral to a dermatologist, who may be able to help you find other ways to control your itching.

Itching is a common and very frustrating symptom for both patients and healthcare professionals to manage. If the self-management tips described here do not seem to help, it might be time to seek the advice of your GP, who can prescribe medications that can help with certain types of itching.

Urinary Incontinence: Loss of Bladder Control

Urinary incontinence is when you have trouble controlling your bladder and accidentally leak urine. If you have trouble controlling your bladder, you are not alone. Many people are coping with this problem. Although urinary incontinence can occur in both men and women, it is more common in women.

It is common to have some incontinence during or after pregnancy or with menopause, ageing, or weight gain. Activities that put increased pressure on the bladder, such as coughing, laughing, sneezing, and physical activity, can cause urine leakage. Incontinence can be related to changes in hormones, weakening muscles or ligaments in the pelvic area, or the use of certain medications. In men, incontinence can be related to an enlarged prostate. Infections in the bladder can also cause temporary incontinence.

Urinary incontinence can affect your quality of life and lead to other health problems. Feeling embarrassed by urinary incontinence causes some people to avoid social activities or sex. Some people experience loss of confidence or depression as a result of incontinence. Leaked urine may also cause skin irritation and infections. The frequent urge to urinate can interfere with sleep. And slipping on leaked urine when rushing to the bathroom can result in injury.

In many cases, incontinence can be controlled, if not cured outright. Many of these are small things you can do at home. If none of the following solves the problem, talk to your GP about other treatments. Don't be embarrassed. Your doctor has heard it all before.

There are three types of persistent or long-term loss of bladder control:

■ **Stress incontinence** refers to small amounts of urine leaking out during exercise, coughing, laughing, sneezing, or other movements that squeeze the bladder. Pelvic floor (also known as Kegel) exercises (described under

'Home Treatments' below) often improve this condition.

- **Urge incontinence**, or overactive bladder, happens when the need to urinate comes on so quickly that you don't have enough time to get to the toilet.

- **Overflow incontinence** is leakage from an overfilled bladder due to a weak bladder or, in men, blockage from an enlarged prostate.

Home Treatments for Incontinence

Small, effective changes to your lifestyle or behaviour are the first treatments for urinary incontinence. For many people, these treatments effectively control or cure the problem.

Pelvic floor exercises strengthen your pelvic floor muscles. This allows better control of your urine flow and prevents leaking. Learning pelvic floor exercises takes a bit of practice and patience. It may take a few weeks to feel an improvement in your symptoms.

Follow these steps to do pelvic floor exercises:

1. First, find the muscles that stop your urine. Do this by repeatedly stopping your urine in midstream and starting again. Focus on the muscles that you feel squeezing around your urethra (opening for the urine) and anus (opening for your bowels).

2. Practice squeezing these muscles when urinating or even when you are not urinating. If your stomach or buttocks move, you're not using the right muscles.

3. Squeeze the muscles, hold for 3 seconds, and then relax for 3 seconds.

4. Repeat the exercise 10 to 15 times per session.

Complete at least 30 pelvic floor exercises every day. The wonderful thing about pelvic floor exercises is that you can do them anywhere and anytime. How about during television commercials or when sitting at traffic lights? No one will know what you are doing except you.

With urge incontinence, retraining your bladder may help. Take the following steps to retrain your bladder:

- Practice 'double-voiding'. Empty your bladder as much as possible, relax for a minute, and try to empty it again. This helps empty your bladder completely.

- Practice waiting a specified amount of time before urinating. This gradually retrains your bladder to require emptying less often.

- Train yourself to urinate on a regular schedule, about every 2 to 4 hours during the day, whether or not you feel the urge. If you now need to urinate every 30 minutes, perhaps you can start by waiting to every 40 minutes and gradually work your way up to every 2 to 4 hours.

Some lifestyle changes can also help with incontinence, including the following:

- Drink fewer beverages that stimulate the bladder and urine production, such as alcohol, coffee, tea, and other drinks that contain caffeine. This can reduce your trips to the toilet.

- If you have extra weight, losing weight can reduce the pressure on your bladder.

Studies show that losing just 10% of total body weight improves incontinence problems for many people.

■ Wearing absorbent pads or briefs does not cure incontinence, but it helps manage the condition.

Treatments and Medications for Incontinence

If changes in your lifestyle or behaviour do not relieve your urinary incontinence, other treatments may help, including the use of medication, a pessary (a thin, flexible ring that can be worn inside the vagina to support the pelvic area), or, in some cases, surgery. You don't have to suffer in silence if you have urinary incontinence. Talk with your GP.

Oral Health Concerns*

A healthy mouth is important to overall health. Many long-term conditions and medications can make oral health problems worse. And evidence suggests that oral conditions, such as inflammation of the gums (gingivitis), may contribute to diabetes, heart disease, and stroke. Good oral health also makes it easier to get good nutrition and eat a healthy diet.

These preventive steps can help keep your mouth and teeth healthy throughout your life:

1. Brush with a soft-bristled brush or electric toothbrush twice a day for at least two minutes each time. If you have problems with grip, use a large-handled toothbrush.

2. Clean between your teeth using interdental brushes such as 'TePe' or dental floss at least once a day. Using an angled floss holder can make flossing easier.

3. Choose a fluoride toothpaste to prevent cavities. Your dentist may also recommend

fluoride rinses or prescription toothpaste for added protection against tooth decay.

4. Every 6 months (or more often if recommended), book a dental hygienist appointment and tooth cleaning. Have your dentist or dental hygienist show you how to brush and floss for best results.

5. Avoid smoking and chewing tobacco, which can cause oral cancers.

6. If you experience tooth pain; hot or cold sensitivity; red, swollen, or bleeding gums; a lump on your tongue or cheeks; or a persistent dry mouth, seek care from a dentist right away. These may be early signs of decay, infection, or even oral cancer. Early detection and treatment is very important.

7. If you have a dry mouth, discuss this condition with your dentist. Many medications can cause this. Sip water frequently during the day. Your dentist may also have recommendations.

---

*Special thanks to Andrew D. Sewell, DDS, for contributions to this section.

In this chapter we have discussed common causes of some of the most common symptoms experienced by people with long-term conditions. We have described some of the tools in your self-management toolbox that you can use to cope with your symptoms. Taking action to manage your symptoms needs to happen on a daily basis. But sometimes this just doesn't seem to be enough. There are times when you may wish to escape from your surroundings and just have 'your time'. This time allows you to clear your mind and gain a fresh perspective. The next chapter discusses different ways to complement the management tools in this chapter with thinking tools. Using the power of your mind can help reduce and even prevent some of your symptoms.

■ ■ ■

As we noted in this chapter, the misuse of prescription medications is a growing problem. Misuse of pain medications is a complicated issue. To learn more about this topic, you might like to explore the following resource from the United States: Beth Darnall, *Less Pain, Fewer Pills: Avoid the Dangers of Prescription Opioids and Gain Control over Chronic Pain* (Boulder, CO: Bull Publishing, 2014). This book is available from Bull Publishing, https://www.bullpub.com/less-pain-fewer-pills.html.

Useful Websites

Alcoholics Anonymous: https://www.alcoholics-anonymous.org.uk/Home

Alzheimer's Society: https://www.alzheimers.org.uk/get-support

Anxiety UK: https://www.anxietyuk.org.uk/

Bladder Health UK: https://bladderhealthuk.org/

British Lung Foundation (Managing breathlessness): https://www.blf.org.uk/support-for-you
/breathlessness/how-to-manage-breathlessness

Dementia UK: https://www.dementiauk.org/

Mind: https://www.mind.org.uk/

NHS (Alcohol support services): https://www.nhs.uk/live-well/alcohol-support/

NHS (Advice on shielding for people at high risk from coronavirus): https://www.nhs.uk
/conditions/coronavirus-covid-19/people-at-higher-risk/advice-for-people-at-high-risk/

NHS (Help with suicidal thoughts): https://www.nhs.uk/conditions/suicide/

NHS (Insomnia): https://www.nhs.uk/conditions/insomnia/

NHS (Medicines A–Z): https://www.nhs.uk/medicines/

NHS (Mindfulness – breathing, dealing with stress, anger): https://www.nhs.uk/conditions
/stress-anxiety-depression/mindfulness/

NHS (Stop smoking services): https://www.nhs.uk/live-well/quit-smoking
/nhs-stop-smoking-services-help-you-quit/

NHS (Stop smoking services – local): https://www.nhs.uk/smokefree/help-and-advice
/local-support-services-helplines/

NHS (Who's at higher risk from coronavirus): https://www.nhs.uk/conditions
/coronavirus-covid-19/people-at-higher-risk/whos-at-higher-risk-from-coronavirus/

Pain UK: https://painuk.org/

Public Health England (Advice for smokers and vapers): https://www.gov.uk/government
/publications/covid-19-advice-for-smokers-and-vapers/covid-19-advice-for-smokers-and-vapers

Rethink Mental Illness (Support groups): https://www.rethink.org/help-in-your-area
/support-groups/

Samaritans: https://www.samaritans.org/

Stroke Association: https://www.stroke.org.uk/

The Sleep Council: https://sleepcouncil.org.uk/

UK Air Information Resource (Daily Air Quality Index – DAQI): https://uk-air.defra.gov.uk
/air-pollution/daqi

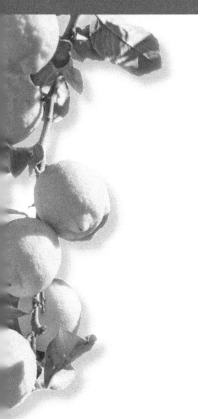

CHAPTER 6

Using Your Mind to Manage Symptoms

THERE IS A STRONG LINK BETWEEN thoughts, attitudes, and emotions and mental and physical health. One of our self-managers said, 'It's not always mind over matter, but mind matters.' Your body is not a mindless machine. Your thoughts, feelings, moods, and actions have important health effects. They determine the start of some conditions, the course of many, and the management of nearly all. What goes on in your mind helps shape your symptoms, overall happiness, and sense of well-being.

Research has shown that thoughts and emotions trigger hormones or other chemicals that send messages throughout the body. These messages affect how the body functions; for example, thoughts and emotions can change heart rate, blood pressure, breathing, blood glucose levels, muscle responses, immune response, concentration, the

Special thanks to Rick Seidel, PhD, for contributions to this chapter.

137

ability to get pregnant, and even the ability to fight off illness.

All people, at one time or another, experience the power of the mind and its effects on the body. Both pleasant and unpleasant thoughts and emotions can cause your body to react in different ways. Your heart rate and breathing can increase or slow down; you may sweat (warm or cold), blush, or cry. Sometimes just a memory or an image can trigger these responses. For example, imagine that you are holding a big, bright yellow lemon slice. You hold it close to your nose and smell its strong citrus aroma. Now you bite into the lemon. It's juicy! The juice fills your mouth and dribbles down your chin. Now you begin to suck on the lemon and its tart juice. What happens? The body responds. Your mouth puckers and starts to water. You may even smell the scent of the lemon. You are not really tasting and smelling a real lemon. All these reactions are triggered by the mind and your memories of a real lemon.

This example shows the power of your mind and its effects. It also gives you a good reason to work to develop ways of using your mind to help manage your symptoms. With training and practice, you can learn to use your mind to relax your body, to reduce stress and anxiety, and to reduce the discomfort or unpleasantness caused by your physical and emotional symptoms. The mind can also help relieve the pain and shortness of breath associated with various diseases and can even make people depend less on some medications. Many of the most powerful prescriptions are ready for you to use right now. They are in the pharmacy of your own brain. In this chapter we describe several means of using your mind to manage symptoms. These are sometimes referred to as 'thinking' or 'cognitive'

tools because they involve the use of your thinking abilities to make changes in the body.

As you read, keep the following in mind:

- **Symptoms have many causes.** This means that there are many ways to manage most symptoms. If you understand the nature and causes of your symptoms, you will be able to manage them better. But remember, mind cannot always triumph over matter. You are not responsible for causing your condition or failing to cure it. But you are responsible for taking action to help manage your condition.

- **Not all management techniques work for everyone.** It is up to you to experiment and find out what works best for you. Be flexible. This includes trying different tools and checking the results to learn which management tool is most helpful for which symptoms and when. Experiment. Don't be frustrated if you don't have time or energy to try out all the suggestions and advice in this book. Even the authors can't practice all they preach!

- **New skills can take time to acquire and master.** Give yourself several weeks to practice before you decide if a new tool is working for you. For any prescription to work, you must take it. Just knowing a technique is not enough. If you want to learn, grow, and become healthier, you need to take action and take some risks. You must actually do something different. Learning requires new actions, not just new information. As you read this book, if the thought 'I already know that' or 'that's too simple to work' crosses your mind, reconsider it.

Knowing something and putting it into daily practice are two different things.

■ **Some of these tools may seem silly, repetitive, or not for you.** Don't worry – not everyone likes the same type of biscuit, but that does not mean that one cannot like any biscuits. The tools in this chapter are like biscuits. You will like some and not like others. Pick and choose. If you don't like one tool, try another.

■ **Don't give up too easily.** As with exercise and other new skills, using your mind to manage your health condition will take both practice and time before you notice the benefits. So even if you feel you are not getting the results you want, don't give up. Also, along the way, remember to give yourself credit for all your efforts.

■ **These techniques should not have negative effects.** If you become frightened, angry, or depressed when using one of these tools, do not continue to use it. Try another tool instead.

■ **These tools are designed to use along with regular medical treatments.** Fortunately, you don't have to choose between medications or mind-body medicine. You can use either or both. The mind-body techniques described here can improve the effectiveness of appropriate medications and other medical treatments.

Mind-body techniques are generally safe. They don't have negative side effects or cause adverse reactions, and there is no risk of overdosing. The most common 'side effects' are a positive sense of well-being, increased self-confidence, better mood, and often better sleep. Since the mind-body approach involves learning and practicing new skills, the benefits may also be long lasting. This is because you can safely use them whenever you need them for the rest of your life. With many medications, the improvement may stop as soon as you stop the medicine. The tools described in this chapter give you more control.

Relaxation Techniques

Relaxation involves using thinking techniques to reduce or eliminate tension from both the body and the mind. This usually results in improved sleep quality and less stress, pain, and shortness of breath. Relaxation is not a cure-all, but it can be an important part of a treatment plan.

There are different types of relaxation techniques. Each has specific guidelines and uses. Some techniques are for muscle relaxation, while others are aimed at reducing anxiety and emotional stress or diverting attention. All of these aid in symptom management.

The term *relaxation* means different things to different people. Most people can identify things they do to relax. For example, you may walk, watch TV, listen to music, knit, or garden. These can be great relaxation strategies. You can also learn specific relaxation skills to quiet the mind, relax the body, and lessen symptoms. In the next sections, we discuss daily activities you can use to relax as well as tried and trusted relaxation techniques and skills.

Pleasurable Activities

Some types of relaxation are so easy, natural, and effective that people do not think of them as 'relaxation techniques'. Savouring all of your senses can be relaxing and restorative. Consider making some of these pleasurable activities part of your week:

- Take a nap or a hot, soothing bath.
- Curl up and read or listen to a good book.
- Watch a funny film.
- Make a paper aeroplane and fly it across the room.
- Get a massage (or give one).
- Enjoy an occasional glass of wine or savour a cup of tea.
- Start a small garden or grow a beautiful plant indoors.
- Do crafts such as knitting, pottery, or woodwork.
- Watch a favourite TV show.
- Listen to an interesting podcast.
- Read a poem or an inspirational saying.
- Go for a walk.
- Start a collection (coins, folk art, shells, or something in miniature).
- Listen to your favourite music or nature sounds (for example, wind, water, crackling fire, or birds twittering).
- Sing or dance around the house.
- Crumple paper into a ball and use a waste-paper bin as a basketball hoop.

- Look at water (an ocean, a lake, a stream, or a fountain).
- Watch the clouds or stars in the sky.
- Put your head down on your desk and close your eyes for 5 minutes.
- Rub your hands together until they're warm, and then cup them over your closed eyes.
- Vigorously shake your hands and arms for 10 seconds.
- Call up a friend or family member to chat.
- Smile and introduce yourself to someone new.
- Do something nice and unexpected for someone else.
- Play with a pet.
- Visit a favourite holiday spot in your mind.

Did we miss some of your favourite pleasurable activities? Don't worry! You can add your favourites to the list.

Nature Therapy

If you live in a city or spend most of your time indoors, you may suffer from what has been called 'nature deficit disorder'. The good news is that you can cure yourself of this condition. All you need to do is get outdoors. For thousands of years, people have been told to expose themselves to natural environments for healing. Get away from artificial lighting, take a break from excessive computer and TV screen time, leave your phone in your pocket, and go outdoors. A brief walk in a park or a longer planned visit to a beautiful outdoor place can restore your mind and body.

If you take the time to look, almost every outdoor place has something of interest or beauty. Something as small as a dandelion pushing its way through a crack in the pavement can be inspiring. You can also bring nature indoors with plants, pets, a fish tank, a rock collection, or pine forest scents. Hang a bird feeder outside your window, or check out a book of nature photography from your library. Visit websites with nature stories and photos. Even a few minutes of playing with or stroking a pet can lower blood pressure and calm a restless mind.

Relaxation Self-Management Tools

The following are some general tips for using relaxation tools:

- **Pick a quiet place and time** when you will not be disturbed for at least 15 to 20 minutes. (If this seems too long, start with 5 minutes. By the way, in some homes the only quiet place is the bathroom. That is just fine.)

- **Try to practice the technique once or twice a day or every other day.**

- **Do not try relaxation techniques that involve concentration while driving or doing other activities that require close attention.**

- **Don't expect miracles.** With some techniques you may notice rapid results, but others may take several weeks of practice before you start to notice benefits.

- **Relaxation should be helpful.** At worst, you may find it boring, but if it is an unpleasant experience or makes you more nervous or anxious, switch to one

of the other symptom management tools described in this chapter.

In the following sections you will learn about several techniques you can use every day to quiet your mind and body.

Body scan

To relax muscles, you need to know how to scan your body and recognise where you are tense. Doing this helps you know how to release the tension. The first step is to become familiar with the difference between the feeling of tension and the feeling of relaxation. This body scan exercise teaches you to compare those sensations and, with practice, to spot and release tension anywhere in your body. It is best to do a body scan lying down on your back, but feel free to do it in any comfortable position. You can find a body scan script on page 142. Follow the script to identify where in your body you are holding tension.

Relaxation response

According to Herbert Benson, a doctor who studied what he called the 'relaxation response', our bodies have several natural states. Perhaps you have heard of the 'fight or flight' response. When you are faced with a great danger, your body becomes quite tense. After the danger passes, you tend to relax. This is the relaxation response. As people's lives become more and more hectic, their bodies tend to stay tense for longer stretches. You can lose the ability to relax. Learning how to prompt your body to start the relaxation response helps you regain this abilty.

To create your own relaxation response, first find a quiet place where there are few or no

Body-Scan Script

As you get into a comfortable position, allowing yourself to begin to sink comfortably into the surface below you, you may perhaps begin to allow your eyes gradually to close … From there, turn your attention to your breath … Breathing in, allowing the breath gradually to go all the way down to your belly, and then breathing out … And again, breathing in … and out … noticing the natural rhythm of your breathing …

Now allowing your attention to focus on your feet. Starting with your toes, notice whatever sensations are there – warmth, coolness, whatever is there … simply feel it. Using your mind's eye, imagine that as you breathe in, the breath goes all the way down into your toes, bringing with it new, refreshing air … And now notice the sensations elsewhere in your feet. Not judging or thinking about what you're feeling, but simply becoming aware of the experience of your feet as you allow yourself to be fully supported by the surface below you …

Next focus on your lower legs and knees. These muscles and joints do a lot of work for us, but we don't often give them the attention they deserve. So now breathe down into the knees, calves, and ankles, noticing whatever sensations appear … See if you can simply stay with the sensations … breathing in new, fresh air, and as you exhale, releasing tension and stress and allowing the muscles to relax and soften …

Now move your attention to the muscles, bones, and joints of the thighs, buttocks, and hips … breathing down into the upper legs, noticing whatever sensations you experience. It may be warmth, coolness, a heaviness or lightness. You may become aware of the contact with the surface beneath you, or perhaps the pulsing of your blood. Whatever is there … what matters is that you are taking time to learn to relax … deeper and deeper, as you breathe … in … and out.

Move your attention now to your back and chest. Feeling the breath fill the abdomen and chest … noticing whatever sensations are there … not judging or thinking, but simply observing what is right here, right now. Allow the fresh air to nourish the muscles, bones, and joints as you breathe in, and then exhaling any tension and stress.

Now focus on the neck, shoulders, arms, and hands. Inhaling down through the neck and shoulders, all the way down to the fingertips. Not trying too hard to relax, but simply becoming aware of your experience of these parts of your body in the present moment …

Turning now to your face and head, notice the sensations beginning at the back of your head, up along your scalp, and down into your forehead … then become aware of the sensations in and around your eyes and down into your cheeks and jaw … continue to allow your muscles to release and soften as you breathe in nourishing fresh air, and allow tension and stress to leave as you breathe out …

As you drink in fresh air, allow it to spread throughout your body, from the soles of your feet all the way up through the top of your head … and then exhale any remaining stress and tension … and now take a few moments to enjoy the stillness as you breathe in … and out … awake, relaxed, and still …

Now as the body scan comes to a close, coming back into the room, bringing with you whatever sensations of relaxation … comfort … peace, whatever is there … knowing that you can repeat this exercise at any appropriate time and place of your choosing … and when you're ready, open your eyes.

distractions. Find a position where you can be comfortable and remain for at least 20 minutes. Now focus on the following steps:

■ Close your eyes.

■ Relax all your muscles, beginning at your feet and progressing up to your face.

■ Breathe in through your nose. Become aware of your breathing. Choose a word, object, or pleasant feeling. For example, repeat a word or sound (such as the word *one*,) gaze at a symbol (perhaps a flower), or concentrate on a feeling (such as peace). As you breathe out through your mouth, say the word you chose silently to yourself. Try to concentrate on your word, sound, or symbol.

■ As you breathe, maintain a passive attitude, and let relaxation occur at its own pace. When distracting thoughts, feelings, or images occur, note what they are. Just let them pass on and gently return to your breathing as you repeat the word you chose. Do not worry about whether you are successful in achieving a deep level of relaxation. It will come.

■ Practice this relaxing technique for 10 to 20 minutes. You may open your eyes to check the time, but do not use an alarm. When you finish, continue to sit quietly for several minutes, at first with your eyes closed. Do not stand up for a few minutes.

Quieting reflex

Physician Charles Stroebel developed a relaxation technique called the 'quieting reflex'. This method can help with short-term stress. It can help calm the urge to eat or smoke. It can also help prevent reactions such as road rage and

help you handle the annoyances of daily life. It relieves muscle tightening, jaw clenching, and holding your breath.

You can use the quieting reflex several times a day, whenever you start to feel stressed. It can be done with your eyes opened or closed. To practice this technique, focus on the following steps:

1. Become aware of what is stressing you: a ringing phone, an angry comment, the urge to smoke, a worrying thought – whatever.

2. Repeat the phrase 'alert mind, calm body' to yourself.

3. Smile inwardly with your eyes and your mouth. This stops your facial muscles from making a fearful or angry expression. The inward smile is a feeling. Others cannot see it.

4. Inhale slowly to the count of 3, imagining that the breath comes in through the bottom of your feet. Then exhale slowly. Feel your breath move back down your legs and out through your feet. Let your jaw, tongue, and shoulder muscles go limp.

With several months' practice, the quieting reflex becomes an automatic skill. And it takes just seconds to do!

Mindfulness

When you practice mindfulness, you keep your attention in the present moment, without judging the moment as happy or sad, good or bad. Mindfulness involves living each moment – even painful ones – as fully and as mindfully as possible. Mindfulness is more than a relaxation technique; it is an attitude toward living. It is a way of calmly observing and accepting whatever is happening, moment to moment.

This may sound simple enough, but our restless, judging minds make it surprisingly difficult. Just as a restless monkey jumps from branch to branch, people's minds jump from thought to thought.

When you practice mindfulness, you try to focus the mind on the present moment. The 'goal' of mindfulness is simply to observe – with no intention of changing or improving anything. People are positively changed by this practice. Observing and accepting life just as it is, with all its pleasures, pains, frustrations, disappointments, and insecurities, allows you to become calmer, more confident, and better able to cope with whatever comes along.

To develop your capacity for mindfulness, follow these steps:

■ Sit comfortably on the floor or on a chair with your back, neck, and head straight, but not stiff.

■ Concentrate on a single object or activity, such as your breathing. Focus your attention on the feeling of the air as it passes in and out of your nostrils with each breath. Don't try to control your breathing by speeding it up or slowing it down. Just observe it as it is.

■ Even when you resolve to keep your attention on your breathing, your mind will quickly wander off. When this occurs, observe where your mind goes: perhaps to a memory, a worry about the future, a bodily ache, or a feeling of impatience. Then gently return your attention to your breathing.

■ Use your breath as an anchor. Each time a thought or feeling arises, acknowledge it. Don't analyse it or judge it. Just observe it and return to your breathing.

■ Let go of all thoughts of getting somewhere or having anything special happen. Just keep stringing moments of mindfulness together, breath by breath.

■ At first, practice this for just 5 minutes, or even 1 minute. You may wish to gradually extend the time to 10, 20, or 30 minutes.

The practice of mindfulness is simply the practice of moment-to-moment awareness. You can apply mindfulness to anything: eating, showering, working, talking, running errands, or playing with children. For example, how many baths or showers have you taken in your life? And how often after bathing did you really pay close attention to how wonderful the towel felt on your skin as you dried off? Or was your mind somewhere else, lost in other thoughts? Try making friends with your towel next time you bathe. Give yourself the gift of 1 minute to pay full attention to how the towel feels on your skin, the different motions, the different sensations, and so forth. Or try savouring your food. How does it look? Smell? Feel in your mouth? Notice your impulse to rush through this mouthful to get to the next one. But stay present with the mouthful you already have. Mindfulness takes no extra time. Considerable research has demonstrated the benefits of mindfulness practice in relieving stress, easing pain, improving concentration, and relieving a variety of other symptoms.

Imagery

You may think that 'imagination' is all in your mind. But the thoughts, words, and images from your imagination can have very real effects on your body. Your brain often cannot distinguish whether you are imagining something or if it is really happening. Remember the exercise of imagining the lemon from the beginning of the chapter. Or perhaps you've had a racing heartbeat, rapid breathing, or tension in your neck muscles while watching a thriller. The images and sounds in a film produced these sensations. During your dreams, your body responds with fear, joy, anger, or sadness – all triggered by your imagination. If you close your eyes and vividly imagine yourself by a still, quiet pool or relaxing on a warm beach, your body responds to some degree as though you were actually there.

Guided imagery and visualisation allow you to use your imagination to relieve symptoms. This is done by using healing images and suggestions.

Guided Imagery

This tool is like a guided daydream. Guided imagery refocuses your mind away from your symptoms and takes you to another time and place. You can picture yourself in a peaceful environment and achieve deep relaxation.

With guided imagery, you focus your mind on an image. Think of a waterfall, a crisp autumn day, or a favourite beach. You then add other senses – smells, tastes, and sounds – to make the image more vivid and powerful.

Some people are highly visual and easily see images with their 'mind's eye'. However, if your images aren't as vivid as scenes from a great film, don't worry. It's normal for people's imagery to vary. The important thing is to focus on as much detail as possible and to strengthen the images by using all your senses. Adding real background music can also increase the impact of guided imagery.

With guided imagery, you are always completely in control. You're the film director. You can project whatever thought or feeling you want onto your mental screen. If you don't like a particular image, thought, or feeling, redirect your mind to something more comfortable. You can use images to get rid of unpleasant thoughts. For example, you can put them on a raft and watch them float away, sweep them away with a large broom, or erase them with a giant rubber. And at any time, you can open your eyes and stop the exercise.

The guided imagery scripts on pages 147–148 are sample guides for this mental stroll. Follow these steps to use imagery:

■ Read the script over several times until it is familiar. Then sit or lie down in a quiet place and try to reconstruct the scene in your mind. The script should take 15 to 20 minutes to complete.

■ Have a family member or friend read you the script slowly, pausing for about 10 seconds wherever there is a series of periods (…).

■ Make a recording of yourself or someone else reading the script and play it to yourself whenever convenient.

■ Use a prerecorded tape, CD, or digital audio file that has a similar guided imagery script (see examples in the 'Useful Websites' section at the end of this chapter).

■ Feel free to edit or change the script to create your own imaginary journey.

Visualisation

This visualisation technique is similar to guided imagery. Visualisation allows you to create your own images, which is different from guided imagery, where the images are suggested to you. Visualisation is another way to create a picture of yourself in any way you want, doing the things you want to do. You already use a form of visualisation every day – when you dream, worry, read a book, or listen to a story. In all these activities the mind creates images for you to see. You also use visualisation when making plans for the day, considering the possible outcomes of a decision you have to make, or rehearsing for an event or activity. You can use visualisation in different ways, for longer periods of time, or while you are doing other things. Do not try visualisation while driving or doing other activities that require close attention.

One way to use visualisation to manage symptoms is to remember pleasant scenes from your past or to create new scenes. Try to remember every detail of a special holiday or party that made you happy. Who was there? What happened? What did you do or talk about? You can use visualisation by remembering a holiday or some other memorable and pleasant event.

You can also use visualisation to plan the details of a future event or to fill in the details of a fantasy. For example, think about the answers to these questions: How would you spend a million pounds? What would be your ideal romantic encounter? What would your ideal home or garden look like? Where would you go and what would you do on your dream holiday?

Another form of visualisation involves using your mind to think of symbols that represent the discomfort or pain felt in different parts of your body. For example, you might visualise a painful joint as red, or a tight chest with a constricting band around it. After forming these images, you then try to change them. Imagine the red colour fading until there is no more colour, or visualise the constricting band stretching and stretching until it falls off. These images can change the way you experience the pain or discomfort.

Imagery for Different Conditions

You have the ability to create special imagery to help specific symptoms or illnesses. Use any image that is strong, meaningful, and vivid for you – if possible, use all your senses to create the image. The image does not have to be accurate for it to work. Just use your imagination and trust yourself. Here are examples of images that some people have found useful:

For Tension and Stress

A tight, twisted rope slowly untwists.

Wax softens and melts.

Tension swirls out of your body and down the drain.

For Healing of Cuts and Injuries

Plaster covers over a crack in a wall. Cells and fibres stick together with very strong glue.

A shoe is laced up tight.

Jigsaw puzzle pieces come together.

For Arteries and Heart Disease

A miniature Dyno-Rod lorry speeds through your arteries and cleans out the clogged pipes.

Guided-Imagery Script: A Walk in the Country

You're giving yourself some time to quiet your mind and body. Allow yourself to settle comfortably, wherever you are right now. If you wish, you can close your eyes. Breathe in deeply, through your nose, expanding your abdomen and filling your lungs. Pursing your lips, exhale through your mouth slowly and completely, allowing your body to sink heavily into the surface beneath you … and once again breathe in through your nose and all the way down to your abdomen, and then breathe out slowly through pursed lips – letting go of tension, letting go of anything that is on your mind right now and just allowing yourself to be present in this moment …

Imagine yourself walking along a peaceful old country lane. The sun is gently warming your back … the birds are singing … the air is calm and fragrant …

With no need to hurry, you notice that your walking is relaxed and easy. As you walk along in this way, taking in your surroundings, you come across an old gate. It looks inviting and you decide to take the path through the gate. The gate creaks as you open it and go through.

You find yourself in an old, overgrown garden – flowers growing where they've seeded themselves, vines climbing over a fallen tree, soft green wild grasses grow and trees stand silently casting shade.

You notice yourself breathing deeply … smelling the flowers … listening to the birds and insects … feeling a gentle breeze cool against your skin. All of your senses are alive and responding with pleasure to this peaceful time and place …

When you are ready to move on, you leisurely follow the path out behind the garden, eventually coming to a more wooded area. As you enter this area, your eyes find the trees and plant life restful. The sunlight is filtered through the leaves. The air feels mild and a little cooler … you savour the fragrance of trees and earth … and gradually become aware of the sound of a nearby stream. Pausing, you allow yourself to take in the sights and sounds, breathing in the cool and fragrant air several times … and with each breath, you notice how refreshed you are feeling …

Continuing along the path for a while, you come to the stream. It's clear and clean as it flows and tumbles over the rocks and some fallen logs. You follow the path easily along the creek for a way, until you come out into a sunlit clearing, where you discover a small waterfall emptying into a quiet pool of water.

You find a comfortable place to sit for a while, a perfect niche where you can feel completely relaxed.

You feel good as you allow yourself to just enjoy the warmth and solitude of this peaceful place … Gradually, you become aware that it is time to return. You arise and walk back down the path in a relaxed and comfortable way, through the cool and fragrant trees, out into the sun-drenched overgrown garden … You take one last smell of the flowers, and walk out the creaky gate.

You leave this country retreat for now and return down the lane. You notice that you feel calm and rested. You feel grateful and remind yourself that you can visit this special place whenever you wish to take some time to refresh yourself and renew your energy.

And now, preparing to bring this period of relaxation to a close, you may want to take a moment to picture yourself carrying this experience of calm and refreshment with you into the ordinary activities of your life … and when you are ready, take a nice deep breath and open your eyes.

Guided-Imagery Script: A Walk on the Beach

Begin by getting into a comfortable position, whether you are seated or lying down. Loosen any tight clothing to allow yourself to be as comfortable as possible. Uncross your legs and allow your hands to fall by your sides or rest in your lap, and if you are at all uncomfortable, shift to a more comfortable position.

When you are ready, you may allow your eyes to close gradually and turn your attention to your breathing. Allow your belly to expand as you breathe in, bringing in fresh new air to nourish your body. And then breathing out. Notice the rhythm of your breathing – in … and out … without trying to control it in any way at all. Simply attend to the natural rhythm of your breath …

And now in your mind's eye, imagine yourself standing on a beautiful beach. The sky is a brilliant blue, and as some fluffy white clouds float slowly by, you drink in the beautiful colours … the temperature is not too hot and not too cold. The sun is shining, and you close your eyes, allowing the warmth of the sun to wash over you … You notice a gentle breeze caressing your face, the perfect complement to the sunshine.

Then you find yourself turning and looking out over the vastness of the ocean … You become aware of the sound of the waves gently washing up on shore … You notice the firmness of the wet sand beneath your shoes, or, if you decide to take off your shoes, you may enjoy the feeling of standing in the cool, wet sand … Perhaps you allow the surf to roll up and gently wash across your feet, or perhaps you stay just out of its reach …

In the distance you hear some seagulls calling to one another and look out to see the birds gracefully gliding through the air. And as you stand there, notice how easy it is to be here, perhaps noticing some sensations of relaxation, comfort, or peace – whatever is there …

Now take a walk along the shore. Turn and begin to stroll casually along the beach, enjoying the sounds of the surf, the warmth of the sun, and the gentle massage of the breeze. As you move along, taking your time, your stride becomes lighter, easier … You notice the scent of the ocean … you pause to take in the freshness of the air … and then you continue on your way, enjoying the peacefulness of this place.

After a time, you decide to rest for awhile, and you find a comfortable place to sit or lie down … and simply allow yourself to take some time to enjoy this, your special place …

And now, when you feel ready to return, you stand and begin walking back down the beach in a comfortable, leisurely way, taking with you any sensations of relaxation, comfort, peace, joy – whatever is there … noticing how easy it is to be here. Continuing back until you reach the place where you began your walk …

And now pause to take one last long look around. Enjoying the vibrant colours of the sky and the sea … the gentle sound of the waves washing up on the shore. The warmth of the sun, the cool of the breeze …

And as you prepare to leave this special place, take with you any sensations of joy, relaxation, comfort, peace – whatever is there – knowing that you can return at any appropriate time and place of your choosing.

And now bring your awareness back into the room, focusing on your breathing … in and out … taking a few more breaths … and when you are ready, opening your eyes.

Water flows freely through a wide, open river.

A crew in a small boat rows in sync, easily and efficiently pulling the slender boat across the smooth water surface.

For Asthma and Lung Conditions

The tiny elastic rubber bands that constrict your airways pop open.

A vacuum cleaner gently sucks the mucus from your airways.

Waves calmly rise and fall on the ocean surface.

For Diabetes

Small insulin keys unlock doors to hungry cells and allow nourishing blood glucose in.

An alarm goes off, and a sleeping pancreas gland awakens to the smell of freshly brewed coffee.

For Cancer

A shark gobbles up the cancer cells.

Tumours shrivel up like raisins in the hot sun and then evaporate completely into the air.

The tap that controls the blood supply to the tumour is turned off, and the cancer cells starve.

Radiation or chemotherapy enters your body like healing rays of light and destroys cancer cells.

For Infections

White blood cells with flashing red sirens arrest and imprison harmful germs.

An army equipped with powerful antibiotic missiles attacks enemy germs.

A hot flame chases germs out of your entire body.

For a Weakened Immune System

Sluggish, sleepy white blood cells awaken, put on protective armour, and enter the fight against the virus.

White blood cells rapidly multiply like millions of seeds bursting from a single ripe seedpod.

For an Overactive Immune System (allergies, arthritis, psoriasis, etc.)

Overly alert immune cells in the fire station are reassured that the allergens have triggered a false alarm, and they go back to playing their game of cards.

A civil war ends with the warring sides agreeing not to attack their fellow citizens.

For Pain

All of the pain is placed in a large, strong metal box that is closed, sealed tightly, and locked with a huge, strong padlock.

You grasp the TV remote control and slowly turn down the pain volume until you can barely hear it; then it disappears entirely.

A cool, calm river flowing through your entire body washes the pain away.

For Depression

Your troubles and feelings of sadness are attached to big, colourful helium balloons and they float off into a clear blue sky.

A strong, warm sun breaks through dark clouds.

You feel a sense of detachment and lightness, enabling you to float easily through your day.

Use any of these images or make up your own. Remember, the best ones are vivid and have meaning to you. Use your imagination for health and healing.

Distraction

Minds have trouble focusing on more than one thing at a time. You can lessen your symptoms by training your mind to focus attention on something other than that symptom. This method is called distraction or attention refocusing. Distraction is particularly helpful for people who feel that their symptoms are painful or overwhelming. It is also good if you worry that every bodily sensation is a new or worsening symptom or health problem.

With distraction you are not ignoring the symptoms but choosing not to dwell on them. Trying to push anxious thoughts out of your mind may result in your thinking more about them. For example, try not thinking about a tiger charging at you. Whatever you do, don't let the thought of a tiger enter your mind. You'll probably find it nearly impossible not to think about the tiger.

Although you can't easily stop thinking about something, you can distract yourself and redirect your attention elsewhere. For example, think about the charging tiger again. Now stand up suddenly, slam your hand on the table, and shout 'Stop!' What happened to the tiger? Gone – at least for the moment.

Distraction works best for short periods or times when you anticipate symptoms. For example, distraction works if you know climbing stairs will be painful or that falling asleep at night is difficult. Try one of the following distraction techniques:

■ Make plans for exactly what you will do after the unpleasant activity passes. For example, if climbing stairs is uncomfortable or painful, think about what you need to do once you get to the top. If you have trouble falling asleep, try making plans for some future event. Be as detailed as possible.

■ Think of a person's name, a bird, a flower, or whatever for every letter of the alphabet. If you get stuck on one letter, go on to the next. (This is a good technique for distraction from pain as well as for sleep problems.)

■ Count backward from 100 by threes (100, 97, 94 …).

■ To get through unpleasant daily chores (such as sweeping, mopping, or hoovering), imagine your floor as a map of the UK. Try naming all the countries and counties, moving east to west or north to south. If geography does not appeal to you, imagine your favourite shop and where each department is located.

■ Try to remember words to favourite songs or the events in an old story.

■ Try the 'Stop!' technique. If you find yourself worrying or entrapped in endlessly repeating negative thoughts, stand up suddenly, slap your hand on the table or your thigh, and shout 'Stop!' With practice, you won't have to shout out loud. Just whispering 'Stop!' or tightening your vocal cords and moving your tongue as if saying 'Stop!' can work too. Some people imagine a large stop sign. Others put a rubber band on their wrist and snap it hard to break the chain of negative thought. Or pinch yourself. Do anything that redirects your attention.

- Redirect your attention to a pleasurable experience:
  - ▸ Look outside at something in nature.
  - ▸ Try to identify all the sounds around you.
  - ▸ Massage your hand.
  - ▸ Smell a sweet or pungent odour.

So far, we have discussed short-term refocusing tools that involve using only the mind.

Distraction also works well for long-term projects or symptoms that tend to last longer, such as depression and some forms of long-term pain.

In these cases, you focus your mind externally on some type of activity. If you are somewhat depressed or have continuous unpleasant symptoms, find an activity that interests you, and use it to distract yourself from the problem. The activity can be almost anything, from gardening to cooking to reading or going to the cinema or doing volunteer work. One of the marks of successful self-managers is that they have a variety of interests and always seem to be doing something.

Positive Thinking and Self-Talk

The following example discusses the same situation and three different responses. Each person's response has a different result.

Mohammed, Angela, and Jackie make a sales presentation after weeks of preparation. The response from their new manager: *'Lousy. You've completely missed the boat.'*

- Mohammed gets angry and rages about his boss. *'He doesn't know anything about the client or this product. He hates everything I do. I could do his job better than he does. It's not fair.'* Mohammed becomes more and more difficult to work with and develops frequent stomach pain.

- Angela worries. *'I knew he wouldn't understand what I was trying to do',* she thinks. *'I don't fit here anymore. I'll probably be fired soon. I'll never get anything right. I'm a*

failure.' Angela finds it harder to go to the office in the morning, can't concentrate on her work, and has trouble sleeping.

- Jackie feels disappointed at first; then challenged. *'He certainly sees things differently',* she reflects. *'I'd better find out what he was expecting.'* Jackie sets up a meeting with the boss to discuss changes to the presentation.

Before reading on, take a moment to reflect honestly on how you would have responded in this situation. How would you 'explain' it to yourself? What would you feel? What do you think the consequences of your response would be?

Mohammed, Angela, and Jackie each interpreted the same event in different ways, and each one led to very different feelings, actions, and consequences. Mohammed's and Angela's responses illustrate two different forms of negative thinking. Mohammed blamed unfair circumstances, and Angela blamed herself. Both of these attitudes are most likely to result in more negative feedback and more bad feelings.

Jackie's response was much more optimistic and allowed her to take positive action. Though she didn't like being criticised, she didn't let it keep her down. She saw herself as having some control over the situation, and that made her feel stronger.

This example shows how people's responses, thoughts, and self-talk can guide how a situation affects them.

You Feel What You Think

People often assume that outside events are the cause of our moods and symptoms. But it's remarkable how different people have such different reactions when faced with the same event. Even when you experience the exact same situation at different times or in different moods, it's surprising how differently you can feel and respond to it.

People are constantly talking to themselves. This 'self-talk' is how you explain the events of your life to yourself. Self-talk controls the way your mind interprets events, how you feel, and what actions you take. Some explanations are positive and empowering. Others cause anger, feed frustration, or lead to depression and despair. How well you communicate with others also affects your self-talk, thoughts, moods, and well-being (see Chapter 11, *Communicating with Family, Friends, and Healthcare Professionals*).

Most people are usually not aware of the ongoing chatter in their heads. You may feel anger, depression, or anxiety, but you don't connect these feelings with the negative thoughts that are going on in your mind and body. You don't notice how these thoughts shape your mood. For example, when waking up in the morning, you may think to yourself, 'I really don't want to get out of bed. I'm tired and don't want to go to work today.' Or at the end of an enjoyable evening, you may say to yourself, 'That was fun. I should get out more often.' This is your self-talk. The way you talk to yourself reflects how and what you think about yourself. Thoughts can be positive or negative, and so is self-talk. Self-talk can be an important self-management tool when it's positive. It can also be a weapon that hurts or defeats us when it is negative.

Much of self-talk is learned from others. It becomes part of you as you grow up. It comes in many forms, unfortunately mostly negative. Negative self-statements are usually in the form of phrases that begin with something like 'I just can't do … ', 'If only I could … ', 'If only I didn't … ', 'I just don't have the energy … ', or 'How could I be so stupid?' This thinking represents the doubts and fears you have about yourself and about your abilities to deal with your condition and its symptoms. Thinking can damage self-esteem, attitude, and mood. Negative self-talk makes you feel bad and makes your symptoms worse.

What you say to yourself plays a major role in determining your success or failure in becoming a good self-manager. Negative thinking tends to limit abilities and actions. If you tell yourself 'I'm not very smart' or 'I can't' all the time, you probably won't try to learn new skills. Soon you can become a prisoner of your own negative beliefs.

Fortunately, negative self-talk is not something fixed in anyone's biological make-up, and therefore it is not completely outside your control. You can learn new, healthier ways to think about yourself so that your self-talk can work for you instead of against you. By changing negative, self-defeating statements to positive ones, you can manage symptoms more effectively. This change, like any habit, requires practice and includes the following steps:

1. **Listen carefully to what you say to or about yourself, both out loud and silently.** When you find yourself feeling anxious, depressed, or angry, identify the thoughts you were having just before these feelings started. Pay special attention to the things you say during times that are particularly difficult for you. Write down all the negative self-talk statements. For example, what do you say to yourself when getting up in the morning with pain, while you are doing those exercises you don't really like, or when you are feeling low?

2. **Challenge negative thoughts by asking questions to identify what is true or not true.** For example, are you exaggerating the situation, generalising, worrying too much, or assuming the worst? Are you thinking in terms of black and white? Could it be grey? Maybe you are making an unrealistic or unfair comparison, assuming too much responsibility, taking something too personally, or expecting perfection. What evidence do you really have to support your conclusions? Are you making assumptions about what other people think about you? What do you know for a fact? Are you

discounting or ignoring the positive? How important will this be in an hour, a week, or a year? Look at the evidence so that you are better able to change these negative thoughts and statements.

3. **Change each negative statement to a more positive (and realistic) one, or find a positive statement to replace the negative one.** Write the positive statements down. For example, negative statements such as 'I don't want to get up', 'I'm too tired and I hurt', 'I can't do the things I like anymore, so why bother?' or 'I'm good for nothing' become positive messages such as 'I'm feeling pretty good today, and I'm going to do something I enjoy', 'I may not be able to do everything I used to, but there are still a lot of things I can do', 'People like me, and I feel good about myself', or 'Other people need and depend on me; I'm worthwhile.' Try self-statements that focus on what you can do rather than on what you can't do. Focus also on the next steps in front of you rather than your ultimate goal.

4. **Read and rehearse these positive statements, mentally or with another person.** Repeating the positive self-talk will help you replace old, habitual negative statements.

5. **Practice these new statements in real situations.** This practice, along with time and patience, will help the new positive pattern of thinking become automatic.

6. **Rehearse success.** When you aren't happy with the way you handled a particular situation, try this exercise:

- Write down three ways that it could have gone better.

- Write down three ways it could have gone worse.

- If you can't think of alternatives to the way you handled it, imagine what someone whom you greatly respect would have done.

- Think what advice you would give to someone else facing a similar situation.

Remember that mistakes aren't failures. They're good opportunities to learn. Mistakes give you the chance to rehearse other ways of handling things. This is great practice for future challenges.

At first, you may find it hard to change negative statements into more positive ones. A shortcut is to use either a thought stopper or a positive affirmation. A thought stopper can be anything that is meaningful to you. It can be a puppy, a polar bear, or an oak tree. When you have a negative thought, replace it with your thought stopper. We know it sounds silly, but try it. It really works!

To break the cycle of automatic negative thoughts, many people find it helpful to repeat positive statements called affirmations. Over time, these affirmations can replace negative statements. Think of a few strong, positive statements about yourself. Put them in the present tense, such as 'I take care of my body' or 'I'm good at my job.'

Creating your own affirmations helps make it clear what you really want. They clarify what you want and replace the negative statements that endlessly float around in your mind.

Affirmations are short and simple. Affirmations refer to something that is true now. It is not something that will happen in the future. For example, 'I forgive myself' is a stronger affirmation than 'I will let go of past mistakes and forgive myself.'

Put your affirmations in writing. Make a short list (no more than two or three). During your relaxation or guided imagery exercise, repeat your affirmations several times. You can also put affirmations on individual cards and place them around your house so you can see them throughout the day. Here are some examples:

- *I have a calm mind and a calm body.*

- *My body knows how to heal itself.*

- *I am doing the best I can.*

- *Peace is within me.*

- *At this moment, right now, everything is as it should be.*

- *I love and accept myself unconditionally.*

- *My relationship with _____ is more and more satisfying.*

- *I am in harmony with my life.*

- *I deserve to be treated well.*

- *I can accept my feelings.*

- *I have confidence in myself.*

A Healthy Perspective or Thinking the Worst?

We all worry. Our natural survival instinct alerts us to threats or potential dangers. But worrying can get out of control. When you focus on the worst thing that can happen, that sort of thinking is called catastrophising. This tendency to anticipate the worst triggers negative emotions and can prevent effective action. Any problem or setback can trigger a cascade of negative self-talk: 'I'll never be respected again; I can't even do my job anymore – I'm worthless.' Your mind races automatically down the path of expecting awful and severe consequences – even when there isn't any evidence to support them!

When living with long-term health conditions, you may find yourself thinking the worst about your symptoms. This can make symptoms harder to manage. For example, the common symptom of pain can be made much worse by the way you think about it. Consider Kevin, who has had chronic lower back pain for several years now. One day he overdoes it working in his garden and the next morning cannot go to work. He then starts worrying: 'When will I be able to go back to work? I'll bet this will be worse than the last episode. This is probably going to be permanent. I'm going to lose my job over this!' Kevin continues to focus on the pain and fears that the pain is only going to get worse. These thoughts lead to a helpless feeling. Kevin becomes sure that he can't do anything about his situation. He stays in bed waiting to get the sack.

The good news is that catastrophising, like all negative self-talk, can be halted. Here are a few things to try if you get stuck imagining the worst:

- **Acknowledge that unpleasant things happen.** Life is full of challenges. Just because one day is bad does not mean that all days will be bad.

- **Say '*Stop!*'** This simple distraction technique (see page 150) can sometimes halt the flow of repetitive negative thoughts.

- **Get real.** Most imagined worst-case scenarios do not come true. Challenge your thoughts. Ask: 'How likely is that outcome? And if it did happen, how could I cope?' Instead of general exaggerated thoughts like 'My life is ruined', get very specific. In the case of Kevin and his back pain, for example, he might ask: 'How long did it take for my other episodes of back pain to improve? Perhaps I can call my boss to discuss if any of my work can be done from home. In the unlikely situation that I did lose my job, how might I search for a different job?'

- **Redirect your attention.** Focus on identifying something positive that is working well in your life and that brings you joy and comfort. Or practise one of the simple relaxation techniques or pleasurable activities discussed in this chapter (see page 140–141).

- **Gain perspective.** Try observing your thoughts as an unbiased observer might. 'I'm having the thought that the pain will never go away. OK, I think that way sometimes, usually because of the mood I'm in. But like any thought, this negative thought will eventually pass. It doesn't have to be true or represent who I am. I'm going to sit with it and watch it pass.' If you find yourself upset, ask, 'How important will this be in an hour, a day, a month, or a year?' This helps you separate things that are important and need action from the dramatic catastrophic thoughts that capture your attention.

- **Acknowledge your best effort.** Sometimes despite your good intentions and efforts, things don't work out as you hope.

Everyone runs into roadblocks and sometimes feels a lack of control. It's not the end of the world. Remember that even if you can't always control the results, you can control your effort. You can short-circuit the flow of negative self-talk by acknowledging that 'I gave it my best effort', or as some athletes say, 'I left it all on the pitch.'

- **Practice self-compassion.** Provide yourself with the same support and understanding that you would give to a friend in a similar situation (see the next section and page 155).

These skills can also help identify the cues that trigger your catastrophic thinking. When are you likely to catastrophise? Is it when you are exhausted, feeling lonely, arguing with others, planning an event, or behind in your work? Understanding what your triggers are enables you to recognise when you are moving toward thinking the worst. Then you can act quickly to break the chain of negative self-talk and the anxiety that goes with it.

Be Kinder to Yourself: Practicing Self-Compassion

Think about a time when somebody you cared about was facing a problem, such as a friend losing a job. When friends tell you their stories, you are likely to offer some support and kindness. You may remind them of some of their positive qualities or simply give them a hug. You let them know that no matter what happened with their life challenges, you appreciate them and care about them.

Unfortunately, that is often not what we say to ourselves. When people make a mistake or fail at something, they often say something to themselves that is very critical, such as 'I really messed this up!' Would you say that to comfort a friend? Self-compassion means learning to treat yourself with the same degree of understanding and kindness that you so easily give to others.

No one likes to be embarrassed or humiliated in front of others. We always try to hide or minimise our flaws, mistakes, or failures. Though this may allow you to avoid looking bad, the cost of hiding your distress is an increased isolation from others. The reality is that everyone makes mistakes and everyone suffers, so accepting our flaws can bring us together rather than isolate us. It is part of what makes us human. Showing your vulnerability can often draw people closer to you.

So, how do you tend to respond to difficult times, personal flaws, mistakes, and failures? Do you think the following negative thoughts (even a little)?

- This is happening because I am inadequate, a loser, or a bad person.

- Everyone else has an easier time of it.

- I am embarrassed, humiliated, and ashamed.

- I am stuck in intense swirling negative emotions.

- I'm probably the only one making this kind of mistake or feeling this way.

- People are going to discover I am am fake.

- I really don't like myself.

If you find yourself saying critical things like this to yourself, practice kinder self-talk by reminding yourself of these things and asking yourself these questions:

■ Everyone feels inadequate and has setbacks at certain times in their lives.

■ Everyone suffers – it's one thing that all people have in common.

■ How can I keep this event in a balanced perspective so that I can view things more clearly?

■ How can I be more patient, caring, and tender with myself?

■ How can I approach my feelings with more curiosity and openness?

■ How can this experience help me have more realistic expectations?

These questions can help you reduce overly critical thoughts and emotions and allow you to be open to new information. In addition, practicing mindfulness (see pages 143–144) can help you focus on the present, rather than focusing on the past or worrying about the future.

More Self-Management Tools to Shift Your Mind and Your Mood

The following material includes additional tools that can help you clear your mind, positively shift your emotions, and reduce tension and stress.

Worry Time

Worry and negative thoughts feed anxiety. Ignored problems have a way of coming back into our consciousness. You will find it easier to set aside worries if you make time to deal with them.

Set aside 20 to 30 minutes a day as your 'worry time'. Whenever a worry pops into your mind, write it down and tell yourself that you'll deal with it during worry time. Jot down the little things (Did Maria forget to tidy up her room?) along with the big ones (Will our children be able to find jobs?). During your scheduled worry time, don't do anything except worry, free-think, and write down possible solutions.

For each of your worries, ask yourself the following questions:

■ What is the problem?

■ How likely is it that the problem will occur?

■ What's the worst that could happen?

■ What's the best that could happen?

■ How would I cope with the problem?

■ What are possible solutions?

■ What is my plan of action?

Be specific. Instead of dwelling on the worst possible outcome, consider, for example, dealing with your worry that you might lose your job. Ask yourself first how likely it is that this will in fact happen. In case it should happen, think concretely about what you will do, with whom, and by when. Write a job search plan.

If you're going on a cruise and you are anxious about getting seasick and not making it to the bathroom in time, imagine how you would manage the situation. Ask yourself if any of this is unbearable. Tell yourself that you might feel uncomfortable or embarrassed, but that you'll survive.

Remember that if a new worry pops up during the rest of the day, refuse to turn to it right away. Instead, jot it down. Then distract yourself by refocusing intently on whatever you are doing.

Scheduling a definite worry time cuts the amount of time spent worrying by at least a third. If you look at your list of worries later, you'll find that most of them will never happen. Or they were not nearly as bad as you thought they would be.

Practice Gratitude

One of the best ways to improve your mood and happiness is to focus on the things in your life that are really going well. What are you grateful for? Research demonstrates that people can increase happiness and physical well-being with gratitude exercises. We encourage you to try these three:

- **Acknowledge at least three good things every day.** Each night before bed, write down at least three things that went well that day. No event or feeling is too small to note … a compliment, a funny film, a message from a friend, or just a good cup of coffee. By putting your gratitude into words, you increase your appreciation and remember your blessings better. Savour and amplify each positive event. Knowing that you will be writing about your day each night changes

your mental filters during the whole day. You will tend to seek out, look for, and specially note the good things that happen. This simple tool can help change your mood *throughout the day*. It doesn't have to be something new every day. If daily is too often, do this once a week.

- **Make a list of the things you take for granted.** For example, if your long-term condition has affected your lungs, you can still be grateful that your kidneys are working. Perhaps you can celebrate a day in which you don't have a headache or backache. Imagine what life would be like *without* the small things you may take for granted: toilet paper, a telephone, a park, clean drinking water, the neighbour's friendly dog, and so on. Counting your blessings can add up to a better mood and more happiness.

- **Write a letter of thanks.** Write a letter of gratitude to someone who had been especially kind to you but had never been properly thanked. Perhaps it's a teacher, a mentor, a friend, or a family member. Express your appreciation for the person's kindness. Include specific examples of what the recipient has done for you. Describe how the actions made you feel. Ideally, read your letter out loud to the person, if possible, face-to-face. Be aware of how you feel and watch the other person's reaction.

Make a List of Your Personal Strengths

Make a personal inventory of your talents, skills, achievements, and qualities, big and small. Personal strengths might include having a sense of humour or being creative, kind, or always on time. Celebrate your accomplishments. When something goes wrong, consult your list of positives and put the problem in perspective. The problem then becomes just one specific experience, not something that defines your whole life.

Practice Acts of Kindness

When something bad happens, it's front-page news. Acts of kindness can be the best relief from the constant parade of bad news. Look for opportunities to give without expecting anything in return. Surprise the people around you, even strangers, by how kind you can be! Here are some examples:

- Hold the door open for the person behind you.

- Write a thank-you note.

- Send an anonymous gift to a friend who needs cheering up.

- Help someone who has their hands full carry a heavy bag or open a door.

- Tell positive stories you know of helping and kindness.

- Cultivate an attitude of gratefulness for the kindness you have received.

- Plant a tree.

- Pick up litter.

- Look up and smile at people serving you in a shop or restaurant.

- Smile and give way to people in a queue or while driving.

- Give another driver your parking space.

Notice the reactions of others. Notice how it makes you feel. Helping others can take the focus off your own problems and give you a sense of accomplishment. Kindness is contagious, and it has a ripple effect. In one study, the people who were given an unexpected treat (biscuits) were far more likely to help others. So, help start a wave of kindness!

Write Away Stress

It's hard work to keep deep negative feelings hidden. Over time, stress can undermine your body's defences and weaken your immunity. Telling your feelings to others or writing them down puts them into words and helps you sort them out. Words help people understand and absorb a traumatic event and eventually put it behind them. Telling your own story can give you a sense of release and control.

In a research study, the psychologist Jamie Pennebaker looked at the healing effects of confiding or writing. In the study, one group was asked to express their deepest thoughts and feelings about something bad that had happened to them. A second group was asked to write about ordinary matters, such as their plans for the day. Both groups wrote for 15 to 20 minutes a day for 3 to 5 consecutive days. No one read what either group had written.

The results were surprising. When compared with the people who wrote about ordinary events, the people who wrote about their bad experiences reported fewer symptoms, fewer visits to the doctor, fewer days off from work, improved mood, and a more positive outlook. Their immune function was enhanced for at least 6 weeks after writing. This was especially true for those who wrote about previously undisclosed painful feelings.

The 'write' thing can help in many situations, including the following:

- when something is bothering you

- when you find yourself thinking (or dreaming) too much about an experience

- when you avoid thinking about something because it is too upsetting

- when there's something you would like to tell others but don't feel able to do so for fear of embarrassment or punishment

Here are some guidelines for writing as a way to deal with troubling or traumatic experiences:

- Set a specific time for writing. For example, you might write 15 minutes a day for 4 consecutive days, or 1 day a week for 4 weeks.

- Write in a place where you won't be interrupted or distracted.

- Don't plan to share your writing – that could stop your honest expression. Save what you write or destroy it, as you wish.

- Explore your very deepest thoughts and feelings and analyse why you feel the way you do. Write about your negative feelings such as sadness, hurt, hate, anger, fear, guilt, or resentment.

- Write continuously. Don't worry about grammar, spelling, or making sense. If your writing is clear and coherent, so much the better, but it doesn't have to be. If you run out of things to say, just repeat what you have already written.

- Even if you find the writing awkward, keep going. It gets easier. If you just cannot write, try talking into a tape recorder for 15 minutes about your deepest thoughts and feelings.

- Don't expect to feel better immediately. At first you may feel sad or depressed. This usually fades within an hour or two or a day or two. Most people report feelings of relief, happiness, and contentment a few days after they begin to write.

- Writing may help you clarify what actions you need to take. But don't use writing as a substitute for taking action or as a way of avoiding things.

Prayer and Spirituality

There is strong evidence in the medical literature of the relationship between spirituality and health. Recent studies find that people who belong to a religious or spiritual community or who regularly engage in religious activities, such as prayer or study, have improved health. According to the American Academy of Family Physicians, spirituality is the way people can find meaning, hope, comfort, and inner peace in their lives. Some find it through music, art, or a connection with nature. Others find it in their values and principles. Spirituality, in whatever form, connects us to something larger, outside of ourselves.

Adapted from the American Academy of Family Physicians, http://www.aafp.org/afp/2001/0101/p89.html.

Many people share their religion with others. Other people do not have a specific religion or practice but do have spiritual beliefs. Your religion and beliefs can bring a sense of meaning and purpose to your life, help put things into perspective, and set priorities. Your beliefs may bring comfort during difficult times. Beliefs can help with acceptance and motivate you to make difficult changes. Being part of a spiritual or religious community can offer a source of support when needed and the opportunity to help others.

There are many types of prayer. Asking for help, direction, or forgiveness; offering words of gratitude; and praising or blessing others are all different forms of prayer. In addition, many religions have a tradition of contemplation or meditation. Prayer does not need a scientific explanation. It is probably the oldest of all self-management tools.

Although religion and spirituality cannot be 'prescribed', we encourage you to explore your own beliefs. If you are not religious, consider practicing some form of reflection or meditative practice. If you are religious, consider telling your doctor and healthcare team. Most healthcare professionals won't ask about your beliefs. Help them understand the importance of your beliefs in managing your health and life. Most hospitals have chaplains or pastoral counsellors. Even if you are not in the hospital, these spiritual counsellors may be available to talk with you. Choose someone with whom you feel comfortable. Their advice and counsel can supplement your medical and psychological care.

■ ■ ■

In this chapter we discussed some of the most powerful tools you can add to your self-management toolbox (see page 92). These tools can help you manage symptoms as well as master the other skills discussed in this book. Remember, you do not need to use all the tools in this chapter. Some may seem difficult, not useful, or just not for you. Pick and choose. If one thing is not helpful, try another.

As with exercise and other acquired skills, using your mind to manage your health condition may require both practice and time before you notice the full benefits. But keep in mind that just by practicing these skills, you are accomplishing something to help yourself.

Useful Websites

NHS (For a range of mental health and well-being techniques, tools and services):
https://www.nhs.uk/conditions/stress-anxiety-depression/

NHS Apps Library (Apps and online tools to help you manage your health and well-being):
https://www.nhs.uk/apps-library/

Other Mindfulness and Relaxation Apps: There are now dozens of apps on the market to help you start, or continue, on your path to mindfulness and relaxation. The vast majority of these apps are free (at least at first).

Search the App Store for Apple devices (https://www.apple.com/uk/ios/app-store/).

Google Play is the official app store for the Android operating system. The Play Store app comes pre-installed on Android devices that support Google Play (https://play.google.com/store/apps?hl=en_GB).

"Activity and rest are two vital aspects of life. To find a balance in them is a skill in itself. Wisdom is knowing when to have rest, when to have activity, and how much of each to have. Finding them in each other – activity in rest and rest in activity – is the ultimate freedom."

— Sri Ravi Shankar, *Celebrating Silence: Excerpts from Five Years of Weekly Knowledge, 1995–2000*

CHAPTER 7

Being Physically Active

PHYSICALLY ACTIVE PEOPLE ARE HEALTHIER AND HAPPIER than people who are not. This is true for people of all ages and conditions. When pain or long-term health issues slow you down and complicate your life, it is very easy to move less and be less physically active and give up other meaningful activities such as socialising, participating in your hobbies, travelling, and working. Even if you know that regular physical activity and exercise are important, with a long-term condition you may not know what to do, or you may worry that you will do the wrong thing. When there are so many concerns and questions, it is easy to give up before you even start. In the past, it was a challenge for people with arthritis, diabetes, or lung conditions to learn how to exercise. But now there are

For the UK edition, special thanks to Nitin Sharma, MCSP, PGDip, MACPOM-IT, AACP, Advanced Physiotherapy Practitioner, for contributions to this chapter.

163

proven ways for you to successfully exercise, no matter what your age and long-term condition, and the research continues to show the physical and psychological benefits for everyone of being physically active and exercising regularly.

Becoming Healthier and Happier with Physical Activity

In this section of the chapter, we tell the stories of two people with long-term conditions who created enjoyable activity routines and discovered how being more active could make their lives better. As you read these stories and this chapter, think about your own situation and how you can learn enjoyable ways to increase your physical activity to become healthier and happier.

Thomas gave up driving six years after he was diagnosed with Parkinson's disease. He soon felt isolated and lonely being home alone all day. Thomas thought about his past activities and remembered that he was happier when he got out and about regularly. He especially enjoyed working out at the local health club and going to museums and outdoor fairs. Doing those things without a driver's licence meant doing things differently. First, he needed transportation. Thomas had trouble finding a solution until a family friend mentioned a concessionary bus pass scheme for older people.

With a way to get around again, Thomas decided to commit to a one-month trial at his local health club. At the end of the month of visiting the club, he had more energy and felt less stiff. He joined as a regular member at a senior citizen rate. Then he learned that the local community centre had weekly outings. Feeling fit enough to participate, he signed up. With his health club exercise and his community centre outings, Thomas feels happier, healthier, and motivated to be more active.

Precious has been living with diabetes for five years. A year ago, a doctor diagnosed her with rheumatoid arthritis. When her joints were sore and painful she avoided moving. Within 6 months, her HbA1c was 73 mmol/mol. Diabetes UK recommends that people with diabetes should have a HbA1c level of 48 mmol/mol or below. Precious' doctor encouraged her to think about ways she could lower her blood glucose.

Precious realised that when her joints were sore, she soothed herself with unhealthy foods and ate a less healthy diet. She also sat around the house more, moved her body less, and she let go of favourite hobbies. She started trying to eat better and move more, but her joints hurt and she felt tired all the time. At first, Precious made backward progress, not forward progress. She realised that her first step to moving more and being healthier was to gain better control of her arthritis. She met with a specialist and started a new medication. Soon, her joints started feeling better. She met with an occupational therapist and a physiotherapist and learned tips for reducing pain and being active.

Once she was on track, Precious decided to get more active and return to her hobby of painting. Painting had always been a stress reducer, but she knew she would need more energy to paint like she used to. She started walking for 15 minutes 3 days a week during her lunch hour. She felt refreshed, and it didn't make her joints sore. So she increased her walking until she did it most days of the week. She wanted to do more than walk, though – she wanted to paint! She found a brush with a larger handle and started doing hand stretches to keep supple. She is now painting again. She even includes her daughters in her hobby, and they love to paint together at weekends. Now that she feels better physically and is more active, she has noticed her eating has also improved. At her last GP visit the doctor said her HbA1c had dropped to 63 mmol/mol and she encouraged Precious to continue her walking and painting.

Problem Solving to Become More Active

How can the stories of Thomas and Precious help you overcome the things that may be getting in the way of being active? Let's review their stories and think about the problem-solving steps from Chapter 2, *Becoming an Active Self-Manager.*

1. Identify the problem.

Focus on a specific problem that you want to solve right now. These individuals targeted problems that were interfering with their life right now. Both Precious and Thomas had a personal desire to overcome the problem, which helped them succeed. Sometimes you also need to look closely at the situation to better understand the problem. Problems can be more complicated than they appear. Thomas wanted to get out of the house more, but he needed to find transportation first. Precious was motivated to improve her blood glucose levels, but she had to learn how to manage her joint pain and swelling so that she could exercise regularly.

2. List ideas to solve the problem.

Many people find it useful to list their ideas to overcome the problem. Thomas and Precious reviewed prior successes and identified several possible solutions to enhance their health and wellness. Freethinking ideas or thinking about past successes offers a good start to solving a problem. Thomas and Precious and many others like them feel healthier and happier when engaging in regular physical activity. You may find it useful to add physical activity ideas to your problem-solving list. In the remainder of this chapter and the next one, there are several strategies to help you get active as well as information on exercises.

3. Select one idea to try.

Choose a possible solution and try it out for a while. Review your ideas and decide what you want to test first. Try it! Some people even make a specific action plan. (See 'Making Short-Term Plans: Action Planning', pages 30–32.)

4. Check the results.

Assess the outcome. Testing your own possible solutions makes you a more active participant in promoting your health. Often, it builds confidence for solving future problems.

5. Pick another idea if the first didn't work.

Solving problems often involves some struggle, and first attempts don't always work. You may need to try out another idea to solve the problem. Precious first gained control of her joint pain, then tried out exercise, and then was able to return to a hobby.

There is a lot to learn from the stories of Thomas and Precious and others like them. We hope you will feel inspired by the possibilities to live a healthier, more active life with long-term health conditions. Although situations differ, the common elements of problem solving are useful for you to consider.

For these individuals, physical activity and exercise helped them overcome problems in their daily life. Precious used exercise to improve blood glucose control. Thomas participated in exercise and found as a result that he had enough energy to participate in community centre activities. Each of them did different types of exercise for different time frames and met different goals. It is important for you to think about how movement might play a role in enhancing your participation in activities you enjoy.

Kinds of Exercise

Just as different foods (such as carbohydrates, protein, fats, and fibre) provide different benefits, different kinds of exercise have different effects on your body. There are four major types of exercise. We list them here:

- **Endurance (aerobic).** Your endurance depends on the fitness of your heart, lungs, and muscles. The heart and lungs must work efficiently to send enough oxygen-rich blood to your muscles. Your muscles must be fit enough to use the oxygen. Aerobic ('with oxygen') exercise involves the large muscles of your body in continuous activity, such as walking, swimming, dancing, mowing the lawn, or riding a bike. Many studies show that aerobic exercise

lessens fatigue, promotes a sense of well-being, eases depression and anxiety, promotes restful sleep, and improves mood and energy levels.

- **Flexibility.** Being flexible helps you move comfortably and safely. Limited flexibility can cause pain, lead to injury, and make muscles work harder and tire more quickly. You lose flexibility when you are inactive or your daily movement is limited. Certain illnesses and diseases can also result in a loss of flexibility. However, even if you have a long-term condition, you can improve flexibility by doing gentle stretching exercises.

- **Strength.** Muscles need to be used to be strong. Inactive muscles weaken and atrophy (shrink). When your muscles get weak, you feel weak and tire quickly. For many people, disability and lack of mobility is due to muscle weakness. Exercises strengthen muscles when they require your muscles to do more work than those muscles are used to doing.

- **Balance.** For good balance, you need strong and coordinated muscles in your trunk (from your neck to your groin but not including your head, neck, arms, or legs) and legs, flexibility, and good posture. Though there are many causes of falls (such as poor vision, poor lighting, obstacles such as rugs on the floor, dizziness, and being tired or distracted), being strong and coordinated is very important and can help prevent falls.

What Exercise Can Do for You

When you are physically active and exercise, you improve your strength, flexibility, and endurance and are able to participate in more meaningful activities. You also reduce your risk of falls and other injuries from strained muscles, overstressed joints, fatigue, and poor balance. Regular exercise improves self-confidence and lessens feelings of stress, anxiety, and depression. In addition, regular exercise can help you sleep better and feel more relaxed and happier. Exercise can help you maintain a good weight, which takes stress off your back and legs. Exercise is also part of keeping bones strong.

The rest of this chapter is about physical activity and endurance exercise. The following chapter, Chapter 8, *Exercising to Make Life Easier*, is about selecting exercises to solve specific problems such as getting up from a chair or reaching up to a shelf. Chapter 8 also contains descriptions and illustrations of different exercises to increase strength, flexibility, and balance and provides suggestions for which exercises might be best for you.

Physical Activity Guidelines*

Many countries and some institutions, including the World Health Organization (WHO), have guidelines for what and how much physical activity you need to do to be healthy. The guidelines are pretty much the same all over the world and apply to adults with and without long-term conditions and disability. When you read the guidelines, it is important to remember

*For the UK edition, special thanks to Brid Cronin, Senior Physiotherapist Cardiac Rehabilitation, for contributions to this section.

that they are goals to work toward; they are not the starting point. On average, only about 25% of people exercise enough to meet these guidelines. Don't worry that everyone else can meet these goals and only you can't.

Your goal is to gradually and safely increase your physical activity to a level that is right for you. You may be able to exercise as much as the guidelines indicate, but maybe you won't. The important point is to use the information to start being more active and healthier in a way that is right for you. Start doing what you can do now. Even a few minutes of activity several times a day is a good beginning. The important thing is to do something that works for you, make it a habit, and gradually increase your time or the number of days a week as you can.

The following guidelines are recommended by the NHS for adults aged 19 to 64 (this includes disabled people, pregnant women, and new mothers). Remember, they are a guide to where you could go, not a requirement for where you should be right now. *You also need to take into account any medical advice you have been given in relation to your long-term condition. For example, it is not recommended that people with heart conditions take part in vigorous exercise. So always check with your healthcare professionals before undertaking a new exercise regime.*

Adults should:

- aim to be physically active every day – any activity is better than none, and more is better still

- do strengthening activities that work all the major muscles (legs, hips, back, abdomen, chest, shoulders and arms) on at least 2 days a week

- do at least 150 minutes of moderate intensity activity a week or 75 minutes of vigorous intensity activity a week

- reduce time spent sitting or lying down and break up long periods of not moving with some activity

---

Endurance Exercise*

Endurance exercise can help you to have more energy and be able to be more active. There are many kinds of endurance exercises. Any physical activity that involves your arms and legs and that you can keep up for at least 10 minutes can be an endurance exercise and qualifies as physical activity. Most of the time we think of activities such as walking, swimming, cycling, dancing, or exercise classes as endurance activities. How-ever, doing household chores or working in the garden can also be endurance exercises. Some regular activity is better than none. Remember that your chosen activity should be comfortable enough that you can keep it up for a while. It is better to begin by underdoing rather than overdoing.

How often you exercise (frequency), how long you are active each session (time), and how

---

*For the UK edition, special thanks to Brid Cronin, Senior Physiotherapist Cardiac Rehabilitation, for contributions to this section.

hard you work (intensity) all work together. You can adjust frequency, time, and intensity to adjust your exercise effort.

Frequency

Frequency refers to how often you exercise. Every other day is a good way to start. NHS guidelines suggest that you can do your weekly target of physical activity on a single day or over 2 or more days. If possible, do not go more than 2 days without exercising.

Time

Time is the length of each exercise session. According to the guidelines, it is best if you can exercise at least 10 minutes at a time. As you build your endurance, you can increase the time of each session and do several 10-minute sessions in a day.

Intensity

Intensity is your exercise effort – how hard you are working. Moderate intensity is safe and effective. When you exercise at moderate intensity, you feel that you are working but you also feel that you can continue for a while and you can talk normally. High-intensity exercise is not necessary to get benefits, and it increases chances for injuries. You are exercising at a high intensity if you feel breathless, have difficulty talking while you are exercising, or feel you can continue only for a few seconds. How hard you work to do a particular exercise depends on how fit you are now. For example, a 10-minute brisk walk may be low intensity for an athlete but may be high intensity for someone who hasn't been active for a while.

Figure out what is moderate intensity for you so that you don't work too hard. There are several easy ways to do this, including the following:

- **Talk Test.** When exercising, talk to another person or yourself, or recite poems out loud. Moderate-intensity exercise allows you to speak comfortably. If you can't carry on a conversation because you are breathing too hard or are short of breath, you're working at a high intensity. Slow down. The talk test is an easy and quick way to recognise your effort. If you have lung condition, the talk test might not work for you. If that is the case, try using the perceived scale of breathlessness as outlined next.

- **Perceived scale of breathlessness.** Rate how hard you're working on a scale of 6 to 20. At the low end of the scale, 6 is sitting down, doing no work at all, and 20 is working as hard as possible – in other words, very hard work that you couldn't do for more than a few seconds. A good level for moderate aerobic exercise is around 13, because at this level you are working 'somewhat hard' but it still feels OK to continue. When you are exercising, ask yourself where you are on the scale.

- **Heart Rate.** Unless you're taking heart-regulating medicine (such as beta-blockers), checking your heart rate is another way to measure exercise intensity. The faster the heart beats, the harder you're working. (Your heart also beats fast when you are frightened or nervous, but here we're talking about how your heart responds to physical activity.) According to the British Heart Foundation your target heart rate is between 50% and 70% of your safe maximum heart rate. To calculate your target heart rate you first need to know your safe maximum heart rate. However, there are a number of factors that can influence your safe maximum heart rate, including your age (the safe maximum heart rate goes down with age), your long-term condition, the kind of medication you are taking, and your resting heart rate (which can vary hugely between people). The British Heart Foundation has a tool on its website that you can use to calculate your target heart rate (see the 'Useful Websites' section at the end of this chapter), or you can ask for help from a healthcare professional. Knowing your target heart rate will

help you increase your fitness and strength safely. Once you know your target heart rate there are a number of ways to monitor your heart beat. Gym equipment often has handgrips that take your pulse. Mobile phone apps, smart watches, and monitors you wear on your wrist or belt can also measure your heart rate. However, you need to be aware that many heart rate monitors can be inaccurate. You can also take your own pulse (the NHS website provides a guide to checking your pulse – see the 'Useful Websites' section at the end of this chapter). It is your job to know what exercise heart rate is best for you, and this is especially important for people with heart conditions, who can get advice on heart rate monitoring from their local cardiac rehab team.

Putting Together Your Own Endurance Programme

You can build your exercise programme by varying frequency, time, and activities. We recommend that you start slowly with moderate-intensity exercise and increase frequency and time as you work toward the recommended guideline of 150 minutes each week. A good way to meet the guideline goals for physical activity is to accumulate 30 minutes of moderate physical activity on most days of the week. This is just 10 minutes, three times each day. This can be a combination of walking, stationary bicycling, dancing, swimming, or chores that require moderate-intensity activity. It is

important to remember that 150 minutes is a goal, not your starting point.

Example Exercise Programmes

If you begin exercising just 2 minutes each time you are active, you will likely be able to build up to meet the recommended goal of 10 minutes, three times a day. Not everyone can reach the guideline goal, but being physically active regularly will bring health benefits. Almost everyone can learn to be active enough to achieve important health benefits.

The following are programmes of moderate intensity that reach 150 minutes aerobic exercise each week:

- a 10-minute walk at moderate intensity three times a day, 5 days a week

- a 30-minute bike ride at moderate intensity (on mostly level ground) 3 days a week plus a 30-minute walk twice a week

- a 45-minute aerobic dance class at moderate intensity twice a week plus two 30-minute walks each week

- gardening (digging, raking, lifting) 30 minutes a day, 5 days a week

If you are just starting, you could begin with:

- a 5-minute walk around the house three times a day, 5 days a week (total 75 minutes)

- a water aerobics class that lasts 40 minutes twice a week and two 10-minute walks on 2 other days a week (total 120 minutes)

- a low-impact aerobics class once a week (50 minutes) and a 15-minute walk on 2 other days a week (total 110 minutes)

Warming Up and Cooling Down

When you do any exercise, it is important to warm up first for 15 minutes and cool down for 10 minutes afterwards. To warm up, do several minutes of a low-intensity activity to allow your muscles, heart, lungs, and circulation to gradually get ready to work harder. Warming up reduces the risk of injuries, soreness, and irregular heartbeat. Cooling down helps your body return to its normal resting state. Repeat your warm-up activity or take a slow walk. Doing gentle flexibility exercises during the cool-down can be relaxing and may help reduce muscle soreness and stiffness.

Choosing Your Endurance Exercise

In this section, we discuss a few common endurance exercises. All of these exercises strengthen your heart, lungs, and muscles as well as relieve tension and help you manage your weight. Most of these exercises also strengthen your bones (water exercise is the exception).

Walking

Walking is easy, inexpensive, safe, and can be done almost anywhere. You can walk by yourself or with companions. Walking is safer than jogging or running and puts less stress on the body. It's an especially good choice if you have been sedentary or have joint or balance problems. If you walk to the shop, visit friends, and do household chores, then you can probably walk for exercise. A walking stick or walker doesn't need to stop you from getting into a walking routine. However, if you are a wheelchair user or use crutches, or you experience more than mild discomfort when you walk a short distance, then you should consider some other type of endurance exercise. Ask your GP or physiotherapist for help. Be cautious during the first two weeks of walking. If you haven't been walking for a while, 5 or 10 minutes may be enough to begin. As you get more comfortable, alternate brisk walks and slow walks and build up your total time. Each week, increase your brisk walking interval by no more than 5 minutes. Try to build to a total of 20 or 30 minutes of brisk walking. Remember that your goal is to walk most days of the week, at moderate intensity, for sessions that are at least 10 minutes long.

Before starting your walking programme, consider these tips:

- Choose your ground. Walk on a flat, level surface. Fitness trails, shopping centres, school tracks, streets with pavements, and quiet neighbourhoods are good places.

- Always warm up and cool down with a stroll.

- Set your own pace. Better to start off slowly than try to go too fast and tire out too quickly.

- Increase your arm work. You can use your arms to raise your heart rate into your target range. However, many people with lung conditions may want to avoid arm exercises, as they can cause more shortness of breath than other exercises.

Suitable shoes

Be sure your shoes fit comfortably and are in good repair. Shoes with laces or Velcro let you adjust width as needed so you get more support than slip-ons. If you have problems tying laces, consider Velcro closures or elastic shoelaces. Many people like shoes with removable insoles

that you can replace with more shock-absorbing insoles. You can find insoles in sports shops, pharmacists, and shoe shops. When you shop for insoles, take your shoes with you. Try on the shoe with the insole inserted to make sure there's still enough room for your foot. Insoles come in different sizes and can be trimmed with scissors for a custom fit. If your toes take up extra room, try the three-quarter insoles that stop just short of your toes. If you have prescribed inserts in your shoes already, ask your podiatrist or physiotherapist about insoles for walking shoes.

Possible problems: walking

If you have pain around your shins when you walk, you may not be warming up long enough. Try some ankle exercises (see Chapter 8, *Exercising to Make Life Easier*) before you start walking. Start your walk at a slow pace for at least 5 minutes. Keep your feet and toes relaxed.

Sore knees are another common problem for walkers. Fast walking puts more stress on knee joints. Slow down at first or walk for shorter distances or shorter intervals. Do the Knee Strengthener and Ready-Go exercises (pages 195 and 197) as part of your warm-up.

You can reduce cramps in the calf and pain in the heel by starting with the Achilles Stretch (page 197). A slow walk to warm up is also helpful. If you have circulation problems in your legs and get cramps or pain in your calves while walking, alternate between comfortably brisk and slow walking. Slow down and give your circulation a chance to catch up before the pain is so intense that you must stop. Exercise may help you gradually walk further with less cramping or pain. If these suggestions don't help, check with your GP or physiotherapist for suggestions.

Swimming

For most people with long-term conditions, swimming is excellent exercise. Swimming uses your whole body. If you haven't been swimming for a while, consider a refresher course. To make swimming an aerobic exercise, you eventually need to swim continuously for 10 minutes. Try different strokes, changing strokes after each lap or two. This lets you exercise all joints and muscles without overtiring any one area.

Swimming is an excellent aerobic exercise, but it does not improve balance or strengthen bones. Because swimming involves the arms, it can lead to excessive shortness of breath. This is especially true for people with lung conditions. However, for people with asthma, swimming may be the preferred exercise, as the moisture helps reduce shortness of breath. People with heart disease who have severely irregular heartbeats and have had an implantable cardioverter defibrillator (ICD) should avoid swimming on their own.

Before starting your swimming programme, consider these tips:

- The breaststroke and freestyle (crawl) normally require a lot of neck motion and may be uncomfortable. To solve this problem, use a mask and snorkel so that you can keep your face in the water and breathe without twisting your neck.

- Wear goggles. The chemicals in the pool may irritate your eyes.

- A hot shower or soak in a hot bath after your workout helps reduce stiffness and muscle soreness.

- Always swim where there are qualified lifeguards, if possible, or with a friend. Never swim alone.

Water Exercise

The buoyancy of water allows you to move and strengthen your muscles and cardiovascular system more easily and with less stress than exercise on land. If you don't like to swim or are uncomfortable learning strokes, you can walk laps or join water exercise classes (aquacise) at the pool. Many local authority leisure centres have swimming pools with classes for those with a disability and for those over 60. The deeper the water you stand in, the less stress there is on joints. However, water above the chest can make it hard to keep your balance. Let the water cover more of your body just by spreading your legs apart or bending your knees a bit. If you have access to a pool and want to exercise on your own, there are many water exercise books available. You can also find water exercise videos online. Water temperature is always a concern with water exercise. Suggestions for swimming pool temperatures for adult recreational swimming and disabled people range from 27C to 32C. Most public swimming pools are regulated at 29C, which is 84F.

Before starting your water exercise programme, consider these tips:

- Wear footgear designed for water. Some styles have Velcro straps to make them easier to put on.

- If you are sensitive to cold or have Raynaud's syndrome, wear water gloves, a wet suit or tights, and a shirt made for use in the water.

- Wearing a flotation belt or life vest adds extra buoyancy and comfort by taking weight off your hips, knees, and feet.

- As on land, moving more slowly makes exercise easier. In the water, regulate exercise intensity by how much water you push when you move. For example, when you move your arms back and forth in front of you underwater, it is hard work if you hold your palms facing each other. It is easier if you turn your palms down and slice your arms back and forth with only the narrow edge of your hands pushing against the water.

- Be aware that additional buoyancy allows for greater joint motion than you may be used to, especially if you are exercising in a warm pool. Start slowly, and do not stay too long in the pool because it feels good. Wait until you know how your body will react or feel the next day.

- If you have asthma, exercising in water can help you avoid the worsening of asthma symptoms that occurs during other types of exercise. This is probably due to the beneficial effect of water vapor on the lungs. Remember, though, that for many people with lung conditions, exercises involving the arms can cause more shortness of breath than leg exercises.

- If you have had a stroke or have another condition that may affect your strength and balance, make sure that you have someone to help you in and out of the pool. You can add to your safety and security by finding a position close to the wall or staying close to a friend who can lend a hand if needed.

- If the pool does not have steps and it is difficult for you to climb up and down a ladder, suggest that pool staff position a three-step kitchen stool in the pool by the ladder rails. This is an inexpensive way to provide steps for easier entry and exit. The steps are easy to remove and store when not needed.

Stationary Bicycling

Stationary bicycles offer the fitness benefits of cycling without the outdoor hazards. The stationary bicycle is a particularly good alternative exercise. It doesn't put excess strain on your hips, knees, and feet; you can easily adjust how hard you work; and weather doesn't matter. Some people with paralysis of one leg or arm can exercise on stationary bicycles with special attachments for their paralysed limb. Use the bicycle on days when you don't want to walk or do more vigorous exercise or when you can't exercise outside.

Before starting your stationary bicycling programme, consider these tips:

- Make it interesting. There are videos to watch or audio books or music to listen to as you pedal along. Some people keep track of their miles and chart their route on a map of a 'bike trip'. Keep a record of the times and distances of your bike trips. You'll be amazed at how much you can do.

- Stationary cycling uses different muscles than walking. Until your leg muscles get used to pedalling, you may be able to ride for only a few minutes. Start with no resistance. Increase resistance slightly as riding gets easier. When you increase resistance, it has the same effect as cycling up hills. If

Stationary-Bicycle Checklist

A safe bike has the following features:

■ The bicycle is steady when you get on and off.

■ The resistance is easy to set and can be set to zero.

■ The seat is comfortable and can be adjusted for nearly full knee extension when the pedal is at its lowest point.

■ The pedals are large and the pedal straps are loose to allow the feet to move slightly while you are pedalling.

■ There is ample clearance from the frame for the knees and ankles.

■ The handlebars allow good posture and comfortable arm positions.

there is too much resistance, your knees are likely to hurt, and you'll have to stop before you get the benefit of endurance.

■ Pedal at a comfortable speed. For most people, 50 to 70 revolutions per minute (rpm) is a good place to start. Some bicycles have an rpm rate readout. You can also count the number of times your right foot reaches its lowest point in a minute. As you get used to cycling, you can increase your speed. However, faster is not necessarily better. Listening to music at the right tempo makes it easier to pedal at a consistent speed. Experience will tell you the best combination of speed and resistance.

■ Set a goal of 20 to 30 minutes of pedalling at a comfortable speed. Build up your time by alternating intervals of brisk pedalling or more resistance with less exertion. Use your heart rate, the perceived scale of breathlessness, or the talk test (see page 169) to make sure you aren't working too hard.

■ On days when you're not feeling your best, maintain your exercise habit by pedalling with no resistance, at a lower rpm, or for a shorter period of time.

Exercising on Other Exercise Equipment

If you have trouble getting on or off a stationary bicycle or don't have room for a bicycle where you live, you might try a restorator. A restorator is a small piece of equipment with foot pedals that you can attach to the foot of a bed or place on the floor in front of a chair. It allows you to exercise by pedalling. You can vary the resistance and adjust for leg length and knee bend. A restorator is a good alternative to an exercise bicycle for people who have problems with balance, weakness, or paralysis. People with other long-term illnesses, such as lung conditions, may also find the restorator to be an enjoyable way to start an exercise programme. Ask your physiotherapist or GP, or contact a medical supply shop.

Arm cranks or arm ergometers are bicycles for the arms. People who are unable to use their legs for active exercise can improve their cardiovascular fitness and upper body strength by using the arm crank. It's important to work closely with a knowledgeable physiotherapist or instructor to set up your programme, because using only your arms for endurance exercise requires different intensity monitoring than using larger leg muscles. Many people with lung conditions may find arm exercises to be less enjoyable than leg exercises because they may experience shortness of breath.

There are many other types of exercise equipment. These include treadmills, self-powered and motor-driven rowing machines, cross-country skiing machines, mini trampolines, stair climbers, and elliptical (cross-trainer) machines. Most are available at gyms and leisure centres. They are sold in both commercial and home models.

If you're thinking about starting to use exercise equipment, know what you want to achieve. For cardiovascular fitness and endurance, choose equipment that will help you exercise as much of your body at one time as possible. The motion should be rhythmic, repetitive, and smooth. The equipment should be comfortable, safe, and not stressful on joints. If you're interested in purchasing a new piece of equipment, try it out for a week or two before buying.

Land-Based Exercise Classes

Exercise classes at a local gym or leisure centre can be fun and safe. You can also get aerobic exercise in classes that include dancing, such as Zumba or Jazzercise. More traditional dancing such as salsa, ballroom, and square dancing also provide good aerobic exercise. Classes in tai chi and some of the martial arts are popular and help with endurance, strength, balance, and relaxation.

When you are new to a class, introduce yourself to the instructor. Let them know who you are, that you may need to modify some movements, and that you will ask for advice. If you don't know other people in a class, try to get acquainted. Be open about why you may do things a little differently. You'll be more comfortable, and you may find others who also have special needs. Ask the instructor to show you how you can modify the routines to better suit you, whether it is to go more slowly, reduce arm work, take breaks, or shorten a routine.

Being different from the group in a room walled with mirrors takes courage, conviction, and a sense of humour. The most important thing you can do for yourself is to choose an instructor who encourages everyone to exercise at their own pace and a class where people are friendly and having fun. Observe classes, speak with instructors, and participate in at least one class session before committing to and paying for a class.

Exercise class tips

Before starting an exercise class, consider these tips:

- Wear comfortable, well-fitting shoes with nonslip soles.
- Protect your knees. Keep your knees relaxed (aerobics instructors call this 'soft knees').

- Don't overstretch. The beginning (warm-up) and end (cool-down) of the session will include stretching and strengthening exercises. Remember to stretch only as far as you comfortably can. Hold the position, and don't bounce. If needed, ask your instructor for an alternative exercise.

- Alternate the kinds of exercise you do. Many exercise facilities have a variety of exercise opportunities: equipment rooms with cardiovascular machines, swimming pools, and aerobics studios. If you have trouble with an hour-long aerobics class, see if you can join the class for the warm-up and cool-down and use a stationary bicycle or treadmill during the aerobics portion. Many people have found that this routine gives them the benefits of both an individualised programme and the social enjoyment of group exercise.

- There are many excellent exercise YouTube videos and DVDs for use at home. The NHS has an online Fitness Studio where you can access a range of exercise videos (see the 'Useful Websites' section at the end of this chapter). These vary in intensity, from very gentle chair exercises to more strenuous aerobic exercise. Ask your GP, physiotherapist, or condition specific charitable organisation for suggestions, or review the videos yourself.

Self-Tests for Endurance: Check Your Progress

For some people, feeling more energetic and healthier are enough to indicate progress with an endurance programme. Others may need proof that their exercise programme is making a measurable difference. To measure your success, use one or both of the endurance fitness tests described in this section. Pick one that works best for you. Record your results before you start. After 2 to 4 weeks of exercise, repeat the test and check your improvement. Talk to your healthcare professionals or exercise instructor to set reasonable and safe goals for yourself.

- **Measure by distance.** For walking and cycling, note how far you go in a set time. See how far you travel in 5 or 10 minutes, for example. Measure distance by counting how many streets you go or keep track of your steps with a step monitor. If you are swimming, count the lengths of the pool. Your goal is to cover more distance in less time or the same distance with less exertion.

- **Measure by time.** Measure a given distance to walk, bike, swim, or water-walk. Estimate how far you think you can go in 3 to 5 minutes. You can pick a number of streets, actual distance, or lengths in a pool. Start timing and move at a moderate pace. At the end of the distance, record how long it took you to cover your course and your perceived exertion (on a scale from 6 to 20). Your goal is to complete the distance in less time or with less exertion.

Exercise Opportunities in Your Community

Many people who exercise regularly do so with at least one other person. Two or more people can keep each other motivated, and a whole class can become a circle of friends. On the other hand, exercising alone gives you the most freedom. You may feel that there are no classes that would work for you, or you don't have a friend to accompany you. If so, start your own programme; as you progress, you may find that these feelings change.

Most communities offer a variety of exercise classes, including special programmes for people over 50, adaptive exercises, walking, fitness trails, tai chi, and yoga. The following are good places to look for classes:

- **Check with the local community centres, parks and recreation programmes, adult education classes, organisations for specific conditions (arthritis, diabetes, cancer, heart disease), and further education colleges.** There is a great deal of variation in these programmes, as well as in the training of the exercise staff. The classes are usually inexpensive, and the staff are responsive to people's needs.

- **Local authorities often sponsor classes that are appropriate for a wide range of ages and needs.**

- **Hospitals often have medically supervised classes for people with heart or lung conditions (cardiac or pulmonary rehabilitation classes).** These programmes have the advantage of medical supervision if that's important to you.

- **Gyms and leisure centres usually offer aerobics or aerobic fitness classes, weight training, cardiovascular equipment, and sometimes a heated pool.** They charge membership fees.

The following list describes things to ask about when you search for community programmes:

- **Classes with moderate and low intensity exercise designed for beginners.** You should be able to observe classes and participate in at least one class before signing up and paying.

- **Qualified instructors who are experienced working with people who have similar abilities as you.** Knowledgeable instructors are more likely to understand special needs and be willing and able to work with you.

- **Membership policies that allow you to pay by the class or for a short series of classes or let you freeze your membership at times when you can't participate.** Some fitness facilities offer different rates depending on how many services you use.

- **Facilities that are easy to get to, park near, and enter.** Exercise sites should be accessible and safe, with professional staff.

- **Staff and other members who are friendly and easy to talk to.**

- **An emergency management protocol and instructors certified in CPR (cardiopulmonary resuscitation, a life-saving medical procedure that is given to someone who is in cardiac arrest) and first aid.**

Your Exercise Programme: Solving Possible Problems

Table 7.1 lists a number of problems that may occur during exercise. Some are serious enough that you should stop your exercise, seek help, and talk to a professional before resuming.

Table 7.1 **If Exercise Problems Occur**

Problem	Advice
Irregular or rapid heartbeat	Stop exercising. Contact your doctor right away.
Pain, tightness, or pressure in the chest, jaw, arms, or neck Shortness of breath lasting past the exercise period	Don't exercise until your doctor has cleared you.
Light-headedness, dizziness, fainting, cold sweat, or confusion	Lie down with your feet up or sit down with your head between your knees. Seek medical advice immediately.
Shortness of breath or calf pain from circulation or breathing problems	Warm up by going slowly at first. Take short rests to recover and keep going.
Excessive tiredness after exercise, especially that continues into the next day	Exercise less hard next time. If tiredness lasts, check with your doctor.

Useful Websites

Asthma UK (Staying active when you have severe asthma): https://www.asthma.org.uk/advice/severe-asthma/making-life-easier-severe-asthma/exercising-when-you-have-severe-asthma/

British Heart Foundation (Your heart rate): file:///C:/Users/User/Downloads/your-heart-rate-is23%20(1).pdf

British Heart Foundation (Understanding your target heart rate): https://extras.bhf.org.uk/patientinfo/heart-rate-calculator/app/index.html

British Lung Foundation Pulmonary Rehabilitation: https://www.blf.org.uk/support-for-you/keep-active/pulmonary-rehabilitation

Cardiac Rehab Programme finder: http://www.cardiac-rehabilitation.net/cardiac-rehab.htm

Living Made Easy (Europe's largest online comparison site for daily living equipment, designed and run by the Disabled Living Foundation): https://www.livingmadeeasy.org.uk/leisure/sport-equipment-3700/

NHS (Cycling for beginners): https://www.nhs.uk/live-well/exercise/cycling-for-beginners/

NHS (Exercise): https://www.nhs.uk/live-well/exercise/

NHS (Fitness Studio exercise videos): https://www.nhs.uk/conditions/nhs-fitness-studio/

NHS (How do I check my pulse?): https://www.nhs.uk/common-health-questions/accidents-first-aid-and-treatments/how-do-i-check-my-pulse/

Parkinson's UK: https://www.parkinsons.org.uk/information-and-support/exercise

Stroke Rehabilitation: https://www.stroke.org.uk/search?key=exercise+classes

Swimming.org: https://www.swimming.org/justswim/get-fitter/aqua-fitness/

Versus Arthritis: https://www.versusarthritis.org/about-arthritis/managing-symptoms/exercise/exercises-to-manage-pain/

'We Are Undefeatable' (Campaign by UK charities and Sport England to support people living with health conditions to build physical activity and exercise into their lives): https://weareundefeatable.co.uk/

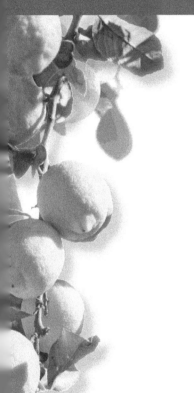

CHAPTER 8

Exercising to Make Life Easier

IN CHAPTER 7, *BEING PHYSICALLY ACTIVE*, YOU LEARNED about the benefits of being more active and trying to fit in 30 minutes of physical activity most days of the week. This goal is achievable for almost everyone. In Chapter 7, we discussed the four major types of exercise: endurance, flexibility, strength, and balance (see page 166–67). In that chapter, you learned how to problem-solve to become more active and how to put together your own endurance programme. This chapter follows up on the information in Chapter 7 with information on flexibility, strength, and balance exercises. You can use these exercises to solve many of the daily problems that result from stiffness, weakness, and poor balance.

When you read this chapter and think about how exercise might help in your life, think about your freedom and safety.

_____

For the UK edition, special thanks to Nitin Sharma MCSP, PGDip, MACPOM-IT, AACP, Advanced Physiotherapy Practitioner, for contributions to this chapter.

181

■ **Freedom is your ability to do things yourself.** If you are free, you can get around more easily. That allows you to be with other people. It also helps you to have the ability to do things that are important and enjoyable. Freedom can be your ability to visit your place of worship or do your own food shopping, to participate in a book club, exercise with friends, or walk your dog.

■ **Safety is avoiding falls and sprains and strains.** For most people, regular, targeted exercise makes the day safer, easier, and more enjoyable.

The exercises in this chapter are listed from head to toe. They are aimed at improving your flexibility and strength. The last section discusses exercises that can help you improve your balance. Choose exercises that you think will help you meet your goal.

Becoming More Free and Safe with Physical Activity

In Chapter 7, *Being Physically Active*, you read some stories about people with long-term health conditions who created enjoyable activity routines and discovered how being more active improved their endurance. In this section of the chapter, we discuss similar stories about how real people incorporated flexibility, strength, and balance exercises to increase freedom and safety. As you read these stories and this chapter, think about your own situation and how you can use the exercises in this chapter to be less uncomfortable and safer and enjoy more personal freedom. The exercises named in these stories are all explained and illustrated later in this chapter.

Samir has been exercising at the gym about three times a week. He would like to stand rather than sit during his exercise class. He decided that his balance was what was holding him back, so he chose four balance exercises: Curl-Up, Ready-Go, Toe Walk, and Heel Walk (see pages 192, 196, and 202). He tried each

exercise for a couple of days. Toe Walking was uncomfortable, so he substituted the Swing and Sway (see page 200). Samir added these exercises to his exercise routine and, after a month, he noticed his balance was better. He now stands during exercise class and uses a chair when he needs support.

Latisha noticed occasional pain in her right knee that kept her from walking more than 10 minutes at a time. She thought this might be because her knees and stomach muscles were weak, so she decided to try the Curl-Up (page 192), Knee Strengthener (page 195), and the Sit-to-Stand exercise (page 196). The Curl-Up strained her neck, so she substituted the Roll-Out (page 193). The Knee Strengthener seemed the most helpful. She now does it every day and can do 20 repetitions on each leg. Latisha has increased her walking from 10 to 20 minutes. She is back to walking her dog every day, walking 15 minutes during her lunch breaks, and walking at the shopping centre with friends at the weekends.

Daniel's family encouraged him to use a wheelchair because he seemed unsteady using a walking stick. He made the change and started using a wheelchair to get around. After a few months, he noticed that it became more difficult for him to get up from his chair or the toilet. He spent more time watching television and left his flat less often. He realised that he missed being with others and decided he needed to get stronger so he could do more. Daniel decided to build his strength by trying the Sit-to-Stand exercise (page 196). He started by doing it just a few times a day. He soon increased to a few times an hour. It got easier to get up from a sitting position. He felt more confident and stronger. Daniel decided to stop using the wheelchair. He was a little shaky with a walking stick at first, so he started using a walker. Daniel now goes to the library and to lunch at the community centre. He is also considering a seated exercise class so he can spend time exercising with others and make new friends.

Which Exercises Are Best for You?

Like Samir, Latisha, and Daniel, you probably have your own reasons to use exercise to solve problems and make life easier. For example:

- If you want to be able to go for a coffee with a friend but don't do it, ask yourself why. Are you worried that you will get too tired or out of breath just getting to the coffee shop? Or are you worried because you have trouble getting up from a chair without arms? To improve your ability to walk a distance and have strong enough legs to get up from a chair, start a walking programme with ideas from Chapter 7 and try the Power Knees and Sit-to-Stand exercises in this chapter on pages 195 and 196.

- Do you want to be able to put on your shoes and socks without working so hard or needing help? Try the Knee-to-Chest Stretch, Low-Back Rock and Roll, and Achilles Stretch exercises on pages 190, 192 and 197.

- Is it getting harder to reach up to shelves in your kitchen or bathroom? Try the Good Morning Stretch and Shoulder-Blade Pinch exercises on pages 188 and 189 to strengthen arms and loosen up shoulders.

- Would you like to take a trip to see friends or family but are afraid that getting around the airport, dealing with your luggage, or getting out of chairs will be too hard? Are you nervous about stepping up and down on curbs? Get in shape for travel with the endurance exercises described in Chapter 7, *Being Physically Active*. And use exercises such as Sit-to-Stand, Roll Out, Straight Leg Raises, and Power Knees on pages 196, 193, 194 and 195 to strengthen your hips and knees.

- If you want to feel steadier on your feet, try the beginning balance exercises on page 200.

What movement or activity is hard or uncomfortable for you? Think about how more strength, flexibility, or better balance might help make things less uncomfortable or painful. Ask yourself what parts of your body keep you from doing what you want. For example, do weak knees make going up a step challenging? Maybe stiff shoulders or elbows make it hard to reach a shelf or do your hair. Does a stiff back or hips make it frustrating to bend over to put on your shoes and socks? Think about what you would like to do better and what is keeping you from doing it.

You can put exercise to work for you using the following problem-solving steps from Chapter 2, *Becoming an Active Self-Manager* (see pages 25 and 26):

1. **Identify the problem.** Identify the part of your body you want to work on.

2. **List ideas to solve the problem.** Look through the exercises in this chapter and find three or four exercises for those parts of your body.

3. **Select one idea to try.** Pick one or more exercises to try a few times a week. Moderate-intensity muscle-strengthening exercise of all major muscle groups should be done at least 2 days a week.

4. **Check the results.** At the end of a week or two, check your progress. Ask yourself if it is easier or more comfortable or if you tire less quickly. If so, you are on the right track.

5. **Pick another idea if the first didn't work.** If things are not going well, try something else. You can add more exercises or continue what you are doing.

General Exercise Suggestions

The exercises in this chapter are for both sides of the body and full joint motion. If you are limited by muscle weakness or joint tightness, go ahead and do the exercise as completely as you can. *The benefit of doing an exercise comes from moving toward a certain position, not from being able to complete the movement perfectly.* In some cases, you may find that after a while you can complete the movement and increase your available range of motion. At other times you will need to keep doing it your own way. The exercises in this chapter are arranged for different parts of your body, starting at the head. The groups contain both stretching and strengthening exercises. There is a separate section for balance practice.

As you begin to exercise for strength, flexibility, and balance, keep the following tips in mind:

■ You can do most of the upper-body exercises either sitting or standing.

■ You can do many of the exercises in this chapter lying down on the floor or on a firm mattress.

■ Move at a comfortable speed. Do not bounce or jerk.

- To loosen tight muscles and joints, stretch just until you feel tension, hold for 10 to 30 seconds, and then relax. Remember to breathe in and out as you stretch.

- Stop if your body starts to hurt. Stretching should feel good, not painful.

- Start with no more than five repetitions of any exercise. Increase the number of repetitions gradually as you make progress.

- Always do the same number of exercises for your left and right sides.

- Breathe naturally. Do not hold your breath. Count out loud to make sure you are breathing.

- If you have pain that lasts after exercising, do fewer repetitions next time, or do fewer kinds of exercises. If an exercise gives you problems, stop and try another exercise.

We have labelled the exercises that are particularly important for breathing and good posture with 'VIP' (Very Important for Posture). Exercises to improve balance by strengthening and loosening legs and ankles are marked 'BB' (Better Balance). There is also a separate selection of balance exercises that are designed to help you practice balance skills.

Neck Exercises

1. Heads-Up (VIP)

This exercise relieves jaw, neck, and upper back tension or pain, and it will help you learn and maintain good posture. You can do the Heads-Up while driving, sitting at a desk, sewing, reading, or exercising. Just sit or stand straight and gently slide your chin back. Keep looking forward as your chin moves backward. You'll feel the back of your neck lengthen and straighten. To help do it correctly, put your finger on your nose and pull your head straight back away from your finger. (Don't worry about a little double chin – you will look much better with your neck straight!)

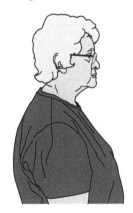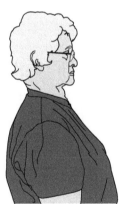

Clues for finding the correct Heads-Up position:

- ears over shoulders, not out in front
- head balanced over neck and trunk, not out in front
- back of neck vertical and straight up and down, not leaning forward
- bit of double chin

2. Neck Stretch

Get into the Heads-Up position (see Exercise 1). With your shoulders relaxed, turn slowly to look over your right shoulder. Then turn slowly to look over your left shoulder. Next, tilt your head to the right and then to the left. Move your ear toward your shoulder. Do not move your shoulder up to your ear.

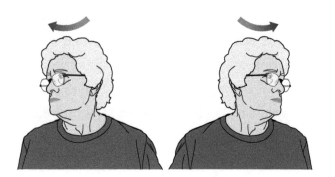 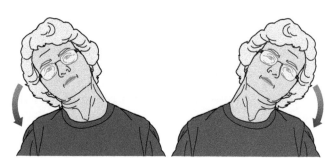

Hand and Wrist Exercises

A good place to do hand exercises is at a table that supports your forearms. Do hand and wrist exercises after washing dishes, after bathing or showering, or when taking a break from handwork such as knitting or wood carving. Your hands are warmer and more supple at these times. The purpose of wrist stretches is to fully extend the muscles that attach to the elbow on the top and the bottom of your forearm. Repetitive tasks can make these muscles stay in a tight and shortened position, resulting in forearm or elbow pain. Stretching them often helps prevent this.

3. Thumb Walk

Holding your wrist straight, form the letter O with one hand by lightly touching your thumb to each fingertip until your thumb has touched each one of your fingers. After you form each O, straighten and spread your fingers. Use the other hand to help if needed. Repeat with the other hand.

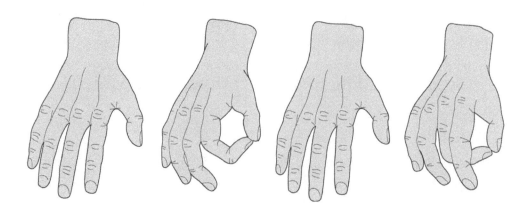

4. Wrist Stretch Down

Start with your elbow straight and palm facing down toward the floor. Make a fist with your hand and bend at the wrist to lower your knuckles down until you feel a stretch in your forearm or elbow. Hold for 5 seconds. Repeat several times.

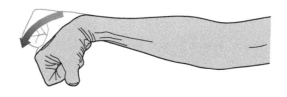

5. Wrist Stretch Up

Start with your elbow straight and palm facing away from you. Put your opposite hand over the away-facing palm. Gently stretch your palm back toward you until you feel a stretch on the underside of your forearm near the elbow. Hold for 5 seconds. Repeat several times.

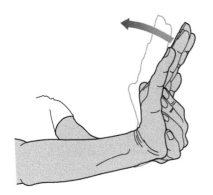

Shoulder Exercises

6. Shoulder Shape-Up

In Heads-Up position (see Exercise 1), slowly raise your shoulders to your ears. Hold this position and then drop your shoulders. Next, raise your shoulders again to the ears and then slowly rotate your shoulders backward by pinching the shoulder blades together. Bring the shoulders down and forward to complete a circle. Return to the Heads-Up position. Reverse the direction of the shoulder circles. This is a good option if the Neck Stretch (Exercise 2) is difficult for you.

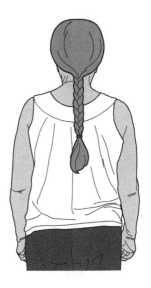
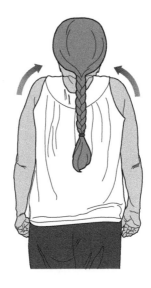
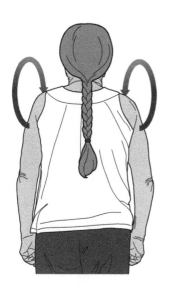

7. Good Morning (VIP)

Start with your hands in gentle fists, palms down and wrists crossed. Breathe in and stretch out your fingers while you uncross your arms and reach up for the sky. Breathe out as you stretch your arms and relax.

If one or both of your shoulders are tight or weak, give yourself a 'helping hand'. In shoulder Exercises 8 (Wand Exercise) and 9 (Pat and Reach), your arms help each other.

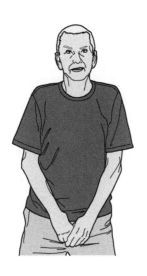
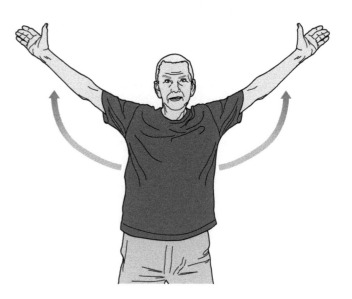

8. Wand Exercise

Use a long-handled broom, mop handle, or walking stick as your wand. Place one hand on each end and raise the wand as high overhead as possible. Try this in front of a mirror. This exercise can be done standing, sitting, or lying down.

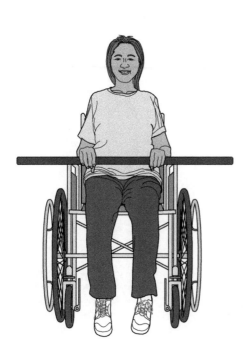
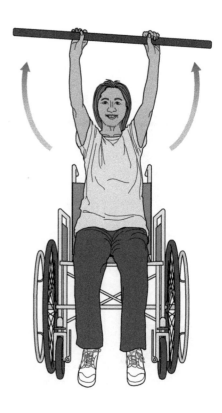

9. Pat and Reach

This double-duty exercise helps increase flexibility and strength for both shoulders. Raise one arm up over your head, and bend your elbow to pat yourself on the back. Move your other arm behind your back, bend your elbow, and reach up toward the other hand. Can your fingertips touch? Do not worry if you cannot touch. Many people cannot touch, but you will improve as you practice. Relax. Switch arm positions. Can you touch on this side? For most people, one side is easier than the other. You can grasp a towel at each end and use it as if you were drying your back. The towel can assist in the motion. Take care not to put too much strain on your shoulders.

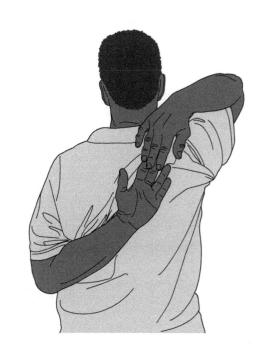

10. Shoulder-Blade Pinch (VIP)

This is a good exercise to strengthen the middle and upper back and to stretch the chest. It can be especially good for individuals with breathing problems. Sit or stand with your head in Heads-Up position (Exercise 1) and your shoulders relaxed. Raise your arms out to the sides with elbows bent. Pinch your shoulder blades together by moving your elbows as far back as you can. Hold that position briefly, and then slowly move your arms forward to touch your elbows. If this position is uncomfortable, lower your arms or rest your hands on your shoulders.

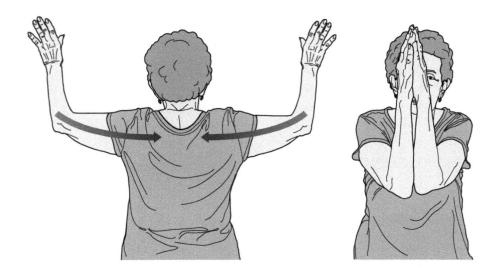

Back and Abdominal Exercises

11. Cat-and-Cow Pose in Seated Position

This two-part exercise stretches and improves flexibility in the entire spine and opens the chest. It is a yoga exercise that can reduce tension and calm the mind. At first, keep your movements small so that you do not strain your lower back. If you have neck problems, make sure to keep your neck in line with your body. Do not let your neck go too far back or too far forward.

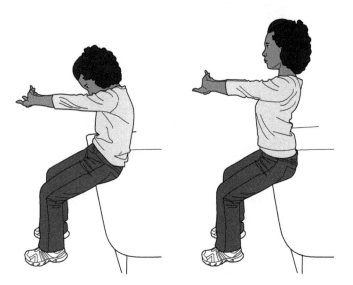

Sit in a straight-backed chair so that your back is not against the back of the chair. Sit with your head over your shoulders and shoulders over your hips. Place your feet flat on the floor with your knees over your heels and your hands rested gently on your thighs.

Imagine a string attached to the top of your head lifting your body to its full length. Start the 'Cat' by exhaling slowly as you bring your belly toward your spine and your back toward the back of the chair. Allow your back and shoulders to round and your head to come forward. Then, move into the 'Cow' by inhaling and bringing the chest forward and up as you let the shoulders come up and back. As you do this, your head raises and gently looks up as far as is comfortable. This puts your back in a gentle back bend. Repeat the Cat-and-Cow several times at your own pace.

12. Knee-to-Chest Stretch

This exercise stretches the low back. Lie on the floor with knees bent and feet flat. Bring one knee toward your chest, using your hands to help. Hold your knee near your chest for 10 seconds and lower your bent leg slowly. Repeat with the other knee. You can also tuck both legs toward your chest at the same time if you wish. Relax and enjoy the stretch.

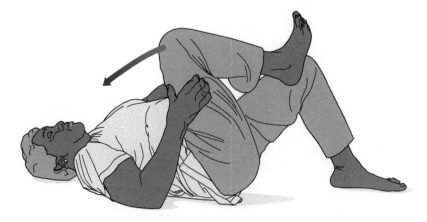

13. Pelvic Tilt (VIP)

The Pelvic Tilt is an excellent exercise for the low back and can help relieve lower back pain. Lie on your back with knees bent, feet flat. Place your hands on your stomach. Flatten the small of your back against the floor by tightening your stomach muscles and your buttocks. Tilt your tailbone forward and pull your stomach back. Think about trying to pull your stomach in enough to zip a tight pair of trousers. Hold the tilt for 5 to 10 seconds. Relax. Arch your back slightly. Relax and repeat. Don't forget to breathe! Count the seconds out loud. Once you've mastered the Pelvic Tilt lying down, practice it sitting, standing, and walking.

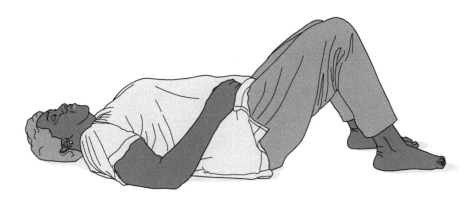

14. Back Lift (VIP)

This two-part exercise improves flexibility along your spine and helps you lift your chest for easier breathing. If you have moderate to severe low back pain, do not do this exercise unless it has been specifically prescribed for you.

Lie on your stomach and rise up onto your forearms. Keep your back relaxed and your stomach and hips down. If this is comfortable, straighten your elbows and raise your chest up away from the surface, arching your back as much as you comfortably can. Breathe naturally and relax for at least 10 seconds.

Lie on your stomach with your arms at your side or overhead. Lift your head, shoulders, and arms. Do not look up. Keep looking down with your chin tucked into a double-chin position. Count out loud to 10 as you hold this position. Relax. You can also lift your legs, instead of your

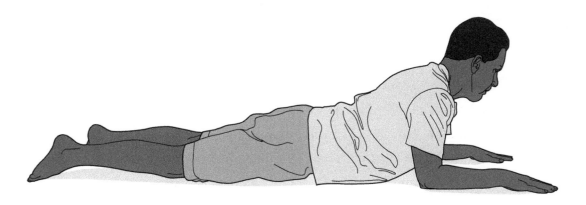

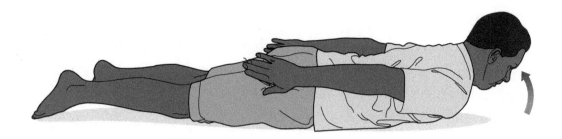

head and shoulders, off the floor. Note that lifting both ends of your body at the same time is a fairly strenuous exercise. It may not be helpful for a person with back pain.

15. Low-Back Rock and Roll

Lie on your back and pull your knees up to your chest. You can keep holding on to your legs with your hands (shown here) or stretch your arms out to your sides to lie on the floor at shoulder level. Rest in this position for 10 seconds. Gently roll your hips and knees first to one side and then to the other. Rest and relax as you roll to each side. Keep your upper back and shoulders flat on the ground.

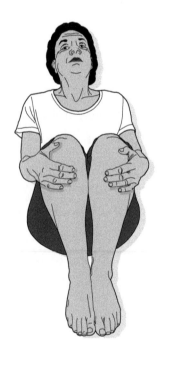 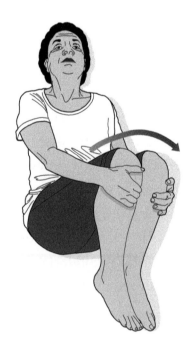

16. Curl-Up (BB)

A Curl-Up, as shown on page 193, is a good way to strengthen stomach muscles. Lie on your back, knees bent, feet flat. Do the Pelvic Tilt (Exercise 13). Slowly curl up in segments. Tuck your chin as you roll your head up and begin to lift your shoulders off the floor. Slowly uncurl back down, or hold for 10 seconds and then slowly uncurl. Breathe out as you curl up,

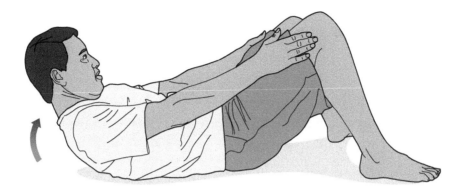

and breathe in as you go back down. Do not hold your breath. If you have neck problems or if your neck hurts when you do this exercise, try the Roll-Out (Exercise 17) instead. Never tuck your feet under a chair or have someone hold your feet when you do a Curl-Up!

17. Roll-Out

The Roll-Out is another good stomach strengthener. It is easy on the neck. Do it instead of the Curl-Up (Exercise 16) if you have neck pain. If neck pain is not a problem for you, do them both.

Lie on your back with knees bent and feet flat. Do the Pelvic Tilt (Exercise 13), holding your lower back firmly against the floor. Slowly and carefully, move one leg away from your chest as you straighten your knee. Move your leg out until you feel your lower back start to arch. When this happens, tuck your knee back to your chest. Resume your Pelvic Tilt and roll your leg out again. Breathe out as your leg rolls out. Do not hold your breath. Repeat with the other leg.

You are strengthening your abdominal muscles by holding your Pelvic Tilt against the weight of your leg. As you get stronger, you'll be able to straighten your legs out farther and move both legs together.

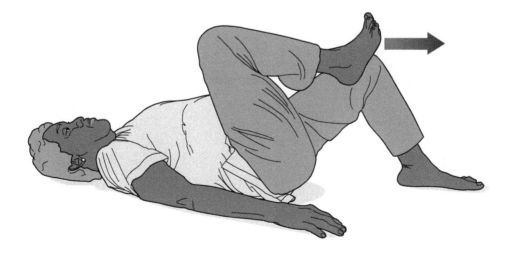

Hip and Leg Exercises

18. Straight-Leg Raises

Straight-Leg Raises strengthen the muscles that bend your hips and straighten your knees. Lie on your back, knees bent, feet flat. Straighten one leg. Tighten the muscle on the top surface of that thigh, and straighten your knee as much as possible. Keeping your knee straight, raise your leg a foot or two (up to 50 cm) off the ground. Do not arch your back. Hold your leg up, and count out loud for 10 seconds. Relax. Repeat with the other leg.

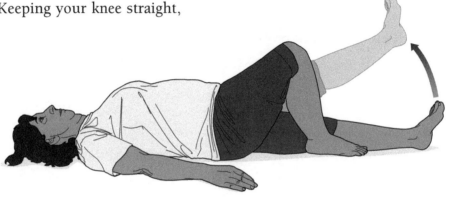

19. Hip Hooray

The Hip Hooray exercise can be done standing or lying on your back. If you lie down, spread your legs as far apart as possible. Roll your legs and feet out like a duck, then in to be pigeon-toed, and then move your legs back together. If you are standing, move one leg out to your side as far as you can. Lead out with the heel and in with the toes. Hold on to a counter for support. You can make the muscles work harder while you are standing by adding a weight to your ankle.

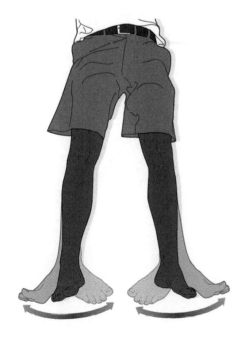
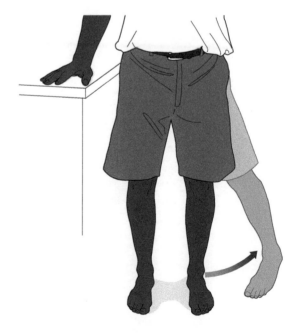

20. Back Kick (VIP) (BB)

The Back Kick increases the backward mobility and strength of your hip. Hold on to a counter for support. Move your leg up and back, knee straight. Stand tall and do not lean forward.

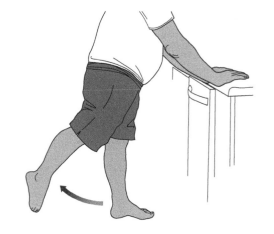

21. Knee Strengthener (BB)

Strong knees are important for walking and standing comfortably. Sitting in a chair, straighten your knee by tightening up the muscle on the top surface of your thigh. Place your hand on your thigh and feel the muscle work. If you wish, make circles with your toes. As your knee strengthens, see if you can build up to holding your leg out for 30 seconds. Count out loud. Do not hold your breath.

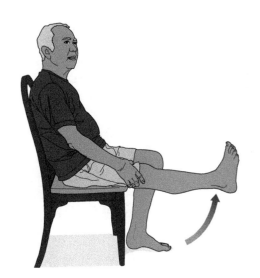

22. Power Knees

The Power Knee exercise strengthens the muscles that bend and straighten your knees. Sit in a chair and cross your legs at the ankles. Your legs can be almost straight, or you can bend your knees as much as you like. Try several positions. Push forward with your back leg and press backward with your front leg. Exert pressure evenly so that your legs do not move. Hold and count out loud for 10 seconds. Relax. Switch leg positions. Be sure to keep breathing. Repeat.

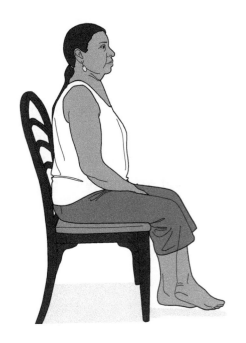

23. Sit-to-Stand

This exercise helps you practice standing up without using your arms. Sit toward the front edge of a straight-backed chair that has arms and a firm seat. Bend your knees so that your feet are flat on the floor and behind your knees. Lean a bit forward and stand up. Practice moving from a sitting to a standing position using your arms as little as possible. At first you may need to push up with your arms. Stand up five times. Rest a bit and do five more. As your hips and legs get stronger, you will be able to stand without using your arms.

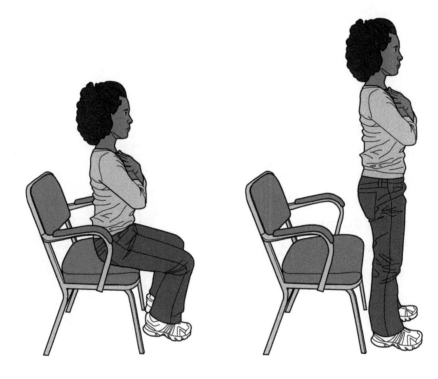

24. Ready-Go (BB)

Stand with one leg slightly in front of the other with your heel on the floor as if you are about to take a step with the front foot. Now tighten the muscles on the front of your thigh, making your knee firm and straight. Hold to a count of 10. Relax. Repeat with the other leg.

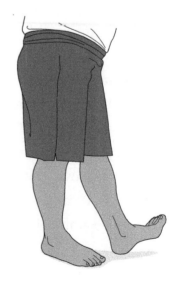

25. Hamstring Stretch

If you have unstable knees or 'back knee' (a knee that curves backward when you stand up), do not do this exercise. Do the self-test for hamstring flexibility (page 204 later in this chapter)

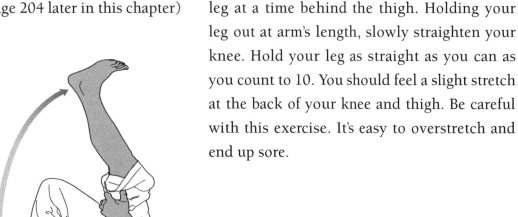

to see if you need to do this exercise. If your hamstrings are tight, this is a good stretch. Lie on your back, knees bent, feet flat. Grasp one leg at a time behind the thigh. Holding your leg out at arm's length, slowly straighten your knee. Hold your leg as straight as you can as you count to 10. You should feel a slight stretch at the back of your knee and thigh. Be careful with this exercise. It's easy to overstretch and end up sore.

26. Achilles Stretch (BB)

This exercise helps keep the Achilles tendon (the large tendon at the back of your ankle) flexible. Good flexibility helps reduce the risk of injury, calf discomfort, and heel pain. The Achilles stretch is especially helpful for cooling down after walking or cycling. It is good for people who get cramps in the calf muscles.

Stand at a counter or against a wall. Place one foot in front of the other, toes pointing forward and heels on the ground. Lean forward, bend the knee of the forward leg, and keep the back knee straight, heel down. You will feel a good stretch in the calf. Hold the stretch for 10 seconds. Do not bounce. Move gently. You can adjust this exercise to reach the other large calf muscle by slightly bending your back knee while you stretch the calf. Can you feel the difference?

If you have trouble with standing balance or spasticity (muscle jerks), you can do a seated

version of this exercise. Sit in a chair with your feet flat on the floor. Keep your heel on the floor and slowly slide your foot (one foot at a time) back to bend your ankle and feel some tension on the back of your calf (lower leg).

It's easy to get sore doing this exercise. If you've worn shoes with high heels for a long time, be particularly careful.

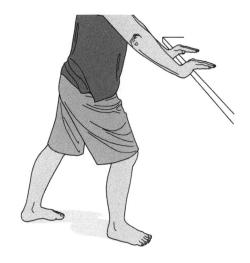

27. Tiptoes (BB)

This exercise helps strengthen calf (lower leg) muscles and makes walking, climbing stairs, and standing less tiring. It may also improve your balance. Hold on to a counter or table for support and rise up on your tiptoes. Hold that position for 10 seconds, then lower slowly. How high you rise up is not as important as keeping your balance and controlling your ankles. It is easier to do both legs at the same time. If your feet are too sore to do this standing, do it while sitting down. If this exercise makes your ankle jerk, stop doing it and talk to your physiotherapist about other ways to strengthen your calf muscles.

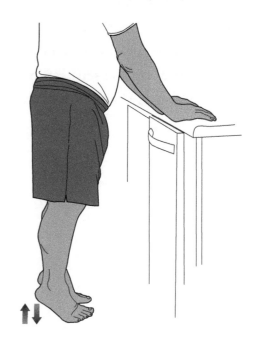

Ankle and Foot Exercises

Do these exercises sitting in a straight-backed chair with your feet bare. Have a bath towel and ten marbles next to you. These exercises can make you more flexible, strong, and comfortable. This is a good time to examine your feet and toes for any signs of circulation or skin problems and to check your nails to see if they need trimming.

28. Towel Grabber

Spread a towel out in front of your chair. Place your feet on the towel, with your heels near the edge closest to you. Keep your heels down and your foot slightly raised. Push the towel back underneath your feet by pulling it with your toes. When you have done as much as you can, reverse the toe motion and push the towel out again.

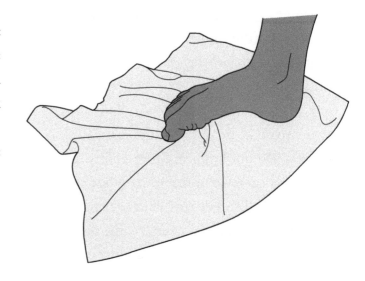

29. Marble Pickup

Place several marbles on the floor between your feet. Do this exercise one foot at a time. Using one foot, keep your heel down and pivot your toes toward the marbles. Pick up a marble with your toes, then pivot your foot to drop the marble as far as possible from where you picked it up. Repeat with the first foot until you have moved all the marbles. Reverse the process, returning all the marbles to the starting position. Repeat the entire exercise with the other foot. If marbles are difficult, try other objects, such as cards, dice, or balls of paper.

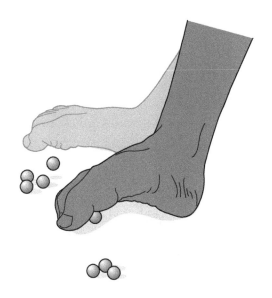

30. Foot Roll

Place a rolling pin (or a similarly shaped stick) under the arch of your foot and roll it back and forth. It feels great and stretches the ligaments in the arch of the foot. Repeat with the other foot.

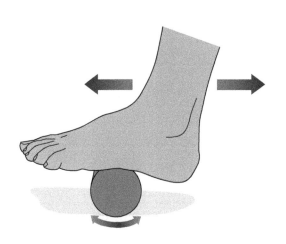

Balance Exercises

The exercises in this section allow you to practice balance activities in a safe and progressive way. We list the exercises in order of difficulty. Start with the first exercises and work up to the more difficult ones as your strength and balance improve. If you feel that your balance is particularly poor, exercise with someone else close by who can give you a supporting hand. Always exercise by a counter or stable chair that you can hold on to if necessary. Signs of improving balance include being able to hold a position longer or without extra support and being able to do the exercise or hold the position with your eyes closed.

Use these exercises to get started. There may also be balance exercise classes in your community. Tai chi, for example, is a wonderful way to improve both balance and strength. It is low impact and gentle on your joints. The NHS and Age UK offer advice and access to a range of resources to support you to exercise, including information on balance exercises (see the 'Useful Websites' section at the end of this chapter for more information).

31. Beginning Balance

Stand with your feet comfortably apart. Place your hands on your hips and turn your head and trunk as far to the left as possible and then to the right. Repeat five to ten times. To increase the difficulty, do the same thing with your eyes closed.

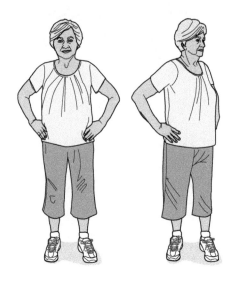
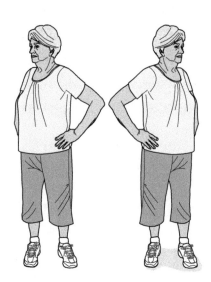

32. Swing and Sway

With both hands on a counter or the back of a stable chair for support, repeat each of the following steps five to ten times:

1. Rock back on your heels and then rise up on your toes.
2. March in place, first with your eyes open and then with your eyes closed.

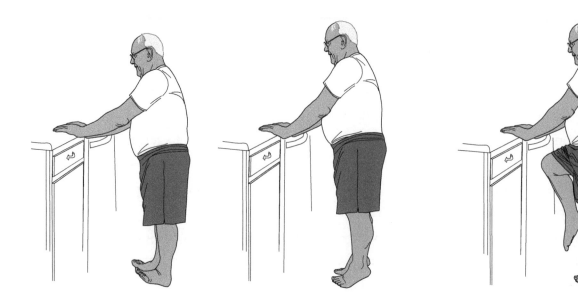

33. Walk the Line

Find a place to walk a few steps next to a kitchen counter or in a hallway with handrails (so you have support if you need it). Walk heel to toe (also called tandem walking). At first you will probably look down to watch your feet. But with practice you will be able to look straight ahead.

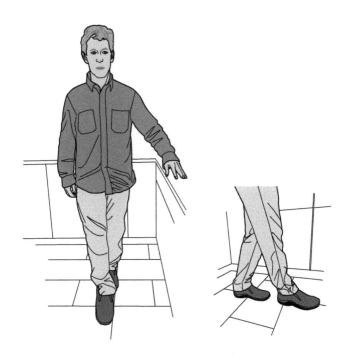

34. Base of Support

Do these exercises with standby assistance or standing close to a counter. The purpose of these exercises is to help you improve your balance by going from a larger to a smaller base of support. Repeat each of the following steps. Try to hold each position for 10 seconds. When you can do it with your eyes open, practice with your eyes closed.

1. Stand with your feet together.

2. Stand with one foot out in front and the other back.

3. Stand heel to toe.

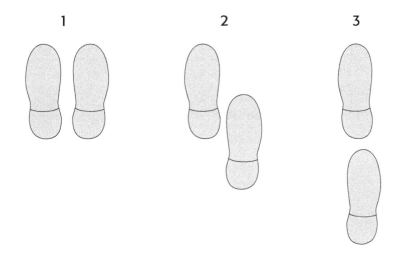

35. Toe Walk

The Toe Walk exercise increases ankle strength. It also helps you practice balancing on a small base of support while moving. Stay close to a counter for support. Rise up on your toes and walk up and back along the counter. Once you are comfortable walking on your toes without support and with your eyes open, try the Toe Walk with your eyes closed.

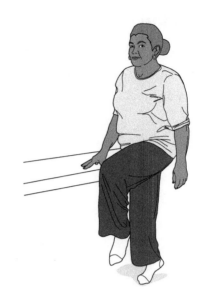

36. Heel Walk

The Heel Walk exercise increases your lower leg strength. It also helps you practice moving on a small base of support. Stay close to a counter for support. Raise your toes and forefoot and walk up and back along the counter on your heels. Once you are comfortable walking on your heels without support and with your eyes open, try the Heel Walk with your eyes closed.

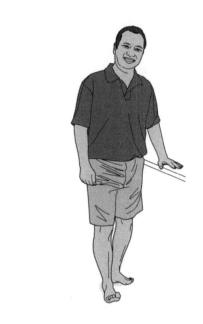

37. One-Legged Stand

Holding on to a counter or chair, lift one foot completely off the ground. Once you are balanced, lift your hand from the counter or chair. The goal is to hold the position for 10 seconds. Once you can do this for 10 seconds without holding on, practice it with your eyes closed. Repeat for the other leg.

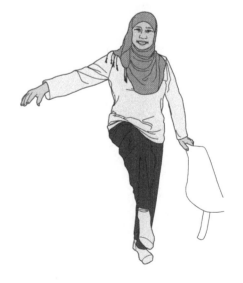

Exercises for Your Whole Body

38. The Stretcher

This exercise is a whole-body stretch that you do while lying on your back. Start the motion at your ankles, as explained here, or reverse the process if you want to start with your arms first. Lying down on your back, perform the following steps:

1. Point your toes, and then pull your toes back towards your nose. Relax.

2. Bend your knees. Then unbend your legs and flatten your knees. Relax.

3. Arch your back. Do the Pelvic Tilt (Exercise 13 on page 189). Relax.

4. Breathe in and stretch your arms above your head. Breathe out and lower your arms. Relax.

5. Stretch your right arm above your head, and stretch your left leg by pushing away with your heel. Hold this position for a count of 10. Switch to the other side and repeat. Relax.

Checking Your Progress: Self-Tests

Everybody needs to know that their efforts are making a difference. But because change is gradual, it's often hard to see improvement. To monitor your progress, you can choose from these self-tests or design your own. Self-tests measure progress toward your goal. Test yourself before you start your exercise program. Record the results. After a week or two, take the test again to check your improvement.

1. Arm Flexibility

Do Exercise 9, Pat and Reach (page 187), on both sides of the body. Ask someone to measure the distance between your fingertips. *Goal:* To decrease the distance between your fingertips.

2. Shoulder Flexibility

Stand facing a wall with your body almost touching the wall. One arm at a time, reach up the wall in front of you. Hold a pencil and mark the highest point you can reach, or have someone mark how far you can reach. Also do this reaching out sideways, standing about 3 inches (8 cm) away from the wall. *Goal:* To reach higher.

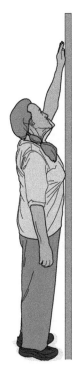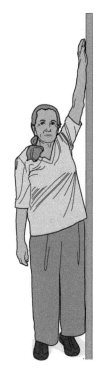

3. Hamstring Flexibility

Do Exercise 25, the Hamstring Stretch (page 197), one leg at a time. Keep your thigh (upper leg) perpendicular to your body. How much does your knee bend? How tight does the back of your leg feel? *Goal:* To have straighter knees and feel less tension in the back of the leg.

4. Ankle Flexibility

Sit in a chair with bare feet flat on the floor and knees bent at a 90-degree angle. Keep your heels on the floor. Raise your toes and the front of your foot. Ask someone to measure the distance between the ball of your foot and the floor. *Goal:* For the distance between your foot and the floor to be 1 to 2 inches (2.5 to 5 cm).

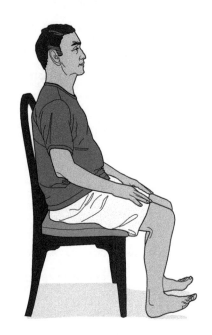

5. Ankle Strength

This test has two parts.

1. Stand at a table or counter for support. Do as many Exercise 27 Tiptoes (page 198) as quickly as you can. How many can you do before you tire?

2. Stand with your feet flat. Put most of your weight on one foot and quickly tap the floor with the front part of your other foot. How many taps can you do before you tire?

Goal: To do a total of 10 to 15 repetitions of each movement without stopping.

6. Balance

Do Exercise 37, One-Legged Stand (page 202). Time yourself and write down how long you can stand on each foot without needing to reach for support. Try with your eyes open and with your eyes closed. When you are ready to test your balance again, see if you can stand on one foot longer than you did last time. Also see if you can stand without support or balance with your eyes closed.

Goal: To be able to balance on one foot with your eyes open for 30 seconds.

Making Your Exercise Programme Work for You

The best way to enjoy and stick with regular physical activity is to suit yourself! Choose what you want to do, a place where you feel comfortable, and an exercise time that fits your schedule. If you want to have dinner on the table at 6:00 p.m., don't choose a 5:00 p.m. exercise class. If you are retired and enjoy lunch with friends and an afternoon nap, choose an early or mid-morning exercise time.

Having fun and enjoying yourself are important benefits of exercise. Too often people think of exercise as serious business. It is fun too! Most people who stick with a programme do so because they enjoy it or feel better. Physically active people think of exercise as recreation or a positive part of life rather than a chore. Start off with success in mind. Allow yourself time to get used to something new. You'll probably find that you look forward to exercise and enjoy the benefits. Experience, practice, and success help build a habit.

Being an Exercise Self-Manager

Follow the steps in Chapter 2, *Becoming an Active Self-Manager*, to make starting and staying with your programme easier. And keep the following tips in mind:

■ **Set an exercise goal and keep it in mind.**

■ **Choose exercises you want to do.** Combine activities that move you toward your goal and activities your healthcare professionals suggest.

■ **Choose the time and place to exercise.** Choose a place where you feel comfortable and an exercise time that fits your schedule.

■ **Tell your family and friends about your plan.** They can support your efforts.

■ **Make an action plan with yourself.** Decide how long you'll stick with these particular exercises; 3 to 4 weeks is a reasonable time for any new programme.

■ **Start your program.** Remember to begin doing what you can and go slowly, especially if you haven't exercised in a while.

■ **Keep an exercise diary or calendar.** Some people enjoy having a record of what they did and how they felt. Others like a simple calendar on which they note each exercise session.

■ **Use self-tests to keep track of your initial fitness and your progress.** Record the date and results.

■ **Repeat self-tests at regular intervals, record the results, and check your progress.**

■ **Revise your programme.** At the end of 3 to 4 weeks, decide what you liked, what worked, and what made exercising difficult. Make changes and draw up an action plan for another few weeks. You may decide to change some exercises, the place or time you exercise, or your exercise partner or group. You may also have to cut back a little.

- **Be patient when there are setbacks.** If you get sick, have to change your routine, or add caring responsibilities to your day and can't exercise as much for a while, know that these things happen and you can pick up again when you can. If you have had to stop exercise for more than 2 weeks, start back at a lower level and gradually move back to where you were before.

- **Reward yourself for a job well done.** The rewards of physical activity include improved health and endurance. But you can also reward yourself with enjoyable family outings, refreshing walks, trips to a concert or museum, or a day out fishing. Pats on the back and a new exercise top can be fun rewards too.

Useful Websites

Age UK (Exercise): https://www.ageuk.org.uk/information-advice/health-wellbeing/exercise/

Chartered Society of Physiotherapy (Helping older people stay active at home): https://www.csp.org.uk/public-patient/keeping-active-and-healthy/staying-healthy-you-age /staying-strong-you-age/strength

Escape pain (Rehabilitation programme for people with chronic joint pain): https://escape-pain.org

NHS (Balance exercises): https://www.nhs.uk/live-well/exercise/balance-exercises

'We are Undefeatable' (Campaign by UK charities and Sport England to support people living with health conditions to build physical activity and exercise into their lives): https://weareundefeatable .co.uk/ways-to-move

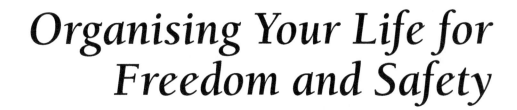

CHAPTER 9

Organising Your Life for Freedom and Safety

IN THE PREVIOUS TWO CHAPTERS WE TALKED ABOUT the benefits of exercise, how to get moving, and how to stay active. In this chapter you'll learn how to use exercise and other tools to avoid injury and reduce your risk of falling. Read on to hear two stories about making changes for safer living.

Nadia had a stroke. After rehabilitation, she returned to work part-time. Everything took longer. She walked slower and felt unsteady – especially when she was tired. After a few hours on the computer, she noticed back and neck pain. At home she was overwhelmed by cooking and housework. Nadia felt she couldn't keep up. She stopped exercising and attending her book club. Soon she was lonely as well as frustrated and unsteady.

Special thanks to Runa Mishra, BSC (Hons) Occupational Therapist, HCPC registered, for reviewing this chapter.

Nadia spoke with her husband. Together, they decided to share household tasks and make the house safer. She improved the arrangement of her computer desk and decided to use a walking stick, especially when she was tired. She asked her physiotherapist for a referral to a community exercise class. Attending the class and doing the group exercises improved her posture. After several weeks of class, Nadia was able to walk faster. In time, she had the energy to return to her book club.

Matthew lives in the city and uses public transport. Although he is in his seventies, he loves his job and continues to work. Five years ago, he was diagnosed with COPD (chronic obstructive pulmonary disease such as long-term bronchitis or emphysema). At first, Matthew was short of breath only when he rushed or when it was cold outside. Then it got worse. Moving was harder on him. He started moving less and was short of breath when he stood up. He began taking a taxi to work. It was much more expensive than the bus, but he felt

weak, and he was afraid he might fall on public transport.

Matthew's GP recommended pulmonary rehabilitation, and he found the rehab programme helpful. He learned to manage his shortness of breath by taking rest breaks at the first signs of difficulty. Since the programme, he began to walk daily and feel stronger. He developed more stamina and began taking the bus again. He leaves his flat in the morning a little earlier because his shortness of breath is worse when he rushes. Matthew started doing relaxation exercises to help with his breathing. Now he is surprised that he feels much calmer and more in control of his breathing. He has more energy and participates in social activities.

This chapter suggests ways you can reduce falls and injury while doing the things you want and need to do. Injury cannot be totally prevented. However, you can reduce the frequency and severity of accidents by being aware of your surroundings and practicing our tips and suggestions.

Understanding the Injury Cycle

If you have a long-term health condition, you can reduce your risk of injury by reviewing the factors in Figure 9.1. The key factors that contribute to injury risk are distraction, poor body mechanics, an unsafe environment, and deconditioning and other physical changes. Each factor of the injury cycle increases risks and influences other factors.

For example, if you are distracted you might not pay enough attention to what you are doing or where you are going. The result

may be a trip or a bruise. Good body mechanics involve moving your body with good posture and coordination. Poor body mechanics mean not using your body in the best and safest possible way. For example, poor body mechanics like poor posture may increase pain. Or using poor body mechanics to try to reach something without standing on a firm surface may result in a fall.

Deconditioning (not being fit) can result in less balance, endurance, and strength. When

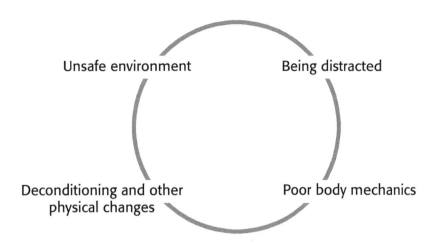

Figure 9.1 **The Injury Cycle**

muscles are weaker, more effort is needed to maintain good posture. Other physical changes, such as numbness in your feet, poor vision, or hearing problems, can make you less aware of your surroundings. These factors may affect your balance and discourage you from exercise. If your surroundings are cluttered, poor balance increases your risk of falling. If you fall and injure yourself, it is even more challenging to remain active. Being inactive results in turn in further deconditioning.

These examples show you how all the parts of the injury cycle affect each other.

Your Tools for Reducing Injury Risk

This chapter offers you some additional tools that give you ways to break the cycle of injury so you can participate in activities that you enjoy with less pain. The following sections describe each tool and how to use it to reduce your injury risk.

■ exercising

■ using good body mechanics

■ becoming less distracted

■ increasing safety with assistive equipment and devices

■ modifying your home and surroundings

■ seeking guidance from healthcare professionals

Exercising to Reduce Your Injury Risk

Long-term conditions can cause pain and lead to injury risks. Exercise is a powerful tool for maintaining your physical abilities. Chapter 7, *Being Physically Active*, and Chapter 8, *Exercising to Make Life Easier*, list many exercise options to build strength, flexibility, endurance, and balance. Researchers have found that exercises to improve strength and balance are the best way to reduce your risk of falling. Building strength in your leg muscles around the hips, knees, and ankles increases stability. If you are stiff, consider exercises to increase your flexibility, and if you feel wobbly, consider balance exercises such as the Heel Walk and Toe Walk (see page 202). Talk with a physiotherapist if you have body pain or a history of falls. Physiotherapists can create an exercise programme for you and help you carry it out. Ask your GP or physiotherapist about local training programmes that can help reduce your risk of having a fall. If you feel that your home is not safe or that you have difficulty carrying out your daily activities, ask your GP to refer you for a home hazard assessment. You can contact your GP or local authority to

---

Treat Hearing Loss to Stay Active and Safe

Hearing loss comes on gradually. Often people don't notice that they are losing their hearing. When you have difficulty hearing, it is common to feel isolated, depressed, and withdrawn from others. Untreated hearing loss increases the risk of dementia, injury, and falls. Some people worry that hearing aids will make them look or feel old. They also know that hearing aids are not perfect. Today, many kinds of hearing aids are hardly noticeable. It is true that hearing aids are not perfect, but not hearing is much worse. Each year, hearing aids are becoming better and better.

See your GP if you're having problems with your hearing. They can refer you to a hearing specialist for an assessment if they think you might need a hearing aid. If your specialist recommends hearing aids, talk to them about the different types available and which is best for you. Hearing aids are available on the NHS for anyone who needs them. The benefits of getting a hearing aid on the NHS include:

- Hearing aids are provided for free as a long-term loan.
- Batteries and repairs are free (there may be a charge if you lose or break your hearing aid and it needs to be replaced).

- You don't have to pay for any follow-up appointments or aftercare.

While several modern hearing aids are available on the NHS, these are usually the BTE (behind the ear) or very occasionally the RITE (receiver in the ear) type. You may need to pay for private treatment if you want one of the other types.

Once you have your hearing aids, be patient. It takes time to get used to hearing aids, and they may need several adjustments. Your hearing will never be 'normal', but hearing aids should allow you to hear those around you and participate in life.

Apps available on your smart phone allow you to adjust the hearing aid settings so you can hear in different settings. You can adjust them to work in different settings from busy restaurants to lecture halls or your TV at home.

Hearing aids are improving every year. Over-the-counter (OTC) hearing aids are expected to be available in the near future. The OTC hearing aids will be sold for less than those fitted and provided by audiologists and are designed for people with mild to moderate hearing loss.

ask about the different kinds of help available in your area (see the 'Useful Websites' section at the end of this chapter for further details available on the NHS website).

Using Good Body Mechanics

Body mechanics refers to the way people move during daily activities. Proper body mechanics can help you reduce the risk of pain and injury. Body mechanics exercises are designed to improve your posture, coordination, and stamina.

Practicing Good Posture

Good posture strengthens your body. There are three natural curves in the spine at the neck, upper back, and lower back. When you maintain these curves, your spine is strongest. These natural curves help the body absorb the 'shock of movement' and hold positions with the least strain. Proper posture involves maintaining these curves. With good posture, all body parts are in alignment. This prevents strain on muscles, ligaments, tendons, and joints. Figures 9.2, 9.3, and 9.4 illustrate good standing and sitting posture.

Good standing posture is characterised by the following:

■ ears over shoulders

■ shoulders over hips (shoulders even and relaxed)

■ hips over knees

■ knees over feet (knees straight but not locked)

■ feet shoulder width apart (even weight on both feet)

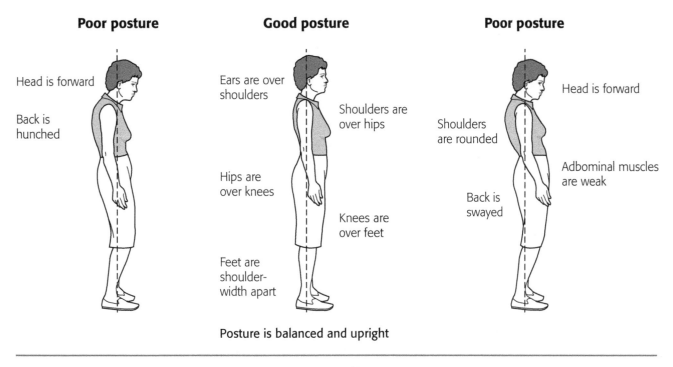

Figure 9.2 **Standing Posture**

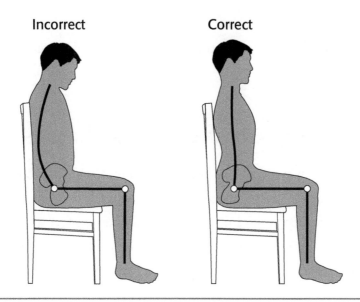

Figure 9.3 **Sitting**

Good sitting posture is characterised by the following:

- ears over shoulders
- shoulders relaxed but not elevated
- upper back relaxed and over hips
- hips bent at 90 degrees
- knees bent at 90 degrees
- buttocks flat on seat with even weight on both hips
- feet flat on the floor or footrest

Posture is also important when you're using computers and electronic devices (phone, laptop, tablet). Figure 9.4 demonstrates proper posture at the computer.

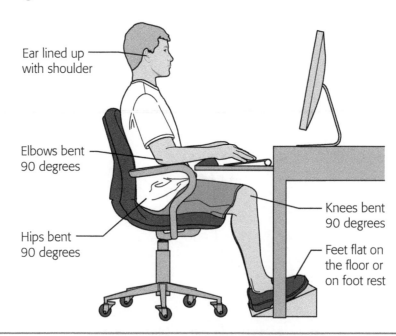

Figure 9.4 **Good Sitting Posture for Computer Use**

Body Mechanics for Daily Activities

Using good posture when you're doing daily activities such as getting dressed, taking a shower, or changing position protects your back and limbs.

- Bend your knees and bend at the hips if you need to lean forward. Do not bend at the waist, as doing that strains your spine.

- Use assistive devices (see pages 222-226) or change your position to avoid awkward body posture. For example, consider putting your feet on a low stool to put on socks, or use a sock aid. Use a long-handled sponge to reduce bending and twisting to wash your back or feet in the shower.

- Reduce twisting, especially while bending forward. One helpful trick is to imagine you are wearing a belt buckle. Make sure to keep your imaginary belt buckle and your feet pointing in the same direction.

- Take time to feel steady before you move. To avoid getting dizzy when moving from a seated or lying position, stand up slowly and remain in one place a moment before you start to move.

- Gently tighten and lift your stomach muscles to support your spine when changing positions.

- If you feel unsteady, allow carers or family members to use a gait belt (which is

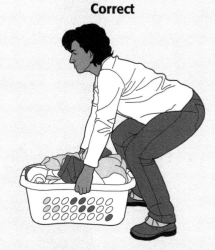

Incorrect

Do not bend at the waist.

Correct

Protect your back by bending your knees and bending at your hips.

a safety device used to help someone move, such as from a bed to a chair) to provide support (see Table 9.2 on pages 223–225).

Changing Positions and Transferring

Posture and body mechanics are especially important when you change positions. This is because when you change positions, you can get into awkward positions or lose your balance. Many people have difficulty changing positions safely. Moving from one position to another, such as from sitting to standing, is often rushed or done with improper positioning. This increases the chance of injury and fall.

This section illustrates step-by-step instructions for a few different transfers. Carefully review the complete instructions and ask a friend or family member to assist or watch you the first time you practice. Adjust the instructions so that you feel safe and steady. If these instructions don't work for you, ask for advice from an occupational therapist or physiotherapist.

Moving from Sitting in an Armchair to Standing

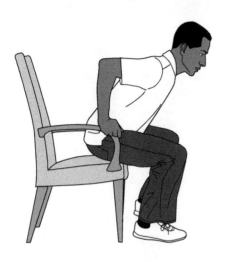

1. Slide your hips forward to sit near the front half of the chair.

2. Make sure your feet are flat on the floor (making a 90-degree angle with your knees).

3. Lean forward (make sure your nose is over your toes).

4. Push from the chair arms and your hips to come to a standing position.

For additional tips see the 'Sit-to-Stand' exercise on page 196.

Getting into Bed

1. Sit on the bed about a foot from the pillow.

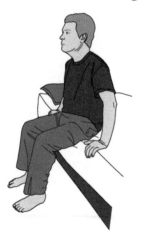

2. Shuffle back so that you are not on the edge of the bed. The back of your knees should be touching the mattress.

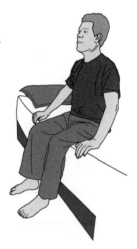

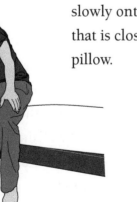

3. Lower your body slowly onto your arm that is closest to the pillow.

4. Ideally, bend your knees and pull into the bed. You may need assistance from a friend, carer, or family member.

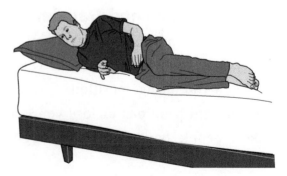

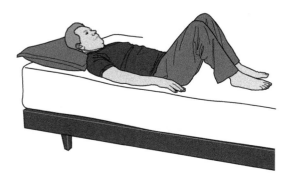 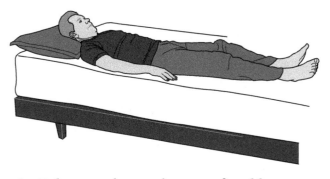

5. Roll onto your back.

6. Relax your legs and get comfortable.

Getting Out of Bed

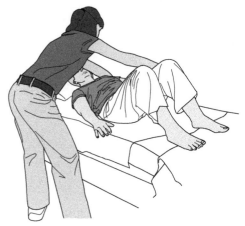 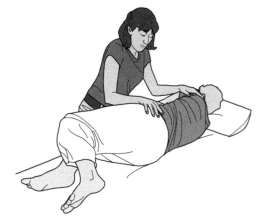

1. While lying on your back, bend your knees.

2. Roll on your side. Many people ask a carer, friend, or family member to stand at the edge of the bed. (If assistance is needed, ask your helper to put one hand on your shoulder and the other on your hip.)

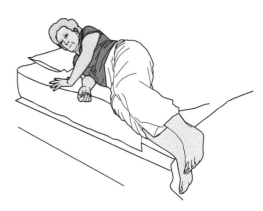 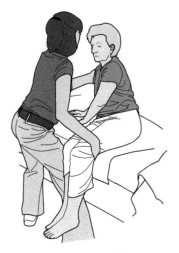

3. Gently move your feet over the edge of the bed while pushing up onto one elbow. (If assistance is needed, ask your helper to put your feet over the edge.)

4. Move to a sitting position. (If assistance is needed, ask your helper to cradle your shoulders in one hand and knees in the other while they guide you up to a sitting position.)

Staying safe during transfers and daily activities

You may need assistance to do a transfer some or all the time. Here are some helpful tips from people who need assistance while transferring:

- 'I can't get up from a low couch, so I request a straight-back chair when visiting friends.'

- 'I used to need a lot of help to get up from a chair without armrests. I started doing the Sit-to-Stand exercise (see Chapter 8, Exercising to Make Life Easier, page 196) and now I need less help.'

- 'I get very stressed during transfers because I am a large person. It has helped me to take two deep breaths before I start.'

- 'I live in a nursing home. When I don't feel safe transferring with a new and inexperienced staff member, I ask them to get additional help so that we both stay safe. I say it in a kind voice; otherwise we get into a fight.'

- 'When I transfer with help from my spouse, I use a gait belt (see page 223) and it helps us both feel safe.'

- 'I use a wheelchair and almost tripped on the leg rests several times. Now I ask those helping me to swing them away or remove them when I transfer.' (See the box on page 217.)

- 'My condition varies. Some days I need someone to stand by and other days I need a lot of help. I check in with my body, figure out how much help I need, and tell my carer. Transfers have gone smoother since.'

- 'My partner and I have a system. We review what we are going to do and use the one-word commands we agreed on: "shuffle, push up, turn, reach, lower." This created better rhythm during the transfer, and we both know what is going on.'

- 'My spouse had back strain after transfers. Last time I needed a few physiotherapy sessions, the physiotherapist gave us both tips and it helped my spouse to accomplish my transfer safely and pain free.'

- 'I used to let others do all the work to transfer me. It took so many people, and they were so irritated. It was stressful. I have gotten stronger and help now. It all goes better.'

Transfer Tips

- Sometimes one side of the bed is easier than the other.
- Consider installing a mobility bed rail (Table 9.2 on pages 223–225) under your mattress to help you sit up and stand.
- If you are using an assistive device (for example, a walker or a walking stick), it's safer not to use the device for pushing up.

- Use a permanent surface such as a safety rail, the edge of the bed, or the arms of a stable chair.
- If you feel unsafe during transfers, talk to a healthcare professional or family member.
- If you use a wheelchair, make sure to swing away the legs before doing a transfer. See the box on page 217.

Safely Swinging Away Wheelchair Leg Rests

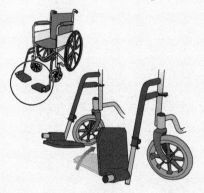 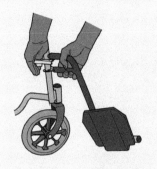 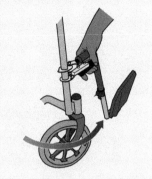

1. Lift the foot rest and calf support so they fold toward the leg rest.

2. Lift/release the lever at the top of the leg rest.

3. Swing away or remove the leg rest.

A Special Type of Transfer: Getting Up from the Floor

Sometimes you may find yourself on the floor. Maybe you fell, or maybe you just had to get down to pick up something or to clean. Here are tips for getting up.

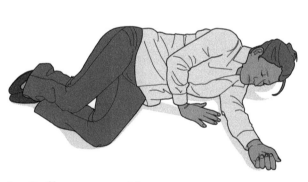

1. Roll onto one side.

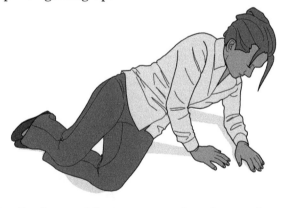

2. Push up with your upper hand enough to get your lower elbow under your body.

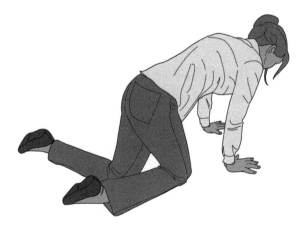

3. Tuck your knees under your body and roll onto all fours.

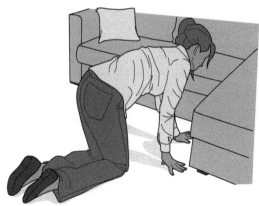

4. Crawl toward a bed, sofa, or sturdy chair.

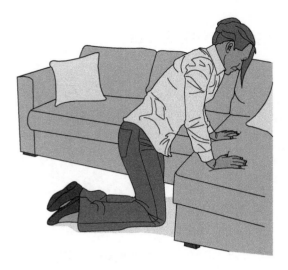

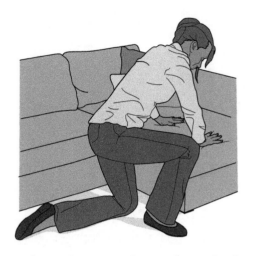

5. Place your hands on a sturdy surface (a sofa, chair, or bed).

6. Bend your stronger leg and put the foot of that leg flat on the floor.

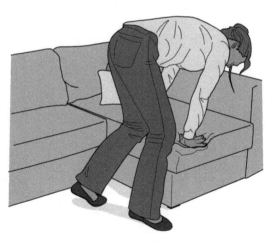

7. Push up to a standing position.

Becoming More Aware and Less Distracted

Distraction is common. Everyone has walked into a room to look for something and forgotten what they were looking for. When people describe why they were involved in an accident or were injured, they commonly say, 'I was rushing', 'I was tired', or 'my mind was somewhere else.' Difficult emotions, such as anger and frustration, can capture your attention and make you less aware of what is going on around you. Recall Matthew from earlier in this chapter. He was surprised that relaxation exercises helped him focus on the present and be less anxious about his shortness of breath. When you're rushing, your attention is focused on the future and not so much on what you are doing right now.

There are many reasons why people rush. Your day may be packed with activity and responsibilities. You may not be allowing the time you need to do things with your long-term health condition. Or you may not be building time into your schedule for the unexpected to occur. Sometimes people have accidents or injuries because they are very tired and have trouble paying attention. When you're tired, it's very easy to lose focus. Though it's unlikely you can stop yourself from ever being distracted, it's possible to gain some control. The first step is understanding how distraction affects you.

The following are suggestions to help you be less distracted and more attentive:

■ **Take control of expected and unexpected tasks.** Allow extra time for self-care, travel, and the unexpected. If you do this, you avoid rushing and blaming yourself when you are late or do not get something done.

■ **Use your mind to turn down the volume on distracting negative emotions.** Review Chapter 6, *Using Your Mind to Manage Symptoms*, to explore relaxation tools such as positive thinking and self-talk, guided imagery, prayer, the quieting reflex, mindfulness, and practicing gratitude.

■ **Cue yourself to pay attention in the present moment.** When you find yourself rushing or thinking about what you have to do next in your day, take a couple of deep breaths to slow down. Check in with yourself to notice your emotions and how your body feels. Give yourself gentle cues quietly or silently such as 'slow down' or 'take a rest' or 'no need to rush'.

Using Assistive Technology to Make Activities Easier and Safer

Assistive technology is a term that includes assistive devices, adaptive or rehabilitation equipment, and other aids that make it easier to do something. The term *adaptive* refers to assistive devices that are *specifically designed* for people with disabilities. Because these terms are often used interchangeably, in this book we will refer to all of them as assistive equipment and devices. Computer software such as voice recognition, hearing aids, ramps, grab bars, mobility aids, and devices to make daily tasks such as dressing, cooking, driving, and grooming easier are all examples of assistive technology.

Assistive equipment and devices can help you do things you can no longer do easily. Using these is not giving in, it is being smarter. All of us have used special equipment all our lives, such as a set of steps to reach high shelves and a fork to keep our fingers clean. There is a device for almost everything. Your job is to find the right one. The important questions to ask are: 'What devices are available?' 'How do I choose the right one?' and 'How do I use the device properly?'

Using Mobility Aids to Get from One Place to Another Safely

Walkers, walking sticks, and wheelchairs are common. Do any of the following apply to you? If so, think about using a mobility aid:

■ Are you touching furniture or steady surfaces to get around the house?

■ Is one leg weaker than the other?

■ Are you unsteady outside of the house or when walking on uneven surfaces?

■ Have you fallen recently due to poor balance, weakness, or slow reaction times?

Falls of almost any type could signal the need for mobility aids. If you have any questions about which mobility aid is right for you or how to use it, ask a healthcare professional, such as a physiotherapist or occupational therapist. Be sure to get proper training. The proper use of aids is not something 'you just know'. You might even want to make a short video on your mobile phone during the training so that you can watch it and better remember how to use your device when you get it home. Using a mobility aid incorrectly or using a poorly fitting mobility aid can lead to falls and injury. If your ability to walk changes, you might need to change aids.

Table 9.1, Mobility Aids and Injury Prevention Tips, lists commonly used mobility aids and tips to prevent injuries. The table is not a substitute for professional help. It just provides information to get you started and may help you think about what questions to ask.

Table 9.1 **Mobility Aids and Injury Prevention Tips**

Mobility Aids	Qualities	Injury Prevention Tips
Walking sticks	◆ Often longer than a conventional walking stick. ◆ You can use one or two sticks. ◆ Use two walking sticks on uneven or rough ground. ◆ Two sticks provide a standing rest break. ◆ Designed for people who have adequate balance on flat ground. ◆ Tend to hold less stigma than a walking stick.	◆ Use of two sticks is helpful when hiking, travelling, or on uneven ground. ◆ Choose cork or moulded rubber handgrips; plastic grips tend to get sweaty.
Single-point or straight walking stick	◆ Good for people who need some stability while walking. ◆ Increases safety and balance compared with no assistive device. ◆ Helps walking when there is pain or weakness on one side of the body.	◆ Hold in hand opposite weak or injured leg; step out with your injured or weak leg and walking stick at same time. Maintain upright posture ◆ Keep the walking stick close to your body. ◆ Don't drag the walking stick. ◆ Not useful if held in the air and not touching the ground.

Table 9.1 **Mobility Aids and Injury Prevention Tips (*continued*)**

Mobility Aids	Qualities	Injury Prevention Tips
Quad walking stick	◆ Good for people who need more stability than a single-point walking stick. ◆ Can stand upright. ◆ Larger base than a standard walking stick.	◆ Hold in the hand opposite weak or injured leg; step out with your injured or weak leg and walking stick at same time. ◆ To be safe, all four feet at walking stick's base must touch the ground. ◆ Pick up the walking stick. Don't drag it.
Rolling walker with seat and four wheels	◆ Good for people who need a little help with balance and can walk steadily but fatigue easily. ◆ Not recommended for people with poor balance. ◆ Fastest walking speed. ◆ Offers a seat for rest breaks and a basket to carry items.	◆ LOCK THE BRAKES BEFORE YOU SIT DOWN OR STAND UP. ◆ Stay close to the rolling walker and stand tall. ◆ Handles of the rolling walker should be at your wrist height (when your arms are hanging straight at your side). ◆ A rolling walker can tip if you put your full weight on the hand rests.
Rolling walker with two wheels	◆ Good for people with some balance issues who need support to walk. ◆ Moves faster than a standard walker. ◆ Less stable than a standard walker.	◆ Stay close to the walker and stand tall. ◆ Handles of the walker should be at your wrist height (when your arms are hanging straight at your side). ◆ Consider attaching tennis balls or glides to the back legs to allow the back legs to slide.
Standard walker	◆ Good for people with limited balance who need a lot of support to walk. ◆ Best choice if you cannot put full weight on both legs (for example, for post-surgery outpatients). ◆ Slow to move. ◆ No wheels. It's the most stable walker. ◆ You must be able to use your arms to pick up the walker to move forward while walking.	◆ Stay close to the walker and stand tall. ◆ Handles of the walker should be at your wrist height (when your arms are hanging straight at your side). ◆ Keep all four walker legs in contact with the ground when walking.

Continues ▶

Table 9.1 **Mobility Aids and Injury Prevention Tips (*continued*)**

Mobility Aids	Qualities	Injury Prevention Tips
Manual wheelchair	◆ Good for people with enough upper body strength to propel the wheelchair. ◆ Good for people who lack the endurance to use a walker or walking stick for outings (museums and outdoor gardens often have wheelchairs available if you call ahead). ◆ Good for people who have someone to push them.	◆ LOCK THE BRAKES BEFORE YOU SIT DOWN, STAND UP, OR TRANSFER. ◆ Swing away the wheelchair legs for a safer transfer (see the box on page 217). ◆ Avoid putting heavy loads on the back of a wheelchair. ◆ Avoid going up or down steep inclines. ◆ If there are no dropped curbs, consider backing up your wheelchair to go up or down a curb.
Scooter	◆ Good for people who don't require a power wheelchair full-time.	◆ Turn the power off before transferring. ◆ Keep track of the battery charge indicator to make sure the battery is fully charged. ◆ Cover handlebars with plastic to protect the electronics from rain. ◆ If your scooter was built before 2016, it should be used on flat surfaces only, and avoid using it in the rain. Contact the manufacturer for details.
Power wheelchair	◆ Good for people who cannot push a wheelchair with their own arm strength. ◆ Power wheelchairs with standing options allow people with paraplegia to stand independently.	◆ Turn the power off before transferring. ◆ Keep track of the battery charge indicator to make sure the battery is fully charged. ◆ Cover the controller or joystick with plastic to protect it from rain. ◆ Contact the manufacturer with questions, read the operating manual, and observe all safety precautions.

Increasing Safety and Reducing Effort with Assistive Devices

Assistive devices can increase your safety and reduce effort. For example, if you can stand up from the toilet by using safety rails, you are safer and more independent. Table 9.2, Assistive Devices, describes devices that make daily tasks easier. Be selective and choose devices that allow you to solve a problem. In addition to the devices listed in Table 9.2, there are many other types of equipment that can increase your independence in daily living tasks.

Table 9.2 **Assistive Devices**

Device	Purpose	Tips
Gait belt	◆ Assists with transfers and unstable walking. ◆ Allows someone to grasp the belt in order to assist you to transfer safely.	◆ Place the gait belt low around the waist. ◆ Fasten the belt tight enough so it does not slide but loose enough so you can slip a finger under the belt. ◆ If you put the belt on while you are sitting, make sure it is fastened tighter than you might think is necessary, as it will loosen when you stand up.
Mobility bed rail	◆ Helps with sitting up or getting out of bed. ◆ Reduces your risk of falls from bed. ◆ Increases independence by allowing you to safely sit up and stand up if you have enough body strength.	◆ Use on your stronger side. ◆ Test that the rail is secure before you use it. ◆ You may need more than a rail if you put excessive weight on it. ◆ The rail is not designed to keep you in bed.
Raised toilet seat/ uplift commode assist	◆ Assists with safely sitting on the toilet seat and coming back to standing position. ◆ Allows you to follow precautions needed after hip replacement.	◆ Make sure the seat fits securely. ◆ Test for stability before you use it. ◆ There are many different models; some types are easier to remove. This is important if the toilet is also used by others.
Toilet safety rails	◆ Assist with safely sitting on the toilet seat and coming back to standing position. ◆ Rails are a good alternative (to the raised toilet seat described above) if you need armrests but not the raised toilet seat.	◆ Test to make sure rails are sturdy enough to hold your weight when pushing up. (You may need to have someone else test this.) ◆ Measure your toilet's width and height to make sure the rails will fit before purchasing rails.

Continues ►

Table 9.2 **Assistive Devices (*continued*)**

Device	Purpose	Tips
Grab bars	◆ Assist with getting in/out of bath/shower. ◆ Assist with slowly and safely assuming a seated position from a standing position. ◆ Provide stability and support longer standing time (for example, so the carer can wash your entire body).	◆ Can be used to enter the shower, to get up from the toilet seat, or to get over a step or a few stairs in a hall (i.e., not just in a bathroom). ◆ See the box "Tips for Installing Grab Bars in the Bathroom" on page 227. ◆ Have grab bars professionally installed so they will not pull out of the wall. ◆ Request assistance and a home visit with an occupational therapist to learn where to place bars. ◆ Avoid suction grab bars; these must be tested every time they are used to ensure that they don't pull away from the wall. ◆ NOTE: a towel bar can unexpectedly pull out of the wall with repeated pressure.
Shower chair/bench	◆ Provides stability and prevents falls in the shower or bath. ◆ A shower stool or folding shower seat is adequate if you get tired but have good balance. ◆ Choose a shower chair with an armrest/back for more support. ◆ Choose a shower chair without arms if you are using a transfer board (described below). ◆ Choose a bath transfer bench if you cannot safely step over the bath edge. ◆ Portable chairs are available for travel.	◆ Measure your bath/shower to make sure the chair or bench fits before purchasing. ◆ Install a handheld showerhead to increase your independence and control water flow. ◆ Test a portable travel chair to make sure it's sturdy enough to be safe.

Table 9.2 **Assistive Devices (*continued*)**

Device	Purpose	Tips
Handy bar	◆ Assists with getting in and out of cars.	◆ Before you use the handy bar, ask a friend or family member to test its sturdiness and then to stand close enough to support you when you first try it.
Swivel cushion	◆ Assists with getting in and out of cars. ◆ Helps you swivel around when you are in a chair or car seat.	◆ Ask someone to test the cushion before you use it.
Transfer board	◆ Assist with chair-to-chair transfer (such as wheelchair-to-car, wheelchair-to-bath bench, wheelchair-to-bed, or wheelchair-to-chair). ◆ Instead of lifting the person being transferred, a carer must make sure to slide them over the board.	◆ Make sure you have good arm and trunk strength before using a transfer board. ◆ Seek instruction from a healthcare professional to make sure you use it safely.

The assistive devices described here help make tasks easier for everyone.

■ There are many commercially available assistive devices for the kitchen, including easy-grip utensils, food processors, and mandolines (utensils with an adjustable blade for slicing foods thinly and evenly).

■ If you struggle to put on clothing, consider buying new items a size larger, and look for clothes designed with a looser fit and a larger neck opening. You can add Velcro closures to clothing or use elastic shoelaces. If you have reduced balance or mobility, use a long-handled shoehorn while sitting to put on your shoes.

■ For bathing, you can use a long-handled sponge to reduce bending and twisting.

■ There are devices to help with wiping after toileting if you have movement restrictions.

■ Install a handheld showerhead or use a pump dispenser for shampoo or body wash to make bathing easier.

■ For eating, use a nonslip mat or material for your plates and other utensils such as Dycem (the brand name for a non-slippery substance you can purchase as a place mat to keep plates from moving). Utensils with built-up handles or other special utensils, such as a rocker knife (a specially designed knife with curved blade that allows users to easily cut food using one hand), can also increase your independence during eating. A scooped plate can prevent food spills. Some of these items are pictured in Figure 9.5.

A good starting point to find these devices and other tools to help you break the cycle of injury is the NHS website (see the 'Useful Websites' section at the end of this chapter). You can also check with your local pharmacy or do an online search of the names of the devices listed in Table 9.2 and Figure 9.5. Or look for a community organisation that rents or loans out equipment such as mobility aids and bathroom safety equipment. Some community organisations give away used equipment. If you have equipment you no longer use, you can donate it.

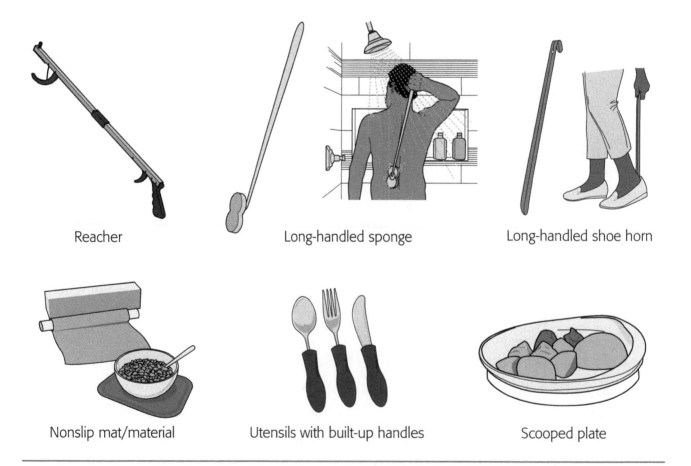

Reacher   Long-handled sponge   Long-handled shoe horn

Nonslip mat/material   Utensils with built-up handles   Scooped plate

Figure 9.5 **Assistive Equipment to Make Tasks Easier**

Tips for Installing Grab Bars in the Bathroom

If you are unsure about the best way to maintain your safety and independence whilst bathing, you are advised to seek a formal assessment of your needs from your local authority social services department or from a private or independent occupational therapist. Correct positioning of grab rails is important to ensure that they provide the support, where necessary, to perform specific tasks. Although there is published guidance for the positioning of rails, you will also need to be guided by:

■ your own requirements

■ the support you require

■ your height and weight

■ the amount of mobility and strength you have in your hands, arms, and shoulders.

There are a number of published documents that can help in the positioning of rails. These are intended to give generic guidance to property developers or housing associations, but the principles and advice may be useful as a starting point. The Disabled Living Foundation (DLF) provides some general guidance to the installation of grab rails in a bathroom (see the 'Useful Websites' section at the end of this chapter).The following are things that you might want to consider:

1. Make sure grab bars are installed where they will be most helpful. Try a 'dry run' in the bathroom to test this out. Notice where you reach out for support. This usually indicates a good location for a grab bar. If you find you put weight on towel bars, replace them with grab bars. Consult with an occupational therapist or physiotherapist to get help with this decision.

2. Consider a vertical bar to help you safely enter the bath or shower. If family or a lodger will also use the bar, consider a longer bar so that people of different heights can use it comfortably.

3. The DLF website provides guidance on funding for adaptations, but if you are paying for the grab bars yourself, hire someone who has experience with grab bar installation. Make sure the installer uses anchors or attaches the grab bar to studs so that it is secure. Ask someone to pull on the grab bar with full strength to test its holding power at the time of installation.

Modifying Your Home and Surroundings

There are many small changes that can make your home safer. After you read this section, take a walk around your home and see how these tips might apply. Increased awareness can help you manage risks outside your home, such as uneven surfaces, damaged pavements, or streets without curbs.

Rearranging Your Home

Your goal is to have clear pathways in the areas where you frequently walk, such as the area between your bed and the bathroom. Pay special attention to the halls and kitchen and areas where you read or watch TV. Take the steps on the next page to clear the high-traffic areas in your home.

▪ **Rearrange furniture and things you use every day.** Rearrange furniture and remove clutter. A straight and wide path means that you don't need to twist to go through a narrow space. Twisting can increase strain and the risk of falls.

▪ **Remove or organise cables and flex wires.** Cables on the floor are major tripping hazards. Use cable or flex wire covers to hide them. Consider having your computer flex wires positioned on the back of your desk and not the floor. Use wireless options.

▪ **Remove or secure rugs.** Rugs tend to slip, slide, or bunch up and are easy to trip over. The best option is to not use them, but if you want to keep one, secure it with non-slip padding or a rug anchor.

▪ **Rearrange the furniture.** While you clear clutter, you can also place furniture so it can be used as a support. Make sure low coffee tables are not in pathways. They are tripping hazards. Place a sturdy chair with arms in your bedroom to use for dressing and one in the kitchen to use for resting while you're waiting for food to cook or water to boil.

▪ **Reorganise items in your cabinets.** This can prevent repetitive movement in an awkward position. Put the most frequently used items in the front of the cabinet and store them between shoulder and hip height. This keeps you from having to bend over or reach every time you use the items.

▪ **Keep frequently used items in each room or, if you live in a multi-storey house, on each floor.** Keep walking sticks, phones, reading glasses, or other important things in the areas where you often use and need them. It is OK to have more than one. Rushing to find and answer the phone often results in a fall. Placing a phone in every room or keeping a mobile phone in a pocket will prevent you from hurrying to answer a ringing phone. You will also have a phone close at hand for emergencies. Check that mobile phones are charged and landline phones are kept on their chargers.

Changing Your Home Lighting

You need to see where you are walking. If your home is dimly lit, it's more likely that you will trip over something.

▪ **Improve lighting.** Check the lighting in all areas in your home and change the bulbs to brighter ones or add more lighting as needed. Do the same for your home entrances. Do not forget the area where you put your rubbish.

▪ **Install nightlights.** Light is particularly important at night. People often fall when they go to the bathroom. Install nightlights or motion-sensitive lights throughout your home, particularly around the path to the bathroom. Consider purchasing lights that are light sensitive and turn on when it's dark, or ones that are motion sensitive and turn on when they sense movement. You don't have to turn these types of lights off and on. You don't even have to think about them.

Choosing Furniture to Reduce Strain

The type of furniture in your home can increase or reduce the amount of assistance you need.

- **Choose sturdy, firm chairs with arms.** Unstable chairs are likely to cause falls. It is far easier to get up from a kitchen chair with arms than from a recliner or sofa.

- **Use beds and chairs at the right height.** Chairs or beds that are too low can be difficult to get out of without help. Chairs that are too high and don't have backs, such as stools, are not safe. Although a high bed is easier to get out of, it is harder to get into independently. Consider purchasing a bed that is height adjustable if this is an issue for you. If you're having difficulty getting out of a bed or a chair, consult with a rehabilitation professional, such as an occupational or physiotherapist.

Adding Environmental Cues

Cues (or prompts) can be reminders to keep you safe. A cue can help anyone in a busy household where it's easy to lose track of things or become careless.

- **Put brightly coloured non-slip tape on stairs.** Stairs are common fall hazards. You can trip over steps or slip because of weakness, balance issues, vision problems, or carelessness. If you wear slippers at home, the risk of falling increases when you are walking on surfaces and stairs that are slippery (such as wooden floors and staircases). To prevent tripping or missing steps, mark the edge of each step (or the last step only) with non-slip brightly coloured grip tape made especially for stairs. There are also glow-in-the-dark tapes that are useful in dimly lit areas such as stairs to the basement or cellar. This tape serves

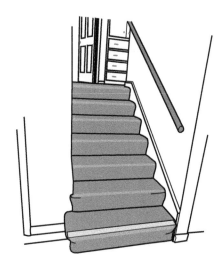

two purposes. It can help you see the stairs better and help prevent your tripping or sliding because it provides traction.

- **Use high-contrasting colours to make it easy to locate items or spaces.** Often, injuries occur at night when using the bathroom. Paint the doors of the bathroom or bedroom with a bright colour. Or use glow-in-the-dark tape to mark the path from the bed to the bathroom. High-contrast colours also help when you're trying to locate items. In a white bathroom, install or use special equipment or bathing items that do not blend in. For example, in the illustration shown here, the bathtub bench is dark, so it stands out in the all-white bathroom environment.

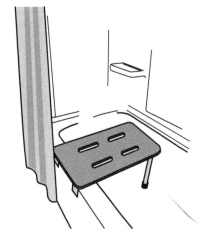

Advocating for Accessibility in Your Neighbourhood or Community

As we mentioned before, fall and injury hazards are not just problems at home. Kerbs, overgrown shrubs, or uneven pavements are common dangerous fall hazards. Being mindful about your surroundings can help you avoid dangerous situations. However, you still may want to make changes so those barriers do not get in your way every time you leave the house. Under the Equality Act 2010 local authorities must take positive steps, or 'reasonable adjustments' to remove the barriers you face because of your disability. For example, they can change the physical feature of pavements and kerbs to make them accessible.

You can ask the local authority to make the necessary changes, or contact your local councillor or Member of Parliament if you need help. If the local authority refuses to make reasonable adjustments, that is unlawful discrimination and you can make a discrimination claim under the Equality Act.

In addition to working with your local authority, you can work with your neighbours to help make the neighbourhood more accessible for all. For example, if you have a neighbour with hedges that extend onto the pavement, ask them kindly to cut or trim them. They are probably unaware of the problem and may be happy to help.

Seeking Guidance from Healthcare Professionals

Self-management is always a good strategy, but you don't have to do everything yourself. Your GP has access to a range of healthcare professionals to support safety and well-being. If you need help, approach your GP with a specific problem. You may even propose some possible solutions. For example, if you have sustained a fall, you might say, 'I've had two falls in the last six months. Do you think I need a walking stick? Can you refer me to someone who can give advice on this?'

Request a medication review to make sure none of your prescribed medications increase your risk of falling. Your GP or a pharmacist can do this. Many pharmacists can also review your medications for fall risk. If you need to adapt your home because of a disability or old age, you can apply to your local council for equipment or

help. A health and social care assessment will be carried out by social services to find out what help and support you need.

If you need rehabilitation services such as occupational therapy, physiotherapy, or speech therapy, ask your GP for a referral. All therapy services begin with an evaluation. The following are services provided by these healthcare professionals:

- **Speech therapy** focuses on helping with talking and understanding and safe eating. Common services offered by speech and language therapists can help you sustain attention, enhance problem solving and understanding, improve speech, and assess swallowing and safe eating practices (to reduce choking risk).

- **Physiotherapy** focuses on restoring normal and safe movement. Common services offered by physiotherapists include instruction in exercise and proper walking; home exercise programmes to increase flexibility, strength, balance, and endurance after you've suffered a fall or injury; transfer training (for example, sitting to standing); selection of mobility aids and training in their proper use; and manual therapy procedures (a form of physical therapy that is used to treat musculoskeletal conditions and associated pain – it involves kneading, muscle manipulation, and joint mobilisation).

- **Occupational therapy** focuses on helping people to regain independence and active participation in everyday activities. Common services offered by an occupational therapist include home safety assessment, transfer training, training and problem solving to improve one's ability to perform daily activities, modifying home and surroundings for convenience and safety, modifying tasks to make them safer and easier, help in selecting and using assistive devices, and guidance to family members and carers.

- **Audiology** focuses on prevention, diagnosis, and treatment of hearing and balance disorders for people of all ages. If you suspect hearing loss or a balance problem, you will likely be referred to an audiologist.

You might be referred to see these healthcare professionals in the community or at a hospital clinic. Many provide home services.

Putting It All Together: Using Your Tools to Reduce Risks

This chapter identified risks that contribute to unintentional accidents and injury and described tools you can use to reduce injury risks. These tools can make it easier for you to participate in activities you enjoy and to stay safe. Although we discussed these tools individually, you can use many of them together to reduce your risk of falls and injury.

What Can You Do to Reduce Injury and Body Pain?

- Exercise regularly.

- Make good posture and good body mechanics a habit in your everyday life.

- Ask healthcare professionals for training and feedback on safe position changes and ways to modify your surroundings and your activities to protect yourself from pain and injury.

- Use practices to reduce rushing and worrying. Pay attention!

What Can You Do to Prevent Falls?

The following are specific ways you can prevent falls. All of these are supported by research.

- Exercise to improve leg strength and balance.

- Have your GP or pharmacist review your medications.

- Have your balance and hearing checked.

- Have regular eye tests and wear glasses according to your current prescription.

- Wear sturdy footwear – do not wear flip-flops or slippers.

- Install and maintain good lighting.

- Remove trip hazards and clutter.

- Install strong railings on all stairs.

- Install and maintain safety equipment and grab bars in the bathroom.

Useful Websites

Age UK: https://www.ageuk.org.uk/information-advice/care/housing-options/adapting-home/

Citizens Advice (Duty to make reasonable adjustments for disabled people): https://www.citizensadvice.org.uk/law-and-courts/discrimination/what-are-the-different-types-of-discrimination/duty-to-make-reasonable-adjustments-for-disabled-people/

Disabled Living Foundation (Choosing and fitting grab rails): https://www.dlf.org.uk/factsheets/grab-rails

Gov.UK (Apply for equipment in your home): https://www.gov.uk/apply-home-equipment-for-disabled

NHS (Falls prevention): https://www.nhs.uk/conditions/falls/prevention/

NHS (Hearing aids): https://www.nhs.uk/live-well/healthy-body/hearing-aids/

NHS (Household mobility aids): https://www.nhs.uk/conditions/social-care-and-support-guide/care-services-equipment-and-care-homes/household-gadgets-and-equipment-to-make-life-easier/

Royal Society for the Prevention of Accidents (RoSPA – Facing up to Falls): https://www.rospa.com/home-safety/Advice/Older-People

Royal Voluntary Service (RVS): https://www.royalvoluntaryservice.org.uk/our-services/advice-and-support/preventing-falls/

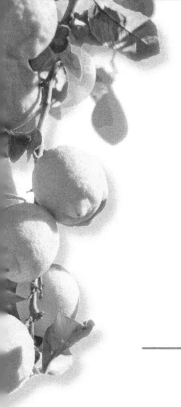

CHAPTER **10**

Healthy Eating

What Is Healthy Eating?

HEALTHY EATING MEANS THAT MOST OF THE TIME you make healthy food and drink choices. It does not mean being rigid or perfect. It can mean finding new or different ways to prepare your meals and snacks. If you have certain long-term health conditions, it may mean that you need to be more mindful about what you eat and how much you eat. Healthy eating seldom means never having your favourite foods. One of the few exceptions to this is where the food may interact with your medication, like eating fresh grapefruit when taking certain

Special thanks to Ann Constance, MA, RDN, CDE, FAADE, Robin Edelman, MS, RDN, CDE, and Yvonne Mullan, MSc, RD, CDE, for contributions to this chapter. For the UK edition, special thanks to Harkesh Verdi, RD (Specialist Weight Management/Renal Dietitian) and Catherine Washbrook-Davies MSc, BSc (Hons), RD (All Wales Dietetic Lead for Diabetes) for contributions to this chapter.

statins. There is more information about these interactions later in this chapter for those with the most common long-term conditions.

In this book we present information about healthy eating, but we do not say there is one best way to apply these guidelines to your life. That is something you decide: 'no one size fits all'. There are different roads to healthy eating, and only you will know the best way to do it for yourself. We offer suggestions that are working for other people and are based on research by nutrition experts. On pages 263–266, you will find information about nutrition for individuals with some of the most common long-term health conditions. (For people with diabetes, this information is in Chapter 14, *Managing Diabetes*.)

Human bodies are complex and marvellous machines. Like a car, you need the proper mix of fuel. Without it, your body might break down, or even stop working. Healthy eating is important to every part of your life. It is linked to how well you move, think, sleep, how much energy you have, and even your enjoyment of life. What you eat may also help with preventing illnesses and healing from illnesses you already have.

When you give your body the right fuel, you:

- have more energy and feel less tired

- increase your chances of preventing health conditions such as heart disease, diabetes, kidney disease, and cancer, and lessen problems linked with health conditions you may already have

- feed your brain, which can help you to better handle life's challenges

- may sleep better

About This Chapter

To write this chapter, we adapted the content of the US 5th edition with guidelines and advice from the NHS and other government-backed websites such as the Food Standards Agency. Information was also gathered from the Association of UK Dietitians, British Heart Foundation, British Lung Foundation, British Nutrition Foundation, Diabetes UK, and other relevant and trusted UK sources, including Action on Salt and Drinkaware. The overall focus is on scientific, evidence-based, nationally established nutrition guidelines.

There are many paths to healthy eating. Some people like a less-detailed, high-level view, and others want to know more details. We have tried to give you a little of both. In many cases we present high-level guidelines before providing more details. You may want to read the chapter from beginning to end, or you may want to look at the topic headings and read only about the topics you find most interesting. If you just want quick tips for healthy eating, read pages 235–238. This information is for you. Use it as you wish.

Guidelines for Healthy Eating

Healthy eating depends on the choices you make. You can be flexible and occasionally enjoy small amounts of foods that may not be so healthy. There is no such thing as a perfect way to eat. Here are some general guidelines about healthy eating:

■ Follow a healthy eating pattern no matter what your age, health conditions, or current weight. Healthy eating is for everyone.

■ Focus on eating a variety of food, especially fruits, vegetables, and whole grains that are rich in vitamins, minerals, and other nutrients.

■ Eat the right amount of food for your weight and health conditions. Refer to the Eatwell Guide handy portion sizes (see page 239) and other guidance developed for people living with long-term conditions. For example, see the British Heart Foundation's *Eat Better* booklet and the British Lung Foundation's web page on eating well for healthier lungs. (See the 'Useful Websites' section at the end of this chapter for more information.)

■ Limit added sugars, saturated fats, trans fats, and salt. Choose healthier fats (see page 243) and salt-free seasonings (herbs and spices).

■ Eat a variety of high-quality protein foods, including fish, eggs, lean meats and poultry, nuts and pulses (dried beans, lentils, and split peas).

■ Quench your thirst with water.

■ If you drink alcohol, the NHS advises men and women not to drink more than 14 units per week on a regular basis. This is equivalent to drinking no more than 6 pints of average-strength beer (4% ABV) or 7 medium-sized glasses of wine (175ml, 12% ABV) or 10 single measures of spirits (35ml, ABV 40%). If you drink regularly, spread your drinking over 3 or more days, and if you are trying to cut down aim for several drink-free days per week. (You can find more information about alcoholic drinks and units, advice, support, and tools to help you manage your relationship with alcohol and improve your health on the drinkaware website, https://www .drinkaware.co.uk/facts).

■ Allow yourself small occasional treats even if they are not the healthiest choices.

■ If you are trying to improve your eating, shift gradually to healthier foods and drinks.

■ Support others by being a model for healthy eating and consider a support group (in person, online, or virtual) to encourage your own healthy eating.

The real issue is not always the healthy foods but the less nutritious foods that people eat in place of healthy foods. You may eat these less healthy foods because they may cost less, are easy to cook, and taste good. The National Diet and Nutrition Survey (NDNS) has shown that the average UK diet is high in sugar, salt, and saturated fat, and lower in fruit and vegetables, oily fish, and fibre. It also estimates that calorie intake exceeds recommended levels for many. In addition to obesity, the average UK diet is a leading factor in many diseases such as heart disease, stroke, type 2 diabetes, and some cancers.

According to the British Nutrition Foundation a good diet is important for our health, but what is a good diet? Apart from breastmilk as a food for babies, no single food contains all the essential nutrients the body needs to stay healthy and work properly. For this reason, your diet should contain a variety of different foods to help you get the wide range of nutrients that your body needs.

The Eatwell Guide was launched in March 2016 and replaced the Eatwell Plate as the UK's healthy eating tool. The guide illustrates the different types of foods and drinks (and the proportions in which they should be consumed), to achieve a healthy balanced diet. Many aspects of the Eatwell Plate remain unchanged, and other elements were adapted following findings from consumer research.

We are not suggesting you change everything you eat overnight. Rather, use this information to gradually make better choices. Read on to learn more about the Eatwell Guide.

The Eatwell Guide

The Eatwell Guide reflects government advice on a healthy balanced diet and applies to most people regardless of weight, dietary restrictions, food preferences, or ethnic origin. However, in some circumstances (for example, people with special dietary requirements or people living with some long-term conditions) you should check with your doctor or a registered dietitian on how to adapt the Eatwell Guide to meet your individual needs.

The Eatwell Guide shows the different types of foods and drinks you should eat (and in what proportions) to have a healthy, balanced diet. The following information has been taken from the *Eatwell Guide* booklet (the booklet can be downloaded from the Internet – see the 'Useful Websites' section at the end of this chapter for more details).

- **Eat at least 5 portions of a variety of fruit and vegetables every day.** Choose from fresh, frozen, canned, dried or juiced. A portion is 80g or any of these: 1 apple, banana, pear, orange, or other similar-size fruit, 3 heaped tablespoons of vegetables, a dessert bowl of salad, 30g of dried fruit (which should be kept to mealtimes) or a 150ml glass of fruit juice or smoothie (counts as a maximum of one portion a day).

- **Base your meals on potatoes, bread, rice, pasta, or other starchy carbohydrates,** choosing wholegrain versions where possible. Starchy food is a really important part of a healthy diet and should make up just over a third of the food we eat. Choose higher-fibre, wholegrain varieties when you can by purchasing wholewheat pasta, brown rice, or simply leaving the skins on potatoes. Wholegrain food contains more fibre than white or refined starchy food, and often more of other nutrients. Some people think starchy food is fattening, but gram for gram it contains less than half the calories of fat.

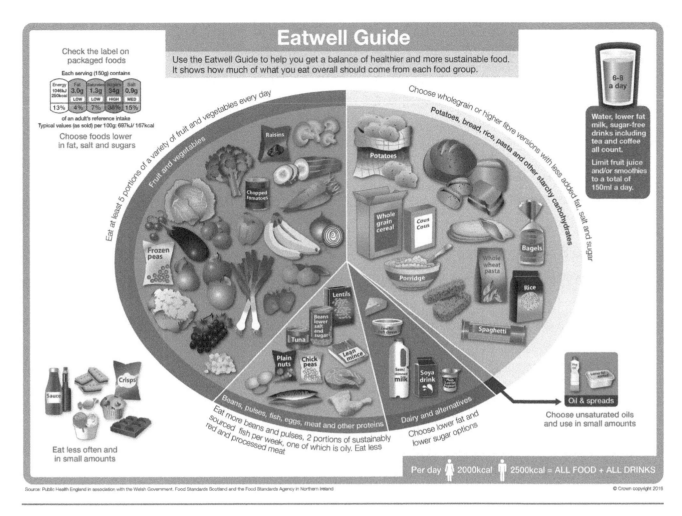

Figure 10.1 **The Eatwell Guide**

■ **Have some dairy or dairy alternatives (such as soya drinks).** Try to have some milk and dairy food (or dairy alternatives) such as cheese, yogurt, and fromage frais. These are good sources of protein and vitamins, and they're also an important source of calcium, which helps to keep your bones strong. Some dairy food can be high in fat and saturated fat, so go for lower fat and lower sugar products where possible.

■ **Eat some beans, pulses, fish, eggs, meat, and other proteins** (including 2 portions of fish every week, one of which should be oily). These foods are sources of protein, vitamins, and minerals, so it is important to eat some foods from this group. Aim for at least two portions (2 × 140g) of fish a week, including a portion of oily fish. Try to cut down on fat by choosing lean cuts of meat and go for leaner mince, cut the fat off meat and the skin off chicken, try to grill meat and fish instead of frying, and have a boiled or poached egg instead of fried. If you eat more than 90g of red or processed meat per day, try to cut down to no more than 70g per day. The term *processed meat* includes sausages, bacon, cured meats, and reformed meat products.

■ **Choose unsaturated oils and spreads and eat them in small amounts.** Unsaturated fats are healthier fats that are usually from plant sources and in liquid form as oil – for example, vegetable oil, rapeseed oil, and olive oil. Swapping to unsaturated fats will help you reduce cholesterol in the blood, so it is important to get most of our fat from unsaturated oils.

■ **Drink 6 to 8 cups or glasses of fluid a day.** Water, lower fat milk, and sugar-free drinks including tea and coffee all count. Fruit juice and smoothies also count toward your fluid consumption, although they are a source of added sugars and so you should limit consumption to no more than a combined total of 150ml per day.

■ **If you do have food and drink high in fat, salt, or sugar, have these less often and in small amounts.** This includes products such as chocolate, cakes, biscuits, full-sugar soft drinks, butter, and ice cream. These foods are not needed in the diet and so, if you include them, eat them only infrequently and in small amounts.

8 Tips for Eating Well	
1	Base your meals on starchy foods.
2	Eat lots of fruit and veg.
3	Eat more fish, including a portion of oily fish each week.
4	Cut down on saturated fat and sugar.
5	Eat no more than 6g (about 1 teaspoon) of salt a day.
6	Get active and be at a healthy weight.
7	Don't get thirsty.
8	Don't skip breakfast.

Knowing What and How Much to Eat

Eating well means knowing something about what you eat. It also means being mindful about how much you eat.

Control Your Portions

Many people make good food choices in terms of nutrients but eat too much or too little food than they need to maintain a healthy weight. To understand healthy eating and to use the food labels on packages and the charts in this book, you also need to know about portions and servings.

The amount of food you **serve** yourself is how much you actually eat. If you eat a small bowl of ice cream, that is your serving. However, if you eat half a large tub of ice cream, that is also your serving (and a likely cause of weight gain, as it contains many more calories than the recommended portion).

Understanding what a recommended portion size is for each food group in the Eatwell Guide can help you to achieve a well-balanced diet (see pages 236–238).

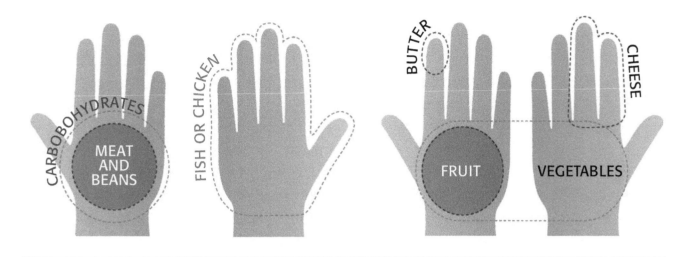

Figure 10.2 **How to Get Portion Sizes Right**

You need to be aware that sometimes the terms *portion* and *serving* are used the other way around, especially in information originating from the United States and on food labels. This can be very confusing! Fortunately, there are some very useful resources available to help you understand and measure portion sizes. For example, the British Heart Foundation website has an interactive portion guide that shows you photos of what single portions of different types of food actually look like. They have also produced a useful booklet of recommended portion sizes called *Taking Control of Food Portions and Labels* which contains a universal visual guide to recommended portion sizes for each of the food groups contained in the Eatwell Guide, see Figure 10.2.

You can find a link to the British Heart Foundation website and downloadable booklet in the 'Useful Websites' section at the of this chapter.

The Importance of Food Labels

Knowing what you are eating means knowing what nutrients are in foods. On pages 242–251, you can find a discussion of specific nutrients. There are several ways to find out what nutrients you are eating:

■ You can read the food labels on food packaging. This is the approach we discuss in this section of the chapter. Food labels can help you to choose between foods and to pick those that are lower in carbohydrates, fat, saturated fat, sugar, and salt. Where colour-coded labels are used you can tell at a glance if foods are high, medium, or low in fat, saturated fat, sugars, and salt.

■ You can follow the Eatwell Guide (see pages 236–238).

■ You can also use the plate method for healthy eating, as explained on page 251.

A Word About Food Labels and Brexit

The UK left the European Union (EU) on 31 January 2020. Following this, the UK entered a transition period during which it remained in both the EU customs union and single market, meaning that most things stayed the same. At the time of writing this book (summer 2020), the UK is still in this transition period, which is due to end on 31 December 2020. Food and drink producers, manufacturers, retailers, and suppliers must change labels from 1 January 2021.

The government has promised to uphold food standards, but some commentators are concerned that the UK's world-leading food standards could be compromised under future trade deals.

The Food Standards Agency (FSA) is an independent government department working across England, Wales, and Northern Ireland to protect public health and consumers' wider interests in food. We suggest you check the FSA website, https://www.food.gov.uk/, after 1 January 2021 to find the most up-to-date food labelling requirements.

Feel free to use one or more of these ways and mix and match as you choose. There are many different ways to help you make healthy food choices.

In the UK all prepacked food requires a food label that displays certain mandatory information. All foods are subject to general food labelling requirements and any labelling provided must be accurate and not misleading. Labels such as the one shown in Figure 10.3, along with the ingredients list, can help you learn more about what is in the packaged foods you eat. These labels are usually shown on the back or side of the pack.

The Association of UK Dietitians (BDA) has produced a useful food fact sheet that explains what information you can expect to find on any prepacked food you buy (see the 'Useful Websites' section at the end of this chapter for more information). A nutrition declaration is required on all packaging larger than 10cm (with specific exemptions for some foods) and must include details of nutrients per 100g,

nutrients per portion/serving, and the number of portions/servings per pack. Nutritional information will appear on the food label as shown in Figure 10.3, alongside other information, including the name of the food, the weight of the food, ingredients listed in order of the quantity used, and nutrition information. The nutritional information on the label can also be repeated to appear on the front of pack, as shown in Figure 10.4.

To help you make a quick decision, this label is based upon our traditional traffic lights, and it shows at a glance whether a product is high, medium, or low for fat, saturates, sugars, and salt. The numbers on the label show you how many calories and how much fat, saturates, sugars, and salt per portion/serving of the food or drink it contains, both in the number of grams (g) and as a share (%) of your daily allowance (RI).

The British Nutrition Foundation has produced a quick guide to understanding nutrition information on food labels to help you make

Chicken & Vegetable Broth

A soup made with vegetables, cooked chicken and pearl barley.

600g ℮

Ingredients

Water, Carrot (10%), Onion, Chicken (6%), Potato (5%), Spinach (2%), Peas (2%), Cabbage (2%), **Celery** (2%), Chicken stock (chicken skin, water, chicken extract, chicken, sugar, salt, cornflour, chicken fat, onion concentrate), Potato starch, Pearl **barley**, Rapeseed oil, Garlic purée, Salt, Black pepper.

! ALLERGY ADVICE

For allergens, including cereals containing gluten, see ingredients in bold.

! Warning

Although every care has been taken to remove bones, some may remain.

Nutrition

Typical values (as consumed)	per 100g	per 1/2 pot (300g)	%RI	your RI*
Energy	167kJ	501kJ		8400kJ
	40 kcal	119kcal	**6%**	2000kcal
Fat	1.2g	3.6g	**5%**	70g
of which saturates	0.2g	0.6g	**3%**	20g
Carbohydrates	4.2g	12.6g		
of which sugars	1.2g	3.6g	**4%**	90g
Fibre	1.1g	3.3g		
Protein	2.5g	7.5g		
Salt	0.5g	1.5g	**25%**	6g

*Reference intake of an average adult (8400kJ/2000kcal) (RI) Contains 2 portions.

Figure 10.3 **UK Back-of-Pack Nutrition Food Label**

Source: The Association of UK Dietitians – https://www.bda.uk.com/resource/food-labelling-nutrition-information.html.

healthy choices next time you're shopping. This guide can be downloaded at

> https://www.nutrition.org.uk/healthyliving /resources/foodlabelling.html

or visit their website (see the 'Useful Websites' section at the end of this chapter).

Portions per container and portion size

You will see that in Figure 10.4 the portion/ serving information is at the very top of the label. All the other information on the label is based on portion size. Remember that the manufacturer's suggested portion/serving size may be more or less than what you usually eat, and so you must compare the suggested portion/ serving size to what you are actually eating. If you eat 250g of cooked rice and the portion size is 125g, this is neither good nor bad. However, it does mean that when you estimate the calories, fats, salt, and carbohydrates in your portion, you must consider that you have eaten twice the quantities as are shown on the label.

Calories

Calories are a measure of energy. Your body weight is largely determined by the number of

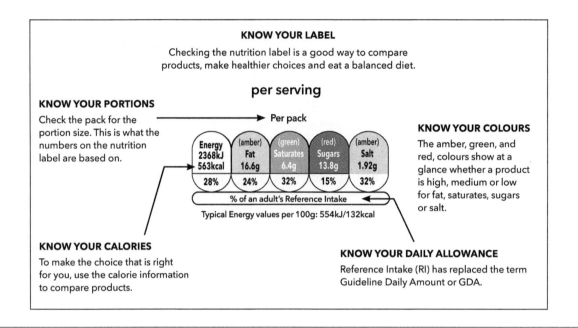

Figure 10.4 **UK Front-of-Pack Food Label**

Source: The Association of UK Dietitians – https://www.bda.uk.com/resource/food-labelling-nutrition-information.html

calories you eat and the number of calories you burn. When a person eats too many calories, the extra energy is stored as fat and the result is being overweight. The number of calories you need per day depends on your age, gender, muscle mass, weight, and height, as well as your physical activity level. On average, to maintain a constant weight, women require 2,000 calories a day and men around 2,500 calories a day. However, that also depends on how active each person is. The calories you need for your body weight goals may be different from those for a person who needs to maintain a constant weight. If you are very active you may need more calories, or if you are very inactive you may need fewer. For example, smaller, older women may need fewer calories, while larger, younger men need more.

Reference intake (%)

The Reference Intake (RI) has replaced the Recommended Daily Amount (RDA). Reference intakes are included in nutrition labels on packaged food and provide useful guidelines on the daily amount of energy and nutrients you need for a healthy balanced diet. The %RI tells you how much of your daily healthy maximum is included in a portion/serving of the product, based on an average female adult. Reference intakes are not individual recommendations, and your needs may well be different from the RI, depending on your age, sex, how physically active you are, and if you have a long-term health condition such as diabetes. They are there to give you a rough idea of how much energy you should be eating each day, and how much fat, sugar, salt, and so on.

NHS guidance on the daily RI for an adult is as follows:

- Energy: 8,400kJ/2,000kcal
- Total fat: less than 70g
- Saturates: less than 20g
- Carbohydrate: at least 260g
- Total sugars: 90g

■ Protein: 50g

■ Salt: less than 6g

Total fat

Fat has a lot of calories, and it's important to check whether the fat is saturated or unsaturated. Unsaturated fats, found in foods such as avocado, nuts, seeds, oily fish, and vegetable oils, are better for your heart health than saturated fats, which are found in foods such as butter, fatty meats, and pastry. Too much saturated fat can increase our cholesterol, which increases risk of coronary heart disease. Saturated fat should be listed on the food label, as well as the total fat. Check the food label information per 100g to see whether the fat content is high, medium, or low (high will be 17.5g or more and low will be 3g or less).

The total fat number listed on the food label includes the healthier fats (polyunsaturated and monounsaturated) and the less healthy fats (saturated and trans). Note that trans fats used to be found in snack food, but the manufacturing industry has removed them from products over time due to their harmful nature and therefore they are no longer included in UK food labels. Some of us think that all fat is bad for us. This is not true. For our bodies to work well we need some fat – about a tablespoon (15 ml) per day. Although all fats have the same number of calories, some fats are healthier than others. In this book we call the healthy fats 'good' and the less healthy fats – which can be harmful – 'bad'. We do this to encourage you to eat healthier fats.

Good fats include oils that are usually liquid at room temperature. These fats help keep our cells healthy, and some of these fats can help reduce blood cholesterol. Good fats include olive, rapeseed, soybean, sesame, corn, peanut, and sunflower oils. Foods rich in good fats include nuts, seeds, and olives (and their oils), as well as avocados.

Another group of good fats – the omega-3s – can be helpful for some people in reducing the risk of heart disease and may help with rheumatoid arthritis symptoms. Omega-3s are found in fatty deep-water fish such as salmon, mackerel, trout, sardines, and pilchards. Other sources of omega-3s include some oils (rapeseed and soybean), chia seeds, flaxseed, and walnuts, although the body may not use omega-3s from plants as well as it uses the omega-3s from fish.

Bad fats (also called saturated fats and trans fats) are usually solid at room temperature. Think about butter, lard, and bacon grease. Bad fats can increase blood cholesterol and the risk of heart disease. Most bad fats are found in animal foods such as butter, beef fat (suet), chicken fat, and pork fat (lard).

Other foods high in bad fats include margarines, red meat, mince, processed meats (sausage, bacon, and luncheon meats), poultry skin, and whole and low-fat milk and cheeses, including cream cheese and sour cream. Palm kernel oil, coconut oil, and cocoa butter are also considered bad fats because they are high in saturated fat.

The worst fats are trans fats. Trans fats are not included in food labels in the UK. Trans fatty acids occur naturally in small amounts in foods produced from ruminant animals (for example, milk, beef, and lamb). However, most of the trans fatty acids are produced during the process of partial hydrogenation (hardening)

Tips for Choosing Good or Healthier Fats

When Choosing Foods

- Eat cooked portions of meat, fish, and poultry that are about the size of a deck of cards or the palm of your hand.

- Do not eat the skin on poultry. It has lots of saturated fat.

- Eat more oily fish, such as salmon, sardines, and mackerel.

- Choose leaner cuts of meat (such as lean minced beef, sirloin, or flank cuts).

- Trim all the fat you can see from meat before cooking.

- Choose low-fat milk and dairy foods (cheese, sour cream, cottage cheese, yogurt, and ice cream).

When Preparing Foods

- Use a non-stick pan or a pan with small amounts of sprayed cooking oil or broth.

- Boil, grill, microwave, poach, bake, or steam when preparing meat or fish.

- Avoid frying or deep-frying foods.

- Skim the fat from stews and soups during cooking. (If you refrigerate them overnight, the solid fat lifts off easily.)

- Use less butter, gravies, meat-based and cream sauces, spreads, and creamy pasta sauces and salad dressings.

- In cooking and baking, use oil (such as olive or rapeseed oil) and soft (tub) margarines instead of lard, butter, or margarine.

- Measure the oil in tablespoons rather than pouring from the container.

- Reduce or cut out spreads like margarine when eating things like beans on toast.

---

of vegetable oils into semi-solid fats. They are therefore found in hard margarines, partially hydrogenated oils, in some bakery products, fried foods, and other processed foods that are made using these. A clue to the presence of trans fat in a food is if 'partially hydrogenated oils' is in that food's ingredients list. Trans fats raise blood cholesterol and the risk of heart disease more than other bad fats. The best advice is to eat as few trans fats as possible. The British Nutrition Foundation has produced a fact sheet about trans fats that can be downloaded from its website (see the 'Useful Websites' section at the end of this chapter).

The daily guidelines recommended by the NHS suggest that the average man should eat no more than 30g of saturated fat a day and that the average woman no more than 20g, and within this, trans fats should be no more than 5g a day.

Cholesterol

Cholesterol is an important part of all our cells. Your body makes cholesterol, and you also get cholesterol from food. Too much cholesterol is a problem because it can clog the blood vessels and cause heart attacks and strokes. Most of the cholesterol that is in your blood comes from the cholesterol your body makes.

Salt and sodium

The Association of UK Dietitians (BDA) has produced a useful salt fact sheet on its website (see the 'Useful Websites' section at the end of this chapter). Salt is the everyday term we use for a chemical compound called sodium chloride; salt is made from two elements, sodium and chloride, which give salt this chemical name. Although no longer required, manufacturers may sometimes still quote sodium content on their labels. When thinking about your salt intake, it's important to know that each 1g of sodium translates to 2.5g of salt, and to take this into account when estimating how much salt you have day to day. Adults should eat no more than 6g of salt (2.4g of sodium) per day, which is about 1 teaspoon. Don't confuse salt and sodium figures. A diet high in salt can cause raised blood pressure, which can increase your risk of heart disease and stroke. Cutting back on salt can help lower blood pressure.

People get salt from most foods we eat – from tiny amounts in some plant foods to higher amounts in some animal foods. You do not have to worry about salt in foods that you eat in their natural, unprocessed form. The foods that contain high amounts of salt are processed foods, which often have different forms of salt added to them in large amounts.

A love of salt comes from eating salty foods. If you eat food with less salt your tastes adjust, and you can learn to like food with less salt. Cutting down takes some getting used to, but over time you will learn to enjoy the natural flavours of food. Here are some tips to help you reduce your salt intake:

- **Avoid using salt substitutes.** Low salt substitutes can be dangerous if you have long-term conditions such as heart disease, kidney disease, and diabetes, as they contain potassium, which in high levels can be harmful to your heart. Using salt substitutes can also raise potassium to risky levels, so always check with your doctor or dietitian.

- **Always taste your food before salting it.** It may taste good without adding more salt.

- **Cut down on the salt in recipes when cooking.** Try adding one half of the recipe's amount. Season with spices, herbs, pepper, garlic, onion, or lemon.

- **Use minimally processed fresh or frozen poultry, fish, and lean meat instead of tinned, breaded, or prepared packaged food.**

- **Choose foods labelled 'low' or 'reduced' salt.** Choose green labels with 0.3g or less of salt per 100g or occasionally amber labels with less than 1.5g of salt per 100g. Avoid red labels with over 1.5g of salt per 100g.

- **Save high-salt food for special occasions.** Eat tinned soups, gravy granules, bacon, luncheon meats, salted snacks (like crisps, nuts, and pretzels), and pepperoni or sausage pizza as part of celebrations or as 'once in a while' foods, not every day.

- **In restaurants, think about the choices you are making from the menu and ask for no added salt to your meal.** Sauces, rice, pasta or potato dishes, stuffing, or foods containing ham, sausage, or bacon are often high in salt. Salad dressings can be high in

How do I know if a food is high in fat, saturated fat, sugar, or salt?

	High	Low
Total fat	More than 17.5g of fat per 100g	3g of fat or less per 100g
Saturated fat	More than 5g of saturated fat per 100g	1.5g of saturated fat or less per 100g
Sugars	More than 22.5g of total sugars per 100g	5g of total sugars or less per 100g
Salt	More than 1.5g of salt per 100g (or 0.6g sodium)	0.3g of salt or less per 100g (or 0.1g sodium)

salt as well. In addition, most soups at restaurants are high in salt.

Total carbohydrates

Carbohydrates are the body's main source of fuel. Your body breaks carbohydrates down (except for fibre) into glucose. Glucose provides energy for your brain and the rest of your body. Carbohydrates – more than protein or fat – largely determine your blood glucose level.

There are two types of carbohydrates: sugars and starches. Carbohydrates are found in plant foods such as grains, fruits, and vegetables. Milk and yogurt also have carbohydrates.

Sugars occur naturally in foods, such as fruits (fructose) and milk/yogurt (lactose). Other foods, such as the ones we buy in boxes, tins, or other packages (for example, fizzy drinks, sweets, and crackers) often have added sugar. The added sugar adds extra carbohydrate and calories, and it is common for healthy nutrients to be missing from these products.

Vegetables such as sweetcorn, green peas, potatoes, winter squash, dried beans, and peas contain starchy carbohydrates. Lentils and other pulses and grains such as rice and wheat also have starchy carbohydrates. This is why rice, pasta, bread, tortillas, and baked goods are high in carbohydrates. In the UK, carbohydrates are typically divided into two categories, simple/free sugars (jam, sweets, fruit juice) and complex/starchy carbohydrates (bread, rice, potato). Some complex/starchy carbohydrates can be highly refined or processed, for example, white bread, whereas others are less refined, typically the wholegrains, for example, wholegrain bread.

Some grain-based foods are more processed (refined) than others. Processing does not change the amount of carbohydrates. However, processing does remove healthy nutrients (phytochemicals) and fibre. It is better to eat foods made from whole grain varieties rather than other processed grains because they are more nutritious. Your body changes some carbohydrates to glucose more quickly than others. The carbohydrates in most high-fibre foods get converted into glucose more slowly than the carbohydrates in low-fibre foods.

If you have diabetes, your body has trouble using all the carbohydrates you eat, and higher levels of glucose build up in the blood. If left untreated, this causes many problems. You can find more about this topic in Chapter 14, *Managing Diabetes*.

Dietary fibre

Fibre is a carbohydrate that is not absorbed by the body. Fibre is found naturally in whole and minimally processed plant foods with skins, seeds, and strings (like those found in celery and string beans). Whole grains, dried beans, peas, lentils, fruits, vegetables, nuts, and seeds all have fibre. Some foods have added fibre (for example, when pulp is added to juice). Animal and refined foods (white flour, bread, many baked and snack foods) have little or no fibre unless the manufacturer adds fibre to the product.

Even though it is not absorbed, fibre helps your body. Wheat bran, some fruits and vegetables, and whole grains act as 'nature's broom'. They keep your digestive system moving and help prevent constipation. The fibre in oat bran, barley, nuts, seeds, beans, all fruits, carrots, and psyllium seed can help manage your blood glucose. This form of fibre, called 'soluble fibre', slows the amount of time it takes for sugar to get into the bloodstream. These foods can help lower blood cholesterol. High-fibre diets may also help reduce the risk of rectal and colon cancers. Government guidelines published in July

Tips for Choosing Healthier Carbohydrates and Increasing Fibre

- Fill at least half of your plate with different kinds of vegetables and whole fruit.

- At least half of the grains you eat should be whole grains (brown rice, whole-grain breads and rolls, whole-grain pasta, and whole grain cereals and oats).

- Choose foods that list whole wheat or a whole grain (such as oats) first on the ingredients list.

- Choose dried beans, split peas, and lentils instead of meat or as a side dish at least a few times a week. Add tinned or cooked dried beans to your vegetable salads and pasta dishes.

- Leave the skin on potatoes.

- Choose whole fruit rather than fruit juice. Whole fruit contains fibre, takes longer to eat, fills you up better than juice, and may help keep you from overeating.

- Aim to eat 5 portions of fruit and vegetables every day.

- Choose wholegrain breakfast cereals (such as shredded wheat, wheat biscuits, or whole porridge oats) and add fruit to your cereal.

- Eat higher-fibre crackers such as whole-rye or multigrain crackers and whole-grain flatbread.

- Snack on whole fruit, raw vegetables, and whole-grain crackers or breads rather than crisps, sweets, or ice cream.

- When you add higher-fibre foods to your diet, do it gradually over a period of a few weeks to allow your gut time to adjust.

- Drink plenty of fluids, the guidelines recommend 6 to 8 glasses per day.

2015 say that our dietary fibre intake should increase to 30g a day, as part of a healthy balanced diet.

Sugar: naturally occurring and added sugar

The sugar information on the food label lists the amount of sugar in one portion/serving of the food. Many foods, such as fruit, have natural sugar. But in many other cases, such as fizzy drinks, sugar is added.

Are natural sugars and added sugars different? No, your body uses natural sugars and added sugars in the same way. They both have the same number of calories for the same weight (grams, ounces, etc.). However processed foods tend to have more added sugars, and added sugars give us extra calories. If you are trying to lose weight or lower your blood glucose, eat as little added sugar as possible. A 330ml can of cola has nearly 40g (almost 8 teaspoons) of added sugar and no beneficial nutrients. Compare this to 150ml of orange juice with no added sugar. The juice has 33g of natural sugar (carbohydrate), but also lots of vitamins and phytochemicals (plant chemicals that have protective or disease preventive properties). For a nutritional perspective, it is clear that the juice is a better choice than the cola. An even better choice is a fresh medium orange. An orange only has approximately 12g of carbohydrate in the form of natural sugar (fructose), and it provides healthy nutrients and fibre. To quench your thirst, choose water, coffee, and tea. These drinks have no added sugar and no carbohydrates (unless you add sugar and milk). A sugar – whether it is natural or added – is a sugar, but foods with natural sugar usually have other healthy ingredients.

Protein

Protein is part of every cell in your body and helps control the way your body works. Protein helps your immune system fight infection and builds and repairs damaged tissues, including muscles and bones. Protein also provides a feeling of comfortable fullness after you eat. It satisfies your appetite and prevents you from getting hungry again too soon after you have eaten. Most people eat more than enough protein. Currently, many people get most of their protein from meat, which tends to be high in bad (saturated) fats. Getting your protein mainly from plant foods along with small amounts of lean meat, poultry, or fish, or eating a variety of plant-based foods, is better for your health.

There are two types of proteins: complete and incomplete. Complete proteins are found in food that contains all 9 essential amino acids in adequate proportions that are needed in your diet.

Your body uses complete proteins just as they are. Complete proteins are found in fish and animal foods – meat, poultry, eggs, milk, and other dairy products – as well as in foods made from soya beans, such as tofu.

Incomplete proteins are low in one or more parts of a complete protein. They are found in plant foods such as grains, dried beans and peas, lentils, nuts, and seeds. Nearly all plant proteins are incomplete proteins. (Most fruits and non-starchy vegetables have little, if any, protein.) That is why it is important for people who are vegetarian or vegan to get a variety of plant-based proteins in their diet over the course of the day to ensure they are more likely to get all of the 9 essential amino acids.

Even though plant proteins are incomplete, they are at the heart of healthy eating. In fact, plant-based diets are becoming more popular, and if they are well planned they can support healthy living at every age and life-stage. The Association of UK Dietitians has produced a fact sheet for anyone considering a meat-free lifestyle (see the 'Useful Websites' section at the end of this chapter).

In addition to containing protein, some plant foods, such as nuts and seeds, are sources of the good fats. Many plant foods are also sources of fibre and phytochemicals. Plant foods have no cholesterol and little to no bad fat. For these reasons, plant foods are often the best choice for healthy eating.

Vitamins and minerals: vitamin D, calcium, iron, and potassium

Vitamins and minerals help keep your body functioning properly and are needed for survival and health. Most people can get all the vitamins and minerals they need from eating healthy foods. Vitamins and minerals must be declared on food labels as % reference intake (%RI) per 100g and only if they are present in significant amounts.

More Is Not Better

When it comes to vitamins and minerals, some people think that if a little is good, then more is better. This is not true. Too much of a good thing can cause harm. This is because everything in your body must be in balance, and too much of anything throws off the balance. (Think of baking. If you put too much of almost any ingredient into biscuits, cakes, or pies, they do not come out right.)

Potassium

The mineral potassium helps regulate our heartbeat and can lower blood pressure. If you follow the Eatwell Guide (see page 237) and eat a balanced diet you will have no problem meeting your potassium requirements.

Many kinds of vegetables and fruits are good potassium sources. These include broccoli, peas, dried beans (such as white, adzuki, and pinto), tomatoes, potatoes, sweet potatoes, avocados, winter squash (such as acorn or butternut), citrus fruits, plantains, bananas, prunes, apricots, and nuts. Some fish (such as salmon, tuna, mackerel, and halibut), milk, and yogurt are also good sources of potassium.

Calcium

Calcium helps build bones, but did you know that it is also needed for blood clotting and helps with blood pressure? It may also protect against colon cancer, kidney stones, and breast cancer.

Unfortunately, some people, especially older women and young children, may not get enough calcium in their diets. You are also more at risk of calcium deficiency if you are on a cow's milk–free or lactose-free diet, have coeliac disease, osteoporosis, are breastfeeding, or are past the menopause. Adults aged 19 to 64 need 700mg of calcium a day. The main sources of calcium in the UK diet are from yogurt, cheese, and milk. Other good sources of calcium are kefir (a fermented beverage that's similar to yogurt); calcium-fortified soy, rice, and almond milks; orange juice; calcium-fortified cereal and breads; and tinned salmon and sardines with bones. Brussels sprouts, kohlrabi, and leafy greens (such as pak choi, kale, greens,

A Word About Vitamin D

We all need some vitamin D to keep our bones healthy. Our bodies cannot use calcium without vitamin D. Beyond this, there is a lot of controversy about how helpful vitamin D is and its role in preventing heart disease and cancer. More recently there have been some news reports about vitamin D reducing the risk of coronavirus (COVID-19). Public Health England advises that adults and children over the age of 1 should consider taking a daily supplement containing 10mcg of vitamin D, particularly during autumn and winter. People who have a higher risk of vitamin D deficiency are being advised to take a supplement all year round. If you do not get much sunlight or you are dark skinned or overweight, you may need a vitamin D supplement. This is especially true if you have a family history of osteoporosis. (Learn more about osteoporosis and healthy eating on pages 265–266.) Some people will have medical conditions that mean they may not be able to safely take as much. If you are not already taking a supplement recommended by your doctor, talk with your GP or a registered dietitian.

beet greens, turnip greens, and spinach) have calcium, but our bodies cannot use some of it. Most fruits are low in calcium. The exceptions are dried figs, although there's not much in fig rolls!

Another reason to eat less salt is because salt can cause your body to lose calcium. If you do not get enough calcium from what you eat and drink, talk to your doctor about calcium supplements (pills).

Iron

Iron is a mineral that helps your body use oxygen. If you do not have enough iron in your diet, you can feel tired, weak, dizzy, and generally unwell. Iron is found in both plant and animal foods. In the UK, white and brown flour is fortified with iron and other vitamins and minerals by law. Other foods like some breakfast cereals are fortified on a voluntary basis. Although iron in animal foods is easier for our bodies to use, our ability to absorb the iron in plant foods is increased when iron-rich plant foods are combined with fruit and vegetable sources of vitamin C, such as citrus fruits.

Water

Water, which makes up more than half of our bodies, is the most important nutrient. Water fills the spaces in and between body cells. All the natural chemical reactions in our bodies require water. Water keeps our kidneys working, helps prevent constipation, and helps us eat less by making us feel full. It also helps prevent medication side effects.

Most adults lose about 10 cups of water a day through urine, sweat, and breathing. However, people usually have no problem getting enough water. The exact amount you need differs depending on the weather, your activity, and your weight. To see if you are drinking enough water, check the colour of your urine. If it is light coloured, you are fine. If it is darker, you probably need more water. When you start to get thirsty, you need more water. Milk, juice, and many fruits and vegetables are good sources of water. Coffee, tea, squashes, and fizzy drinks are also good sources of water. Alcohol is not a good source of water. Do not depend on alcohol to meet your need for water.

If you have kidney disease, congestive heart failure, or are taking special medications, you may be on a fluid restriction and need to drink less water. Talk to a registered dietitian or your doctor if this is the case.

The Ingredients List

An ingredients list is usually found on food labels alongside the nutrition food label (see page 241), but it may be elsewhere on food packaging. The ingredients are listed in the order of quantity used. The last ingredients listed are those that make up the smallest part of the food. The ingredients list uses the common names of the ingredients. Ingredients give you more detailed information about what you are eating. They are especially important if you are trying to avoid certain items, such as soya or gluten.

Another Way to Make Food Choices: The Plate Method

Food labels and ingredient lists inform you about what and how much you are eating and how this compares to a healthy diet. (To learn more about daily recommended intake (RI), see pages 242–243.) However, not all foods have labels, and sometimes we need something easier to help us eat healthier. The plate method developed by the US Department of Agriculture (USDA) is a technique for dividing up your plate to enable you to measure out appropriate portion sizes of different

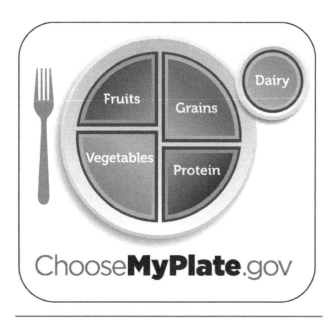

Figure 10.5 **MyPlate: A Map for Healthy Eating from the USDA**.

foods, as shown in Figure 10.5. The plate method can be used to aid weight management and can also be helpful for people with diabetes in managing carbohydrate intake. The plate method is simple to apply and is therefore an easy way to manage your energy intake and ensure a healthy balance of nutrients in your diet.

For the plate method to work well, it helps to begin with a suitably sized plate. Many dinner plates in the UK are up to 12 inches in diameter. Replacing a larger plate with one that has a 10-inch diameter can you help to reduce your meal size.

Put your meal together so that one half of the plate is covered with vegetables and fruit, one quarter with protein (lean meat, fish, or poultry, or better yet, plant foods such as tofu, cooked dry beans, or lentils), and the remaining quarter with grains (preferably at least half from whole grains) or other starches such as potatoes, rice, yams, or winter squash. Finish off your meal with calcium-rich foods. These

On the Internet, there are many people who say they are nutrition experts who may not be. A dietitian is a qualified health professional, who as well as providing general health advice, can also work with people with special dietary needs due to health conditions such as coeliac disease. A nutritionist should be able to provide information about food and healthy eating, but not about special diets for medical conditions. The title 'dietitian' is protected by law. This means that you're not allowed to call yourself a dietitian unless you're properly qualified and registered. The title of nutritionist is not protected by law, meaning that anyone can advertise their services as a nutritionist. So, it's important to find a nutritionist who is appropriately qualified and registered by a trustworthy professional body. As a starting point, contact your GP surgery to find out about a referral to a dietitian in your area and check out the NHS website for more information about the differences between dietitians and nutritionists (see the 'Useful Websites' section at the end of this chapter).

Nutrients: What Does the Body Need?

You now know a lot about healthy eating but may not know how to put it all together. For most people, eating a healthy, balanced diet based on the Eatwell Guide should provide all the nutrients needed to stay healthy. Having a balanced diet is about getting the right types of foods and drinks in the right amounts. The British Nutrition Foundation (BNF) has developed an easy guide to balancing food groups and finding the portion sizes that are right for you. This guide aims to give you an idea of the portion sizes of different foods and drinks and how often to eat foods from different food groups. This guide, called *Find Your Balance – Get Portion Wise!*, can be downloaded from the BNF website,

https://www.nutrition.org.uk/attachments /article/1193/Find%20your%20 balance_%20booklet.pdf.

could be milk or foods made from milk (preferably fat-free or low-fat), such as cheese, yogurt, frozen yogurt, puddings, or calcium-fortified foods such as soya milk. Of course, your food choices and amounts should depend on what you like and need. A small amount of 'good' fat (see pages 243–244) is healthy at each meal. This may come from oil you use while cooking the food, dressing a salad, or seasoning food to add flavour. It could also come from nuts mixed in with a grain, such as brown rice. Read more about suggestions for choosing healthy fats and seasonings on page 244.

Even with the plate method, the amounts of food you eat (your serving size) are important. The Eatwell Guide (see page 237) shows how much of what we eat overall should come from each food group to achieve a healthy, balanced diet. You can also find more information about recommended portion sizes on the Association of UK Dietitians and the British Nutrition Foundation websites (see the 'Useful Websites' section at the end of this chapter). Of course, every person is different and your needs may vary because of your long-term condition, so always check with your GP or dietitian.

Eating for Specific Long-Term Conditions

In the following sections of the chapter, we discuss several long-term conditions and eating considerations related to them. These are general overviews. If you have any of these conditions, it is important to talk to your healthcare professional or a registered dietitian about how to eat healthily.

Overweight and Healthy Eating

Being overweight is a long-term condition for many people. And being overweight makes most long-term health conditions worse. The good news is that you can improve your health by losing even a small amount of weight. Body weight is important for many reasons. Too much weight puts stress on the joints and is linked to arthritis. When you are overweight, the heart works harder and that can lead to high blood pressure, heart disease, and stroke. People with diabetes can have problems keeping blood glucose within target range. Raised blood glucose levels can lead to complications such as heart and nerve problems (see 'Preventing Diabetes Complications' in Chapter 14, *Managing Diabetes*). If you have prediabetes, losing 5% of your body weight can significantly reduce your risk of developing type 2 diabetes.

Losing 5% of your current weight prevents or delays many health problems. A 5% weight loss, for a 11-stone (70kg) person, is losing 7.5 pounds (3.5kg). We are aware that losing weight and maintaining a weight loss of any amount is difficult. Studies show that people who lose weight and maintain their new weight usually have ongoing support. Besides having ongoing support from family, friends, healthcare professionals, or a group, people who lose weight and maintain the loss stick with healthier ways to eat and get regular physical activity.

What Is a Healthy Weight?

There is no such thing as an 'ideal' weight. A healthy weight is a range of pounds. Pinpointing your healthy weight range and deciding whether you want or need to change your weight depends on your age, activity level, your health, how much and where your body fat is located, and your family history of weight-related health problems, such as high blood pressure and diabetes.

One way to understand a healthy weight is to calculate your Body Mass Index (BMI). BMI includes both height and weight in a single number. Although not a perfect measure, BMI is a useful general guide. To get a sense of a healthy weight range take a look at the chart in Table 10.1. Find your height and follow that line to the number nearest to your current weight. The point at which they both meet will tell you what range or group you are in: Underweight, Healthy Weight, Overweight, Obese, or Very Obese. Then refer to Table 10.2. It tells you more about what your BMI score means in terms of your health. Alternatively, you can use the BMI healthy weight calculator on the NHS website, https://www.nhs.uk/live-well/healthy-weight /height-weight-chart/

If you are older than 65, your healthcare professionals may recommend a healthy weight range that is a little higher than the numbers for 'healthy weight' and 'overweight' in Table 10.1.

Remember that pinpointing your healthy weight range depends on several things. These include your age, your long-term conditions, how much body fat you have and where it is located, and your family history of weight-related issues such as high blood pressure or diabetes.

Measuring your waist is a good way to check that you're not carrying too much fat around your stomach. You can have a healthy BMI and still have too much tummy fat, meaning that you're still at risk of developing some long-term conditions. Measure your waist by standing up straight and using a tape measure (one that is

Table 10.1 **BMI Chart**

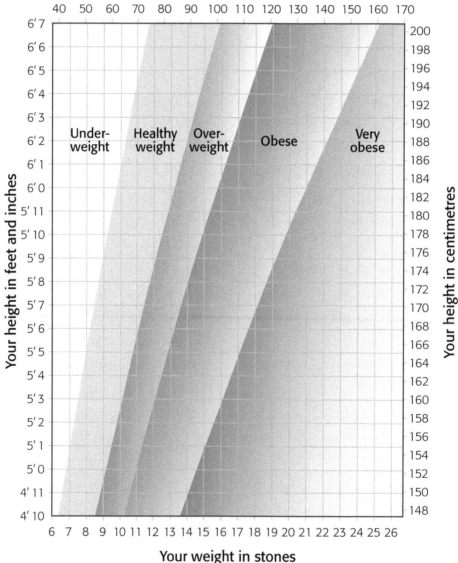

not old and stretched out) to find the bottom of your ribs and the top of your hips. Wrap the tape measure around your waist, midway between these points, and breathe out naturally before checking the number on the tape measure.

Regardless of your height or body mass index (BMI), the NHS recommends that you should try to lose weight if your waist is 94cm (37in) or more for men and 80cm (31.5in) or more for women. You're at very high risk of some serious health conditions and should see a GP if your waist is 102cm (40in) or more for men and 88cm (34.5in) or more for women. This is because your risk of getting some health problems is affected by where you store your body fat, as well as by your weight. Carrying too much fat around your middle (waist) can make it more likely for you to get conditions such as heart disease, type 2 diabetes, cancer, and stroke.

Making the Decision to Change Your Weight

Reaching and maintaining a healthy weight usually means making some changes. Whether or not you make these changes is your decision, not that of your friends, family, or healthcare professionals. If you want to make changes, do it slowly, and only make changes that are realistic for you. The motto 'go for the real, not the ideal' is a good one for weight loss.

To get started, review the information about action planning in Chapter 2, *Becoming an Active Self-Manager*. If you think you want to change your weight, consider asking your GP to refer you to a registered dietitian. You might also join a weight loss support group. You can find a local weight loss support group on the NHS website (see the 'Useful Websites' section at the end of this chapter for more information). Losing weight is

Table 10.2 **Weight Classifications Based on Body Mass Index**

Body Mass Index	Weight Classification	What It Means
Less than 18.5	Underweight	Unless you have other health problems, being in this weight class may not be an issue if you are small or petite.
18.5 to 24.9	Healthy weight	This is the healthy range.
25 to 29.9	Overweight	This range suggests that you are carrying extra pounds. But it may not be of much concern if you are healthy and have few or no other health problems or risk factors or are physically active and have a lot of muscle.
30 to 39.9	Obese	This range signals that it is likely you have a large amount of body fat. It puts you at increased risk for weight-related health problems.
40 and over	Extremely obese	This weight class pinpoints that a high proportion of your body weight is fat. It puts you at very high risk for developing serious health problems.

not something you need to do alone. In fact, people who have ongoing support are usually better able to meet their goals and maintain them.

When you are ready to consider weight loss, ask yourself the following two primary questions:

Why do I want to change my weight? Each of us has personal and different reasons for losing weight. Here are some examples:

- to improve my health symptoms (pain, fatigue, shortness of breath, and so on)
- to manage my diabetes or other long-term condition
- to have more energy to do the things I want to do
- to feel better about myself
- to change the way others think of me
- to take more control of my health or my life

List your reasons here (yes, you can write in this book):

_____

_____

_____

_____

Am I ready to make lifelong changes? The next step is to find out if this is a good time to start making changes. If you are not ready, you may be setting yourself up for failure. But the truth is that there will never be a 'perfect' time. The following additional questions may help you determine whether you are ready:

- Are there other things in my life that might make it easier? To get more exercise, for example, is there a dog that needs walking, or can I get off the bus one stop earlier?
- What things may get in the way of not making eating or activity changes?
- Will worries or concerns about family, friends, work, or other things make it difficult to make changes?
- Do I have support? Is there someone who will make it easier to begin and continue making changes?

Use Table 10.3 on page 257 to help you think about what will help and what will get in the way of making changes. You might also revisit the section on problem solving on pages 25–26 in Chapter 2, *Becoming an Active Self-Manager*. You may find tools there to help you make changes, or you may find that now is not the best time to start. If the latter is true for you, you can revisit this in the future. No matter what you find, accept that this is the right decision for you now.

If you decide to start making changes, start with the changes that are easiest and the most comfortable. Take 'baby steps'. This means working on only one or two things at a time. Do not try to do too much. Action planning tools are great for this. (See pages 30–32 and 36 in Chapter 2, *Becoming an Active Self-Manager*.) Slow and steady wins the race.

Getting Started with Weight Loss

Start by keeping a diary of what you eat now and how much you exercise. Do this for at least one weekday and one weekend day (or one work day and one non-work day). If you can keep it for more days, all the better. Write down

Table 10.3 **Factors Affecting the Decision to Gain or Lose Weight *Now***

Things that Will Enable Me to Make My Desired Changes	Things that Will Make It Difficult for Me to Change
Example: I have the support of family and friends.	*Example:* The festive holidays are coming up, and there are too many parties to prepare for.

what you eat in Table 10.4, or use an app or fitness tracker to note:

■ what you eat and where you are eating

■ why you are eating (are you hungry or just eating because you are bored?)

■ how you feel when eating (your mood or emotions)

■ your exercise (the activities you take part in)

You might also have a section in your diary for ideas about what you would like to do differently. See an example in Table 10.3.

When you have kept a diary for a week or two, look at what you have written. You may be surprised at how much or little you exercise,

that you drink a lot of fizzy drinks, or that you eat ice cream every night. You can use what you learn about yourself and your habits to decide where to start making changes.

Making Eating and Activity Changes

The two basics are first, take 'baby steps', and second, start by making changes you know you can accomplish. There is no getting around it: you will probably need to change the amount of food you eat as well as some of the things you eat and drink. This may seem scary or even impossible, but by following the basics you can do it! For instance, instead of eating a cup of rice or a bowl of ice cream, eat a few tablespoons less. Try eating more slowly. There are many more tips for losing weight on pages 260–262.

Table 10.4 **Lifestyle Tracking Diary**

Date	Time	What I Ate	Where I Ate	Why I Ate	My Mood or Emotions	My Exercise

When you find things you want to change, start by choosing only one or two things at a time. You have heard this before, but we repeat it here because it is important. Allow yourself time to get used to changes and then slowly change more things. If you tell yourself you are going to walk 5 miles (8 km) a day every day of the week and never eat potatoes or bread again, you probably won't be able to do this very long. You won't lose weight, and you will feel frustrated and discouraged. Instead, plan to have only one piece of toast at breakfast instead of two and take two 10-minute walks four times a week. This way you are more likely to stick to it, make long-term changes, and lose weight.

When you change your weight slowly, you have a better chance of keeping the weight off. This is partly because your brain begins to recognise the changes as part of your regular routine and not just a passing fad. Remember, the best plan combines healthy eating and exercise and is a slow, steady plan that feels right to you.

The 200 Plan

One way to get started is the 200 Plan. It involves making small daily changes in your eating and physical activity. You change what you do by 200 calories a day. To lose weight, eat 100 fewer calories a day than you do now and burn off 100 calories a day more with a little bit of extra activity. This may add up to losing about 20 pounds (9kg) a year. The 200 Plan is a good way to balance eating and exercise and helps you achieve long-term weight change.

Eat 100 fewer calories a day

Look at your food diary and see if there is anywhere you can easily cut back. For example, a medium slice of brown bread has close to 100 calories. By not eating one of the slices of bread on your sandwich, you cut out close to 100 calories.

Burn an extra 100 calories a day

Add 20 to 30 minutes to your regular activity routine, which could be walking, cycling, dancing, or gardening. Take the stairs and park farther away from the shops or work. If time is an issue, burning your extra 100 calories in three 5- to 10-minute chunks of time over the day works just as well as doing it all at once. A fitness tracker can help with this.

Physical Activity and Weight Loss

Physical activity can help you lose weight and keep it off. But it is very difficult to exercise enough to lose weight without also changing what you eat. You can learn more about endurance exercises on pages 168–170 in Chapter 7, *Being Physically Active*. These exercises help you lose weight because they use the large muscles that burn the most calories.

The UK Chief Medical Officers' Physical Activity Guidelines published in 2019 recommend that adults (19 to 64 years) should carry out muscle strengthening activities (heavy gardening, carrying heavy shopping, or resistance exercises) at least two days a week. They should also accumulate at least 150 minutes (2.5 hours) of moderate-intensity activity (such as brisk walking or cycling); or 75 minutes of vigorous intensity activity (such as running); or even shorter durations of very vigorous intensity activity (such as sprinting or stair climbing); or a combination of moderate, vigorous, and very vigorous intensity activity.

Older adults (65 years and over) should maintain or improve their physical function by undertaking activities aimed at improving or maintaining muscle strength, balance, and flexibility on at least two days a week. In addition, each week older adults should aim to accumulate 150 minutes (2.5 hours) of moderate intensity aerobic activity, building up gradually from current levels. Those who are already regularly active can achieve these benefits through 75 minutes of vigorous intensity activity, or a combination of moderate and vigorous activity, to achieve greater benefits. Weight-bearing activities that create an impact through the body help to maintain bone health. Exercising in short bouts of 10 minutes or more works as well as longer workouts. If you can add more minutes, that is even better. Don't underestimate the importance of involving some strength training. Muscle-strengthening activities help you maintain your muscles during weight loss, plus muscle burns calories around the clock, even while you are asleep!

These guidelines apply across the general population. However, if you are unsure about the guidelines in respect of your long-term condition (especially if you live with a heart condition) speak to you GP or other healthcare professional.

It is true that the more calories you burn with exercise, the more weight you lose. However, that is only part of the story. It is important to understand that the most success comes from making exercise and eating changes that become part of your daily life. As you think about adding exercise, follow the same guidelines as you did for eating. Take 'baby steps' to make small changes and start with changes you know you can accomplish. See *Appendix A: Healthy Eating Plans for 1,400 and 1,900 Calories* for details of a free 12-week NHS weight-loss support plan (see page 271).

If you exercise too hard or too long, you are more likely to have to stop because of an injury, fatigue, frustration, or loss of interest. You don't have to do it all at once. Whatever you do to increase your physical activity will be helpful. Do your physical activities of choice four or five times a week. Try not go more than two days without exercising. And add to your activities a little each week.

At some point you might become discouraged. The pounds may stop coming off. There are many reasons why this might happen. Exercise may be building muscle as well as reducing fat. Muscle weighs more than fat, so you could be losing fat, but the scale is not showing it. If you keep track of body measurements such as waist and hips or notice that your clothes fit better or are looser, this can be a signal that exercise is working. And remember, when you exercise regularly, even if you don't lose weight, you are doing good things for your body. Regular aerobic exercise can help give you more energy. Exercise can also help a person who has prediabetes avoid getting diabetes. Exercise can reduce blood glucose, blood pressure, and blood fat levels as well as increase good cholesterol, reduce the risk of heart disease, and help with depression and anxiety.

Tips for Losing Weight

The following are some additional tips to help you lose weight:

- **Set small, gradual weight loss goals.** Break the total amount of weight you want to lose into small, reachable goals. For most people, aiming to lose 1 to 2 pounds (0.5 to 1kg) a week is realistic and doable, especially in the first several weeks. After a while, a smaller goal (such as 0.5 pounds or 0.25 kilograms per week) may be more doable. You may also consider yourself successful if you hold your lower weight steady without gaining any pounds back.

- **Identify your specific actions to lose weight.** For example, walking 20 minutes a day 5 days a week, not eating between meals, and eating more slowly. Review the information about action planning in Chapter 2, *Becoming an Active Self-Manager.*

- **Pay attention to what you eat.** Overeating is common when we are with friends, using the computer, or watching television. Set out your serving and keep the other food out of sight. By focusing on what you are eating and not what you are doing (such as watching television), you will be more satisfied, and you will eat less.

■ **Know a portion size when you see one and choose appropriate amounts.** Foods that come pre-packaged as single portions/servings can help you learn what you eat. When eating away from home, consider selecting appetizers or first courses over main entrées, or order a child's meal. This will help you eat fewer calories. Don't eat 'family style' by putting food on large serving dishes on the table. Put your meal on a plate and leave everything else in the kitchen. Put leftovers away as soon as you have finished eating or after you have dished out your meal. Knowing what a single portion of food actually looks like can be tricky. Have a look back at Figure 10.2 to check what single portions of different types of food actually look like in relation to your hands.

■ **Watch out for supersizing and portion inflation.** Research carried out by the British Heart Foundation suggests that portion sizes for certain foods in the UK have grown since the early 1990s. For example, portion sizes for white bread slices have increased, particularly for medium-sized bread. There has been a clear increase in individual portion/servings for ready meals by as much as 98 per cent. There is also wide variation in portion/serving sizes for chips and roast potatoes. Smaller crisp

packets are now only available in multi-pack form, while larger sharing packs have also been introduced. In addition, there is wide variation in portion/serving sizes, which can make it difficult to compare like-for-like foods across different brands. Pay attention to the nutritional information printed on food packages to see if you are eating one or more portions from the servng size you choose when eating at home. Ask for calorie information about menu choices when eating out.

■ **Do not skip meals.** Eat three meals per day, including breakfast. If you skip a meal, you may feel hungrier later and end up eating more than you need to satisfy your larger appetite.

■ **Eat slowly.** If you take less than 15 or 20 minutes to eat a meal, you are probably eating too fast. Give your brain time to catch up with your stomach. If you find it hard to slow down, try putting your fork down on the table between bites, and pick it up only after you have swallowed. Try not to be the first person at the table to be finished.

■ **Clock yourself.** Make it a habit to wait about 15 minutes before either taking another portion or starting to eat dessert or a snack. You'll often find that the urge to eat or to continue eating will go away.

■ **Keep on top of what is happening.** Check your weight on a schedule that works for you. You may not need to check it every day. If you check your weight at the same time of day (usually first thing in the morning), it is easier to note changes.

- **Make sure you are drinking enough water.** Sometimes people think they are hungry when they are actually thirsty.

- **Join a support group (either in person or online) and stay with it for at least 4 to 6 months.** Look for a group that does the following:
  - emphasises healthy eating
  - emphasises lifelong changes in eating habits and lifestyle patterns
  - gives support in the form of ongoing meetings or long-term follow-up
  - does not make miraculous claims or guarantees – remember, if something sounds too good to be true, it probably is
  - does not rely on special meals or supplements

Tips for Keeping Weight Off

If you begin to lose weight, make sure to keep your weight loss within healthy guidelines. If you are feeling well, have good blood glucose and cholesterol levels, and are managing other health issues well, you may not need to lose more weight. Maintaining weight loss also requires effort. The following are some tips to help you move from weight loss to keeping the weight off:

- **Instead of focusing on weight loss,** focus on staying at the same weight and not gaining any weight for a few weeks; then reconsider your weight-loss plan.

- **Increase your physical activity.** Your body may have adjusted to your lower weight and therefore needs fewer calories, so you may need to exercise more to burn more calories.

- **Plan your meals ahead.** Dinner is usually the largest meal. Dinner planning helps you make sure you have the ingredients you need when you want them. Take time once a week to plan meals for the week and make a shopping list. This can reduce food waste and save money.

- **Log your foods in a food diary periodically to get back on track.**

- **Try different fruits to end your meals with something sweet but light and refreshing.**

- **Allow yourself an occasional treat so you don't feel deprived.** This is a higher-calorie food you don't usually eat. Be sure the treat is a small portion.

- **Keep thinking positively.** Remind yourself of what you have already done on sticky notes and post them where you will see them.

- **Set a personal weight gain 'upper limit'.** This could be perhaps 3 pounds (1.4kg) higher than your current weight. Knowing where your weight is at can help you take action, if needed. Some people decide that when they regain, say, 3 pounds (1.4kg), it is a signal to get back into eating less or moving more. If you hit this mark, go back on your weight loss programme. The sooner you start, the faster the newly added pounds will come off.

- **Plan to be active on most days.** Once you have lost some weight, exercising most days of the week improves your chances of keeping the weight off.

- **If something big is happening in your life,** weight management may need to take a back seat for a while. Set a date when you will restart your weight management program.

■ **If you have not already done so, join a support group.**

Heart Disease and Stroke and Healthy Eating

Healthy eating if you have heart disease or had a stroke involves lowering weight if overweight, lowering blood pressure, and lowering cholesterol so your arteries do not harden or become clogged. Losing just a little weight often results in making it easier for the heart to work and lowers blood pressure. Watch the amount of food, the types of fats, and the amount of salt you eat and the amount of alcohol you drink. Drinking more than two drinks in one sitting raises blood pressure. If you are a heavy drinker and want to cut back, do so slowly over a 1- to 2-week period. Stopping drinking suddenly can also raise blood pressure. The definition of heavy drinking is drinking more than 8 units of alcohol (equivalent to 4 pints of lower-strength lager – 3.6% ABV) in a single session for men or 6 units of alcohol (just under 3 x 175ml glasses of wine – 12% ABV) in a single session for women. There is not an exact definition for binge drinking that applies to everyone, as tolerance to alcohol can vary from person to person. The speed of drinking in a session can also alter alcohol's effects. Most people don't drink alcohol every day, but if you do, you should aim to have some days off. Just make sure you don't increase the amount you drink on the other days. The Chief Medical Officers' low-risk drinking guidelines advise that men and women are safest not to regularly drink more than 14 units a week (this is equivalent to 6 pints of average strength beer, or 6 175ml glasses of average strength wine). If people do choose to drink as much as 14 units, it is best to spread them evenly over three days or more.

The British Heart Foundation website says that it's usually fine for most people with a heart condition to drink alcohol within the recommended limits (14 units per week for both men and women). However, they recommend that you check with your doctor for advice on whether it is safe for you to drink alcohol and how much.

The British Heart Foundation has produced an excellent *Eat Better* booklet, which can be downloaded free of charge at

https://www.bhf.org.uk/informationsupport /publications/healthy-eating-and-drinking /eat-better.

It contains a summary of many of the things we have talked about in this chapter, including the following:

■ **Use the Eatwell Guide.** It includes advice on the types of foods to eat and in what proportions to maintain a healthy balanced diet.

■ **Watch your portion sizes.**

■ **Cut back on sugar by using food labels to identify exactly how much you are eating.** Read more about sugar on page 248.

■ **The type of fat you eat is important.** Most of the fat you eat should be good fat (unsaturated fat). Avoid bad (saturated) fats. Eat little to no trans fat. See pages 243–244 for suggestions for ways to make healthy fat choices.

■ **Increase the amount of fibre you eat.** Fibre – especially from oats, barley, dried beans and peas, lentils, apples, citrus fruits, carrots, and psyllium seed – can be helpful in managing high blood cholesterol, a major risk factor for heart disease. See page 247 for suggestions for ways to increase fibre in your diet.

■ **Eat less salt to help prevent or control high blood pressure.** Try to limit the daily total amount of salt you get to no more than that found in 1 teaspoon of table salt (about 6g). Some people may need to eat less than 6g of salt. Use food labels to learn how much salt is in the processed food you eat. Instead of salt, use herbs, spices, lemon, and vinegar for flavour.

■ **Maintain a healthy lifestyle to control high blood pressure.** Weight loss, limiting alcohol, being physically active, and following a healthy eating plan are also important for controlling high blood pressure. If medication is needed, taking it as directed is also important for controlling cholesterol, blood pressure, and blood glucose.

Lung Disease and Healthy Eating

For people with lung disease, such as emphysema and COPD, it is important to eat a balanced diet that includes fruit and vegetables. Here are some tips to help you achieve this goal:

■ **Limit salt at meals and drink plenty of liquids.**

■ **Avoid carbonated beverages.** They increase the amount of carbon dioxide in the body, which means the lungs and kidneys have to work harder to remove it from the body.

■ **Don't fill up on drinks like coffee and tea.** If you have trouble getting enough calories in your diet, try sipping on a smoothie or a high-calorie liquid supplement.

■ **For some, eating several smaller meals per day and waiting until the end of the meal to drink liquids** may help with breathing.

■ **Although not a part of healthy eating, avoid smoking and secondhand smoke.**

■ **Participating in a pulmonary rehab programme can be helpful to learn about healthy eating as well as exercise and breathing.**

■ **Try eating higher-calorie foods throughout the day, such as dried fruit and nuts,** if it is hard for you to eat enough food (when you have little or no appetite).

■ **Keep healthy, easy-to-eat food near you and available in the kitchen.**

- **If you often don't feel like eating, talk with your doctor** to find out if you are having some problems with depression.

- **A dietitian can help with weight gain or loss.** If you are underweight, you will find tips on how to gain weight on page 268. Lung disease can also cause problems resulting in weight gain, such as from steroid medicines that have this side effect.

The British Lung Foundation website offers comprehensive information about eating well for healthier lungs, including information about foods and fluids with essential nutrients to help prevent infections and keep your lungs healthy (see the 'Useful Websites' section at the end of this chapter).

Osteoporosis and Healthy Eating

Osteoporosis is a condition that causes your bones to become brittle. It has been called a silent disease because its first symptom can be a bone fracture, especially in the spine, hip, or wrist. However, it is never too late to slow the symptoms of osteoporosis. You can help yourself if you have osteoporosis. Include enough calcium and vitamin D in your diet. Regularly do muscle-strengthening and weight-bearing exercises (such as walking; see Chapter 7, *Being Physically Active*). And follow your healthcare professional's recommendations, such as taking prescribed medications for bone loss.

Osteoporosis is technically not a calcium deficiency disease, and after bone has been lost, just including more calcium in your diet will not fix it. But getting vitamin D along with enough calcium can help the body better absorb the calcium and slow down bone loss. Everybody needs some calcium every day. The best sources are milk and foods made from milk. But some people avoid milk products because they don't like them, do not eat animal products, or have problems digesting milk sugar (lactose

intolerance). You can get enough calcium from your diet even if you have problems with milk. Many people can enjoy milk products if they take them in small amounts or eat other foods at the same time. Consider eating cereal with low-fat milk or zero-fat Greek yogurt with berries. If you are lactose intolerant, you can use over-the-counter tablets or drops and lacto-free milk containing lactase enzyme to better digest the lactose. Or you can eat foods that are lower in lactose, such as kefir, yogurt, and hard cheeses. You can also drink non-dairy alternatives such as soy and almond beverages. Just make sure they are fortified with calcium.

Knowing your tolerance level is key to managing your symptoms if you are lactose intolerant. According to the British Nutrition Foundation, people from countries like the UK where milk and dairy products have been a staple of the daily diet for centuries are less likely to be lactose intolerant. Conversely, among Black and Asian communities where milk is not traditionally consumed as part of the typical adult diet, lactase deficiency (low levels of the enzyme) can be almost 100%. Lactose intolerance is also very common in people of West African, Arab, Jewish, Greek, and Italian descent.

Calcium in vegetables is not as well absorbed as calcium in animal (dairy) sources. Some foods and beverages have added calcium, such as tofu and orange juice. Calcium and vitamin D supplements are available without a prescription (over-the-counter). If you think you may not be getting enough calcium, talk to your GP or a registered dietitian about your diet and whether calcium and vitamin D supplements (pills) are needed. It is best to try and meet your calcium needs through diet first.

Kidney Disease and Healthy Eating

Kidneys are organs that rid the body of waste. If your kidneys are not functioning well it is difficult for your body to remove waste. There are different stages of kidney disease. Depending on the stage of kidney disease you have been diagnosed with, there are different suggestions for what is best for you to eat and drink. You may need to limit foods and fluids that are high in potassium, phosphorus, and salt. You many need to change the amount and type of fluids you drink. Some people with kidney disease may also need calcium and vitamin D supplements.

Most people with kidney problems will benefit from a healthy diet. It is important to try to eat the right balance of foods to stay healthy. It will help to control your blood pressure and blood glucose levels and reduce your risk of heart disease. These have a role in protecting your kidneys from further damage. Kidney Care

UK, in collaboration with the Renal Association, has developed a booklet containing information about a healthy lifestyle and diet for your kidneys (this can be downloaded at https://www .kidneycareuk.org/about-kidney-health/living -kidney-disease/lifestyle/, along with booklets containing renal diet recipes). The main thing to remember is that most people with long-term kidney conditions will not need a special diet and are advised to follow a well-balanced diet as set out in the Eatwell Guide (see pages 236–238). However, as kidney function decreases over time they will be asked to limit or avoid certain foods, as advised by their dietitian.

If you are diagnosed with a long-term kidney condition, you will be assigned to a specialist team of doctors and other healthcare professionals. You will receive appropriate dietary advice from them as part of your package of care.

Diabetes and Healthy Eating

If you have diabetes, it is extremely important that you eat a well-balanced diet and manage your intake of carbohydrates, as this will enable you to maintain control of your blood glucose levels. See pages 339–345 in Chapter 14, *Managing Diabetes*, for more information about what to eat, how much to eat, and when to eat when you have diabetes.

More Tips for Healthy Eating

The following sections contain more information for making choices to support your healthy eating habits.

Tips for Choosing Foods

■ **Follow the Eatwell Guide.** Choose a variety of foods from the following five food groups to achieve a well-balanced diet (see pages 236–238 for more information about the Eatwell Guide):

1. Fruit and vegetables

2. Potatoes, bread, rice, pasta, and other starchy carbohydrates

3. Beans, pulses, fish, eggs, meat, and other proteins

4. Dairy and alternatives

5. Oil and spreads

■ **Choose foods that are close to the way nature made them.** Shop in the areas surrounding the middle aisles containing packaged foods. These surrounding areas are where you find fresh fruits, vegetables, meat, seafood, and dairy. Buy fewer items in the middle aisles that contain junk foods, snacks, and highly processed foods. To make processed foods, manufacturers add something (often sugar, salt, or fat) or remove something (often fibre and healthful nutrients).

■ **Eat foods high in phytochemicals.** Plant foods such as fruits, vegetables, whole grains, nuts, and seeds have these naturally occurring healthy chemicals that fight disease. When manufacturers refine or process food, phytochemicals are lost.

■ **Eat a wide variety of colourful, unprocessed foods.** The more variety in your food, the better. The more colours on your plate from vegetables and fruits, the better.

■ **Eat foods that are minimally processed.** For example, choose grilled chicken breast instead of fried breaded chicken nuggets. Choose a baked potato (with skin) rather than frozen chips. And opt for whole grains, such as whole-grain bread, whole-wheat pasta, and brown rice.

■ **Get your nutrients from food, not supplements.** Dietary supplements cannot make up for unhealthy eating. Foods as nature made them have the right nutrient amounts and combinations for our bodies. Nutrients that are not naturally found in foods may be present in amounts that are not healthy, or they may not work the way they should. They may even have harmful side effects.

■ **There is a place for supplements in some diets.** Sometimes we cannot get all the nutrients we need from food. For example, older people may need a larger amount of calcium to help prevent or slow osteoporosis. If you are thinking of taking a supplement, talk to your GP or a registered dietitian first. It is important to know how supplements will interact with any medications you may take.

■ **Eat at regular, preferably evenly spaced times during the day.** This prevents you from getting overly hungry and maintains and balances your blood glucose level. Eating regularly means different things for different people. It can mean three regular-size meals or five small meals, or whatever works for you and your health conditions.

- **Eat what your body needs (not more or less).** This is easy to say but more difficult to put into action. How much you should eat depends on the following:
  - ▸ your age (We need fewer calories as we get older.)
  - ▸ if you are a man or woman (Men usually need more calories than women.)
  - ▸ your body size and shape (In general, if you are taller or have more muscle, you can eat more.)
  - ▸ your health needs (Some conditions affect how your body uses calories.)
  - ▸ your activity level (The more you move or exercise, the more calories you can eat.)

Tips for Gaining Weight (Food Fortification)

- **Eat dried fruit in place of some fresh fruit** or drink nectars instead of regular fruit juice.
- **Choose whole milk** instead of lower-fat dairy products.
- **Add extra whole milk** or milk powder to sauces, gravies, cereals, soups, and casseroles.
- **Drink liquid supplements or smoothies** with or between meals.
- **Drink high-calorie beverages** such as malt drinks, milk-based coffee, hot chocolate, fresh fruit juices, milkshakes, smoothies, or enriched soups.
- **Top salads, soups, and casseroles** with shredded cheese, nuts, dried fruits, or seeds.
- **Eat smaller meals** several times a day.
- **Try waiting to drink beverages** 30 minutes after a meal so you have more room to eat food with higher calories. Or **sip high-calorie drinks with your meal** if you are thirsty. Try it both ways to find what works best for you.
- **Leave some nuts or dried fruit out** and eat a few pieces each time you pass the bowl.
- **Eat the highest-calorie foods first,** saving lower-calorie foods for later (for example, eat buttered bread before cooked spinach).
- **Add melted cheese** to vegetables and other dishes.
- **Use butter, margarine, or sour cream** as toppings. Add a flavoured plant-based oil as a heart-healthy topping.
- **Keep a snack at your bedside** so that you can eat something if you wake in the middle of the night. Dried fruit and nuts are healthy snacks.

Tips for Mindful Eating

Go for the real, not the ideal. Healthy eating is not all or nothing. Healthy eating is making small changes.

- **Be mindful while you eat.** Notice what you eat, how much you eat, and how you are enjoying it. Practice this without things that take your attention away, such as friends, your smart phone, or television.

When you eat, concentrate on eating. When something tastes good, savour the flavour.

- **Replace thoughts that include** *never, always,* **and** *avoid.* Instead, tell yourself that you can enjoy things occasionally, 'but a healthier choice is better for me most of the time'.

- **Think about retraining your taste buds** and know that making healthier choices can help you on the road to healthier eating. This is especially true when cutting back on salt. Your taste buds eventually adjust to less salty flavours and learn to enjoy them.

- **Try a relaxation exercise** before eating or a few deep breaths during eating.

- **Notice your food–mood connection in your diary (Table 10.4).** Read your food diary, especially the notes you took about how you feel when eating (your mood or emotions). Spot patterns. Use what you learn to make small changes.

- **When you are bored** and are thinking about eating, ask yourself, 'Am I really hungry?' If the answer is no, make yourself do something else for a few minutes. Keep your mind and hands busy. Or it might be that you are thirsty – hunger and thirst signals can get mixed up, so try a glass of water first.

Tips for Enjoying Cooking and Eating

- **Cook something new.** Take a cooking class or watch videos on television or on YouTube. If you have odds and ends or leftovers, search the Internet for recipes that can help you figure out what to do with them.

- **If you love to cook but are now cooking for one,** invite someone for dinner, plan a potluck, or prepare food for a local bake sale or charity event.

- **Illness, medicines, and surgery can change how food tastes.** Here are some things you might try if the lack of taste is keeping you from eating enough:
  - Ask your doctor about possible medication changes.
  - Avoid smoking and limit alcohol.
  - Practice good oral care. Ask your dentist or doctor about treatment for dry mouth, if that is a problem.
  - Use herbs (basil, oregano, tarragon) and spices (cinnamon, cumin, curry, ginger, nutmeg).
  - Squirt fresh lemon juice on foods.
  - Use a small amount of vinegar in or on foods. There are many flavoured vinegars – try different ones.
  - Add healthy ingredients (carrots or barley to soup, or dried fruits and nuts to salads) to make them tastier.
  - Chew your food slowly and well to release more flavour.

- **If fatigue gets in the way of cooking or eating, here are some hints.**
  - Cook enough for two or three and freeze for the future.
  - Exchange meals with friends or family.
  - Break your food preparation into steps, resting in between.

- ▸ Ask for help, especially for big festive meals or family gatherings.
- ▸ Use a meal delivery service. Check if you are eligible for your local 'meals on wheels' service (see the 'Useful Websites' section at the end of this chapter) or search for the many new food delivery services you can find on the Internet.

- ■ **If eating causes discomfort or shortness of breath, try these tips.**
  - ▸ Eat four to six small meals a day.
  - ▸ Avoid foods that produce wind or bloating, such as cabbage, broccoli, brussels sprouts, onions, and beans
  - ▸ Eat slowly, take small bites, and chew your food well. Pause occasionally. Eating quickly to avoid shortness of breath can cause shortness of breath.
  - ▸ Choose easy-to-eat foods such as yogurt or rice puddings, shakes, or fruit smoothies.

Tips for Eating Out

The British Heart Foundation website offers 10 tips for healthy eating when dining out (see the 'Useful Websites' section at the end of this chapter for more details).

- ■ How often are you eating out? If this is an occasional treat, then fine – but if it's a regular occurrence, think about how this will fit into your overall diet.

- ■ Check what's on the menu before you arrive.

- ■ Decide before you begin if you are going to have a starter or a dessert, and which one you'll find easier to decline.

- ■ Don't be afraid to ask the restaurant to adapt dishes, such as replacing chips with a jacket potato, salad, or vegetables. Ask for your salad dressing on the side.

- ■ Think about your portions. You can order small plates or appetisers instead of main courses.

- ■ Choose dishes that are based on lean proteins such as chicken or turkey (where you can remove the skin) or lean red meats such as fillet of pork or beef. Choose menu items that are low in fat, salt, and sugar.

- ■ Having a good helping of vegetables with your meal will add vitamins, minerals and fibre and help you toward your five a day.

- ■ Try not to exceed the recommended 2 to 3 units of alcohol a day for women and 3 to 4 for men. Don't forget the calories that drinks, both alcoholic and non-alcoholic, can add. If you can, choose sugar-free drinks or water, and alternate these with any alcoholic drinks you are having.

- ■ Entertain at home. That way you can control what's on the menu, and it will be cheaper, too!

- ■ For dessert, select fruit, zero-fat yogurt, sorbet, or sherbet.

Tips for Snacking

- ■ Stick to a daily treat allowance of 150kcal for women and 200kcal for men. You can then have whatever treat or snack food you fancy, but your portion will be controlled because of your allowance (150kcal = 2 plain chocolate digestives).

- Rather than crackers, crisps, and biscuits, munch on fresh fruit, raw vegetables, or fat-free or plain popcorn.

- Make specific places at home and work 'eating areas', and don't eat anywhere else.

- If you crave something sweet, try a boiled sweet or wine gums (or frozen grapes) in small amounts instead of ice cream or biscuits.

Appendix A: Healthy Eating Plans for 1,400 and 1,900 Calories

The NHS weight loss guide (developed under the supervision and advice of specialist dietitians from the British Dietetic Association) is a free 12-week diet and exercise plan designed to help you lose weight at a safe rate of 0.5kg to 1kg (1lb to 2lb) each week by sticking to a daily calorie allowance. For most men, this means sticking to a calorie limit of no more than 1,900kcal a day, and 1,400kcal for most women.

The NHS weight loss plan:

- promotes safe and sustainable weight loss

- enables you to set your own personal weight loss target

- supports you to make healthier food choices

- records your activity and progress

- contains exercise plans to help you lose weight

- helps you learn skills to prevent weight regain

The plan is broken down into 12 weeks. It is full of healthy eating, diet, and physical activity advice, including weekly challenges.

Each week contains a food and activity chart to help you record your calories, exercise, and weight loss so you can see how well you're doing at a glance. As you work through the weeks, you'll get lots of ideas and structured programmes to help you get active, from easy ways to gradually build activity into your day, to the popular Couch to 5K, 5K+, and Strength and Flex podcasts.

This plan is intended for use by healthy adults with a body mass index (BMI) of 25 and over. The plan is not suitable for children and young people or pregnant women. **People with long-term conditions are advised to consult their GP before starting** as it's always a good idea to get the advice of a healthcare professional before starting on any weight loss programme.

The guide is available as an app on the App Store and Google Play or in the form of printable PDFs. You can find everything you need to know about the NHS weight loss plan at

https://www.nhs.uk/live-well/healthy-weight/start-the-nhs-weight-loss-plan/?tabname=weight-loss-support.

Useful Websites

Action on Salt: http://www.actiononsalt.org.uk/

Association of UK Dietitians (Medical conditions food facts): https://www.bda.uk.com/food-health /food-facts/medical-conditions-food-facts.html

Association of UK Dietitians (Food fact sheets: portion sizes): https://www.bda.uk.com/resource /food-facts-portion-sizes.html

Association of UK Dietitians (Plant-based diet): https://www.bda.uk.com/uploads/assets /3f9e2928-ca7a-4c1e-95b87c839d2ee8a1/Plant-based-diet-food-fact-sheet.pdf

Association of UK Dietitians (Salt: Food fact sheet): https://www.bda.uk.com/resource/salt.html

British Heart Foundation (Heart conditions and alcohol): https://www.bhf.org.uk /informationsupport/support/healthy-living/healthy-eating/alcohol-and-your-heart

British Heart Foundation (10 tips for healthy eating out): https://www.bhf.org.uk /informationsupport/heart-matters-magazine/nutrition/eating-out

British Heart Foundation (*Eat Better* booklet): https://www.bhf.org.uk/informationsupport /publications/healthy-eating-and-drinking/eat-better

British Heart Foundation (Portion size guide): https://extras.bhf.org.uk/patientinfo/portion-size _v1.0/app/

British Heart Foundation (*Taking Control of Food Portions and Labels*): https://www.bhf.org.uk /informationsupport/publications/healthy-eating-and-drinking/taking-control-of-food-portions -and-labels

British Lung Foundation (Eating well for healthier lungs): https://www.blf.org.uk/support-for-you /eating-well/eating-a-healthy-diet

British Nutrition Foundation: https://www.nutrition.org.uk/healthyliving/healthydiet /healthybalanceddiet.html

British Nutrition Foundation (*Facts About Trans Fats*): https://www.nutrition.org.uk /attachments/045

British Nutrition Foundation (*Get Portion Wise*): https://www.nutrition.org.uk/attachments /article/1193/Find%20your%20balance_%20booklet.pdf

Drinkaware: https://www.drinkaware.co.uk/facts

Eatwell Guide booklet: https://assets.publishing.service.gov.uk/government/uploads/system /uploads/attachment_data/file/742750/Eatwell_Guide_booklet_2018v4.pdf

Food Standards Agency (Labelling of prepacked foods): https://www.food.gov.uk/business-guidance
/packaging-and-labelling#the-legislation

GOV.UK (Find local meals on wheels services): https://www.gov.uk/meals-home

NHS (8 tips for healthy eating): https://www.nhs.uk/live-well/eat-well/eight-tips-for-healthy-eating/

NHS (Local weight loss support groups): https://www.nhs.uk/service-search/other-services
/Weight%20loss%20support%20groups/LocationSearch/1429

NHS (Salt: the facts web guide): https://www.nhs.uk/live-well/eat-well/salt-nutrition/

NHS (*The Eatwell Guide*): https://www.nhs.uk/live-well/eat-well/the-eatwell-guide/

NHS (Vitamin D): https://www.nhs.uk/news/food-and-diet/the-new-guidelines
-on-vitamin-d-what-you-need-to-know/

NHS (How do I find a registered dietitian?): https://www.nhs.uk/common-health-questions/food
-and-diet/how-can-i-find-a-registered-dietitian-or-nutritionist/

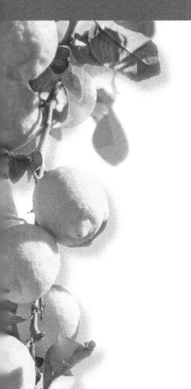

Communicating with Family, Friends, and Healthcare Professionals

'You just don't understand!'

THIS STATEMENT OFTEN SUMS UP A FRUSTRATING DISCUSSION. Whenever you talk, your goal is that another person understands what you are saying. You are frustrated when you feel misunderstood. Poor communication often leads to anger, isolation, and depression. This can be worse when you have a long-term health problem. When communication breaks down, symptoms often get worse. Pain can increase, blood glucose and blood pressure levels may rise, and there is increased strain on the heart. When you are misunderstood, you may become irritable and unable to concentrate. This can lead to accidents. Clearly, poor communication is bad for your physical, mental, and emotional health.

Healthy communication is one of the most important tools in your self-management toolbox. It helps you use the rest of your tools better. And it is important to good relationships. Good relationships help people cope and deal with stress. Poor

275

communication is the biggest reason for poor relationships between spouses or partners, family, friends, colleagues, or healthcare professionals.

Good communication is a necessity when you have a long-term condition. In particular, it is vital that your doctors, nurses, and other healthcare professionals understand you and that equally you understand them. When you don't understand advice or recommendations from your doctor or healthcare team, the resulting lack of clarity can be life-threatening. For a self-manager, effective communication skills are essential.

In this chapter we discuss tools to improve communication. These are tools to help you express your feelings to get positive results and to avoid conflict. We also discuss how to listen, how to recognise body language, and how to get the information you need. Communication is a two-way street. If you are uncomfortable expressing your feelings or asking for help, others probably feel the same. It may be up to you to make sure the lines of communication are open. Here are two keys to better communication:

- Do not make assumptions. We often think, *'They should know.'* But people are not mind readers. If you want to be sure they know, tell them.

- You cannot change how others communicate. What you *can* do is change your communication to be sure you are understood.

Communication Hurdles

When you have a long-term condition, you may face communication problems. You may need support from your family and friends. And getting that support requires communication. At times they may be trying to hide their feelings of anger, grief, and guilt. They may not know how to act toward you. This is especially true if your condition is sudden or even life-threatening, such as cancer or a stroke.

If you have a long-term condition, you might face some of the following communication challenges:

- telling people about the diagnosis
- deciding whom to tell about your condition
- talking about fear of the future
- talking about fear of recurrence
- becoming dependent on others
- being dropped by friends
- dealing with workplace issues
- talking to children about your condition
- talking to elderly parents about your condition
- admitting any financial difficulties you may have
- talking about sexual difficulties
- asking for help
- making decisions
- talking about end of life

The tools in this chapter can help in these situations. Remember that the first time you use them it might feel awkward. It will get easier over time.

Expressing Your Feelings

When communication is difficult, it can help to review the situation. Ask yourself to identify what you are feeling. Identifying feelings and expressing them can make communication better. Consider the following example.

Michael and Tony agreed to go to a football match. When Michael came to pick him up, Tony was not ready. In fact, he was not sure he wanted to go because he was having trouble with the arthritis in his knees.

Tony: *You just don't understand. If you had pain like I do, you wouldn't be so quick to criticise. You don't think of anyone but yourself.*

Michael: *Well, I can see that I should just go by myself.*

In this conversation, neither Michael nor Tony stopped to think about what was really bothering him or how he felt about it. Each blamed the other for an unfortunate situation.

The following is the same conversation using more thoughtful communications.

Michael: *When we have made plans and then at the last minute you are not sure you can go, I feel frustrated and angry. I don't know what to do – go on without you, stay here and change our plans, or just not make plans.*

Tony: *When this arthritis acts up at the last minute, I'm confused too. I keep hoping I can go and so I don't call you. I don't want to disappoint you and I really want to go. I keep hoping that my knees will feel better.*

Michael: *I understand.*

Tony: *Let's go to the match. You can let me off at the gate so I won't have to walk far. I can do the steps slowly and be in our seats when you arrive. I really want to go to the match with you. In the future, I will let you know sooner if my arthritis is acting up.*

Michael: *Sounds good to me. I really do like your company and knowing how I can help. It is just that being caught by surprise sometimes makes me angry.*

In this example, Michael and Tony talked about the situation and how they felt. Neither blamed the other.

Unfortunately, situations where one person blames the other are common. Consider the following example from a workplace.

Corrina: *Why are you always late when you say you are going to do something? I get stuck doing everything myself.*

Sandra: *I understand. Having a deadline makes my anxiety worse. I want to get things done on time, but sometimes I offer to do too much. When my anxiety acts up at the last minute, I am confused. I keep hoping I can get everything done, and I don't tell you I'm behind because I don't want to disappoint you. I keep hoping that I will feel less anxious as the day wears on and I will catch up.*

Corrina: *Well, I hope that in the future you will call. I don't like being caught by surprise.*

Sandra: *I understand. I will start on the report and if the time is short and I get anxious, I will let you know.*

In this example, only Sandra is being thoughtful and expressing her feelings. Corrina continues to blame. The outcome, however, is still positive. Both people got what they wanted.

The following are some suggestions for using good communication and creating supportive relationships:

- **Show respect.** Always show respect. Try not to preach. Avoid demeaning or blaming statements such as *Why are you always late when you say you are going to do something? I get stuck doing everything myself.* The use of the word *you* is a clue that blaming is happening. Courtesy can go a long way toward softening the situation. (See 'Anger' in Chapter 5, *Understanding and Managing Common Symptoms and Emotions*, on pages 122–124.)

- **Be clear.** Describe the situation using facts. Avoid general words like *everything, always,* and *never.* For example, Sandra said, '*I understand. I will start on the report and if the time is short and I get anxious, I will let you know.*'

- **Don't make assumptions.** Ask for more detail. Corrina did not do this. She assumed that Sandra was being rude or inconsiderate and that is why Sandra did not get the report done. It would have been better if she asked Sandra why she hadn't let her know earlier about the delay. Assumptions are the enemy of good communication.

Many arguments arise from one person expecting the other person to be a mind reader. One sign that you are making assumptions is thinking, '*This person should know …*' Don't rely on mind reading; express your own needs and feelings directly and clearly. Ask questions if you don't understand why someone else is acting a certain way.

- **Open up.** Express your feelings openly and honestly. Don't make others guess what you are feeling – their guess might be wrong. Sandra did the right thing. She talked about getting started on the report and letting Corrina know early if she had anxiety problems.

- **Listen first.** Good listeners seldom interrupt. Wait a few seconds when someone is finished talking before you respond. He or she may have more to say.

- **Accept the feelings of others.** It is not always easy to understand or accept what someone else is feeling. Sometimes this takes time and effort. You can stall a bit by saying 'I understand' or 'I'm not sure I understand; could you explain some more?'

- **Use humour carefully.** Sometimes it helps to gently introduce a bit of humour. But don't use sarcasm or hurtful humour. Know when to be serious.

- **Don't play the victim.** You become a victim when you do not express your needs and feelings. Sometimes you may expect that the other person should act in a certain way, but unless you communicate about what you want, they may not act that way. Unless you have done something to hurt another person, do not apologise. Apologising all the time is a sign that you see yourself as a victim. You deserve respect, and you have a right to express your wants and needs.

Using 'I' Messages

Many people have problems expressing feelings. This is especially true when being critical of someone else. When frustration mixes with high emotions, the result is often many 'you' messages. 'You' messages usually start with the word *you*. They often suggest blame. The person being addressed feels attacked and becomes defensive. Communication barriers spring up everywhere. The result is more anger, frustration, and bad feelings. Everyone loses. No one wins.

One way to avoid this is to try using 'I' statements instead of 'you' statements. 'I' statements are strong and direct ways to express your views and feelings. 'I' messages start with the word 'I'.

Here are some examples of 'I' statements you can use instead of 'you' statements:

■ Say 'I try very hard to do the best work I can' rather than 'You always find fault with me.'

■ Say 'I like it when you turn down the television while we talk' rather than 'You never pay attention.'

Sometimes people think they are using 'I' messages when they are really using 'you' message. For example, 'I feel that you are not treating me fairly' is a disguised 'you' statement. A true 'I' statement is 'I feel angry and hurt.'

Here are some more examples of 'I' statements and 'you' statements:

■ 'You' message: *'Why are you always late? We never get anywhere on time.'*

'I' message: *'I get really upset when I'm late. It's important to me to be on time.'*

■ 'You' message: *'There's no way you can understand how lousy I feel.'*

'I' message: *'I'm not feeling well. I could use a little help today.'*

Watch out for hidden 'you' messages. These are 'you' messages with 'I feel …' stuck in front of them:

■ 'You' message: *'You always walk too fast.'*

■ Hidden 'you' message: *'I feel angry when you walk so fast.'*

■ 'I' message: *'I have a hard time walking fast.'*

The trick to 'I' messages is to report your personal feelings using the word "I". Do your best to not use the word "*you*". Of course, like any new skill, using 'I' messages takes practice. Start by listening to yourself and to others. (Supermarkets are a good place to hear lots of 'you' messages as parents talk to their children.) In your head, take some of the 'you' messages and turn them into 'I' messages. You'll be surprised at how fast 'I' messages become a habit.

If using 'I' statements seems difficult, try starting out your sentences with these phrases:

- 'I notice ...' (state just the facts)
- 'I think ...' (state your opinion)
- 'I feel ...' (state what your feelings are)
- 'I want ...' (state exactly what you would like the other person to do)

For example, imagine you make a special cake to bring to a friend as a gift. A family member comes along and cuts out a large slice. You're upset because, with a piece missing, the gift is ruined. You might say to the cake eater: 'You cut into my special cake' (observation). 'You could have asked me first' (opinion). 'I'm really upset and disappointed because I can't give the cake as a gift now' (feeling). 'I'd like an apology, and next time I would like you to ask before you help yourself' (want).' Yes, this contains some 'you' messages, but they state specific observations and opinions. This approach is better than the obvious 'you' messages we talked about earlier. It gives the other person some specific details to help them understand your feelings and how to deal with them.

> ## Exercise: 'I' Messages
>
> Change the following statements into 'I' messages. (Watch out for hidden 'you' messages.)
>
> 1. 'You expect me to wait on you hand and foot!'
> 2. 'Doctor, you never have enough time for me. You're always in a hurry.'
> 3. 'You hardly ever touch me anymore. You haven't paid any attention to me since my heart attack.'
> 4. 'Doctor, you didn't tell me the side effects of all these medications or why I have to take them.'

'I' messages are not a cure-all. Sometimes the listener must have time to hear them. This is especially true if the person is used to hearing blaming 'you' messages. If 'I' messages do not work at first, keep using them. As you gain new communication skills, old patterns of communication will change.

Some people use 'I' messages to manipulate others. They express that they are sad, angry, or frustrated to gain sympathy from others. If you use 'I' messages in this way, your problems

> ## Ensuring Clear Communication
>
> | Words That Help Understanding | Words That Harm Understanding |
> | --- | --- |
> | I, me, mine | you, yours |
> | Right now, at this time, at this point | Never, always, every time, constantly |
> | Who, which, where, when | Obviously ... |
> | What do you mean, please explain, tell me more, I don't understand | Why? |

can get worse. Good 'I' messages report honest feelings.

Finally, note that 'I' messages are also an excellent way to express positive feelings and compliments. For example, 'I really appreciate the extra time you gave me today, doctor.'

Good communication skills help make life easier for everyone, especially those with long-term health problems. The 'Ensuring Clear Communication' box (see page 280) lists some words that can help or harm communication.

Lessening Conflict

Besides 'I' messages, there are other ways to reduce conflict.

■ **Refocus the discussion.** If you get off topic and emotions are running high, shift the focus. Refocus and bring the discussion back to the agreed topic. For example, you might say, 'We're both getting upset and drifting away from what we agreed to discuss.' Or, 'I feel like we are bringing up things other than what we agreed to talk about. I'm getting upset. Can we talk about these other things later and just talk about what we originally agreed to discuss?'

■ **Ask for more time.** For example, you might say, 'I think I understand your concerns, but I need more time to think before I respond.' Or, 'I hear what you are saying, but I am too frustrated to respond now. Let me find out more and then we can talk.'

■ **Make sure you understand the other person's viewpoint.** Do this by summarising what you heard and asking for more clarity. You can also switch roles. Try arguing the other person's position the best you can. This will help you understand all sides of an issue. It also shows that you respect and value the other person's point of view.

■ **Look for compromise.** You may not always find the perfect solution or reach total agreement. Nevertheless, it may be possible to find something on which you can agree (compromise). For example, you can do it your way this time and the other person's way the next time. Agree to part of what you want and part of what the other person wants. Or decide what you'll do and what the other person will do. These are all forms of compromise and can help you through some difficult times.

■ **Say you're sorry.** We have all said or done things that have hurt others. Many relationships are hurt – sometimes for years – because people have not learned the powerful social skill of apologising. Often all it takes to restore a relationship is a simple sincere apology. Rather than a sign of weakness, an apology shows great strength. For an apology to be effective, follow these steps:

  ▸ **Admit the specific mistake and accept responsibility.** Name the offense. Don't gloss over it by saying something general like 'I'm sorry for what I did.' Be specific. You might say, for example, 'I'm very sorry that I spoke behind your back.' Explain what led you to do what you did. Don't offer excuses or sidestep responsibility.

- ▸ **Express your feelings.** A genuine, heart-felt apology involves some suffering. Sadness shows that the relationship matters to you.
- ▸ **Admit to the impact of wrongdoing.** You might say, 'I know that I hurt you and that my behaviour cost you a lot. For that I am very sorry.'
- ▸ **Offer to make amends.** Ask what you can do to make the situation better or volunteer specific suggestions.

Making an apology is not fun, but it is an act of courage, generosity, and healing. It creates the possibility of a renewed and stronger relationship, and it can also bring peace.

- ■ **Forgive others.** There are two sides to making up. When someone offers you an apology, accept it as graciously as possible and be ready to tell them how they can make amends. Sometimes you are wronged and the other person does not apologise. Whatever happened can grow larger and larger in your mind. Maybe the relationship is over but the wrong still upsets you. In this case, you need to work on forgiveness. That does not mean that you have to restart the friendship. What it means is that the past wrong no longer weighs you down.

Asking for Help

Getting and giving help is a part of life. Even though most of us need help, few of us like to ask for it. We may not want to admit that we are unable to do things for ourselves. We may not want to burden others. We may hedge or make a very vague request: 'I'm sorry to have to ask this ... ', 'I know this is asking a lot ... ', and 'I hate to ask this, but ...' Hedging tends to put the other person on the defensive: 'Gosh, what's she going to ask, anyway?' To avoid this, be specific. A general request can lead to misunderstanding. The person being asked to help may react negatively if the request is not clear. This leads to a further breakdown in communication and no help. A specific request is more likely to have a positive result.

Here are some examples of specific requests you can use instead of general requests:

General request: *'I know this is the last thing you want to do, but I need help moving. Will you help me?'*

Reaction: *'Uh ... well ... I don't know. Um ... can I get back to you after I check my diary?'*

Specific request: *'I'm moving next week, and I'd like to move my books and kitchen stuff ahead of time. Would you mind helping me load and unload the boxes in my car Saturday morning? I think it can be done in one trip.'*

Reaction: *'I'm busy Saturday morning, but I could give you a hand Friday night.'*

If you are the kind of person who hesitates to ask for help, you can use a tool discussed in this chapter in 'Expressing Your Feelings' on pages 277–279. Imagine yourself as the person being asked for help by a friend. How do you feel? Probably pretty good. Most of us like to be helpful. It makes us feel useful, and providing help is a way we can show friendship. Now, think again about asking for help. Have you ever considered that maybe you are giving your friend or family member a gift? They want to help, they want to feel good, but they may not know what to do and may not want to offend.

Sometimes you might get offers for help that you don't want or need. In most cases, these offers come from important people in your life. These people care for you and genuinely want to help. A well-worded 'I' message allows you to decline the help without embarrassing the other person. For example: 'Thank you for being so thoughtful, but today I think I can handle it myself. I hope I can take you up on your offer another time.'

Saying No

What about when *you* are asked for help? It is probably best not to answer right away. You may need more information. If a request leaves you feeling negative, trust your feelings.

The example of helping a person move house is a good one. 'Help me move' can mean anything from moving furniture upstairs to picking up the pizza for the hungry helpers. Using communication skills to find out more specific information will help you avoid problems. It is important to understand any request fully before responding. Asking for more information or restating the request will help you understand. Start by saying, 'Before I answer ...' and then ask key questions. This will not only clarify the request but also prevent the person from assuming you are going to say yes.

If you decide to say no, it is important to acknowledge the importance of the request. In this way, people can see that you are rejecting their requests, not rejecting them. Your turndown should not be a putdown. For example, here is a polite way to say no: 'That sounds like a worthwhile project you're doing, but it's beyond what I can do this week.' Again, specifics are the key. Try to be clear about the conditions of your turndown. Give them information. Let them know if you will always turn down this request, or that today or this week or right now is the problem. If you are feeling overwhelmed and imposed upon, saying no can be a useful tool. You may wish to make a counteroffer such as, 'I won't be able to drive today, but I will next week.' But remember, you always have the right to decline a request, even if it is a reasonable one.

Accepting Help

You may often hear, 'How can I help?' And your answer may be 'I don't know' or 'Thank you, but I don't need any help.' All the time you may be thinking, 'They should know …' Next time, accept help by being specific. For example, 'It would be great if we could go for a walk once a week' or 'Could you please take out the rubbish? I can't lift it.' Remember that people cannot read your mind, so you'll need to tell them what help you want and thank them for it. Think about how each person who offers help in your life can help. If possible, give people tasks that they can easily accomplish. You are giving them a gift. People like being helpful and feel rejected when they cannot help you if they care about you. When people help you, do not forget to say thank you. It is important and healthy to express your gratitude. (See 'Practice Gratitude' in Chapter 6, *Using Your Mind to Manage Symptoms*, page 158.)

Listening

Good listening is probably the most important communication skill. Most of us are much better at talking than listening. Sometimes when others talk to us, we are half listening as we prepare a response. The following are steps to good listening:

1. **Listen to tone of voice and observe body language** (see pages 286–287). There may be times when the words don't tell the whole story. Is the person's voice wavering? Is the speaker struggling to find the right words? Do you notice body tension? Are they distracted? Do you hear sarcasm? What is the facial expression? If you see some of these signs, you will pick up what speakers are communicating about beyond just the words they say.

2. **Let the person know you heard.** This may be a simple 'uh-huh'. Many times, the only thing the other person wants is to know is that you are listening. They may just need to talk to a sympathetic listener.

3. **Let the person know you heard both their content and the emotion.** You can do this by restating what you heard. For example, 'Sounds like you are planning a nice trip.' Or you can respond by acknowledging the emotions: 'That must be difficult' or 'How sad you must feel.' When you respond on an emotional level, the results are often startling. These responses tend to open the gates for more expression of feelings and thoughts. Responding to either the content or the emotion can help communication. It discourages the other person from simply repeating what has been said. Don't try to talk people out of their feelings. They are real to them. Just listen and reflect.

4. **Respond by seeking more information** (see page 285). This is especially important if you are not completely clear about what was said or what is wanted.

Getting More Information

Getting more information is an art. The simplest way to find out more information is to ask for it. Simply saying 'tell me more' generally works to get you more information. Other easy phrases are 'I don't understand; please explain', 'I would like to know more about ...', 'Would you say that another way?' 'How do you mean?' 'I'm not sure I got that', and 'Could you expand on that?'

Paraphrasing Questions

Another way to get more information is to paraphrase, which means to repeat what you heard in your own words. Use this tool when you want to make sure you understand. When you paraphrase what someone says, it helps you understand the true meaning of what was said.

But there is a trick to this. Paraphrased *questions* help communications; paraphrased *statements* can harm communications. For example, imagine someone says:

'I *don't know. I'm really not feeling well. This party will be crowded, there'll probably be smokers, and I really don't know the hosts very well.*'

Poorly paraphrased statement:

'Obviously, *you're telling me you don't want to go to the party.*'

People don't like to be told what they meant. This response might get an angry response such as, 'No, I didn't say that! If you're going to be that way, I'll stay home for sure.' Or the response might be no response – a total shutdown because of either anger or despair ('he just doesn't understand').

Better paraphrased question:

'Are *you saying that you'd rather stay home than go to the party?*'

The response to this paraphrased question might be:

'That's *not what I meant. Now that I'm using oxygen, I'm feeling a little nervous about meeting new people. I'd appreciate it if you'd stay near me during the party. I'd feel better about it, and I might have a good time.*'

As you can see, the paraphrased question helps communication. The question gets at the real reason for your friend's hesitation about the party. You get more information when you paraphrase with questions.

Asking Specific Questions

Be specific when you ask questions. If you want specific information, you must ask specific questions. We often speak in generalities. For example:

Doctor: *How have you been feeling?*

Patient: *Not so good.*

The doctor has not gotten much information. 'Not so good' isn't very useful. Here's how the doctor gets more information:

Doctor: *Are you still having those sharp pains in your right shoulder?*

Patient: *Yes. A lot.*

Doctor: *How often?*

Patient: *A couple of times a day.*

Doctor: *How long do they last?*

Patient: *A long time.*

Doctor: *About how many minutes would you say?*

And so on …

Healthcare professionals are trained to get specific information from patients, although they sometimes ask general questions. Most of us are not trained, but we can learn to ask specific questions. Simply asking for specifics often works: 'Can you be more specific about …?' 'Are you thinking of something special?'

Avoid asking, 'Why?' This is too general. 'Why?' makes a person think in terms of cause and effect and can put people on the defensive. Most of us have had the experience of being with a 3-year-old child who just keeps asking 'Why?' over and over again. The poor parent doesn't have the faintest idea what the child has in mind and answers 'Because …' in an increasingly specific order until the child's question is answered. Sometimes, however, the parent's answers are very different from what the child really wants to know, and the child never gets the information she or he wanted. Rather than using *why*, begin your responses with *who*, *which*, *when*, or *where*. These words usually get a more specific response.

We should point out that sometimes we do not get the correct information because we do not know what question to ask. In important situations, consider thinking about and writing down your questions before you ask them. For example, you may be seeking legal advice from Citizens Advice. You call and ask if there is a solicitor on the staff and hang up when the answer is no. If instead you had asked where you might get low-cost legal advice, you might have got some referrals.

Being Aware of Body Language and Conversational Styles

Part of listening to what others are saying includes watching how they say it. Even when people say nothing, their bodies are talking; sometimes they are even shouting. Research shows that people communicate more than half of what they are saying through their body language. If you want to communicate well, be aware of your body language, facial expressions, and tone of voice. These should match the words you say. If you do not do this, you are sending mixed messages and creating misunderstandings.

For example, if you want to make a firm statement, look at the other person and keep your expression friendly. Stand tall and confident, relax your legs and arms, and breathe. You may even lean forward to show your interest. Try not to sneer or bite your lip; this might indicate discomfort or doubt. Don't look away, move away, or slouch, as these movements communicate disinterest and uncertainty.

When you notice that the body language and words of others do not match, gently point this out. Ask for clarification. For example, you might say, 'Dear, I hear you saying that you would like to go with me to the family picnic, but you look tired and you're yawning. Would you rather stay home and rest while I go alone?'

In addition to reading people's body language, it is helpful to recognise and appreciate that everyone expresses themselves differently. Our conversational styles vary according to where we were born, how we were raised, our occupations, and our cultural backgrounds. By accepting that people have different communication styles and not expecting everyone to communicate in the exact same way, you can reduce some of the misunderstanding, frustration, and resentment that sometimes occur when talking with others.

Communicating across cultures can also be confusing. This is true even if everyone is fluent in the same language. In the North West of England tap water is called 'corporation pop'. In Scotland if you say something is 'boggin', that means it is filthy. Body language can also be different. For example, it may be accepted for people from some cultures to stand closer to strangers than you are used to. This might be uncomfortable for you. If you move farther away from them, they might see you as standoffish.

These are a few examples of how communication can differ across cultures. The topic is too complex for this book to address in detail. All we can say is, when you're in doubt about what someone is trying to communicate to you, ask for more information or an explanation.

Communicating with Members of Your Healthcare Team

One of the keys to getting good healthcare is good communication with healthcare professionals. This can be a challenge. You may be afraid to talk freely, or you may feel that there is not enough time whenever you are in a healthcare setting. Healthcare professionals may use words you do not understand. You may not want to share personal and possibly embarrassing information. These fears and feelings can block communication with professionals and harm your health.

Note that in this section we use the terms 'GP', 'doctor', and 'healthcare professional' to refer to the range of primary healthcare professionals you may encounter. Although for many of your healthcare needs, you may be seeing a nurse practitioner or another member of the team, to simplify the discussion and save words we sometimes simply refer to the person who is diagnosing and treating you as 'doctor'.

Healthcare professionals share the responsibility for poor communication. They sometimes seem to feel too busy or important to take the time to talk with and get to know their patients. They may ignore or tune out your questions. Their actions or inactions might hurt or offend you.

Although you do not have to become best friends with your doctors, you should expect them to be attentive, caring, and able to explain things clearly. This is especially important if you have an ongoing health condition. You may think that you can only get the best care from specialists. This may sometimes be true, but it can also greatly complicate your care. You may be seeing several specialists. They may not get to really know you and may not be aware of what the other healthcare professionals are doing, thinking, or prescribing. These are the reasons why we have a GP who is the primary coordinator of our care. A relationship with a GP is much like a business partnership or even a marriage. Establishing and maintaining this long-term relationship may take some effort, but it can make a large difference to your health.

Your GP probably knows more personal details about you than anyone else, except perhaps your spouse, partner, or parents. You, in turn, should feel comfortable expressing your fears, asking questions that you may think are 'stupid', and negotiating a treatment plan that satisfies you both.

To successfully communicate with your doctors, you must be clear about what you want. Many people would like their healthcare professional to be warm-hearted computers with gigantic brains, stuffed with knowledge about the human body and mind. You may want your doctors to analyse the situation, read your mind, make a perfect diagnosis, come up with a treatment plan, and tell you exactly what to expect. At the same time, you may want them to be warm and caring and to make you feel as though you are their most important patient.

Most doctors wish they were just that sort of person. Unfortunately, no one professional can be all things to all patients. Professionals are human. They have bad days, they get headaches, they get tired, and they get sore feet. Many have families who demand their time and attention. Paperwork, electronic record-keeping, and large bureaucracies may frustrate them just like they frustrate you.

Most healthcare professionals entered the healthcare system because they wanted to help sick people. Despite their years of training, many times they must be satisfied with improvements rather than cures for their patients. Sometimes all they can do is slow the decline of someone's condition. Undoubtedly, you have been frustrated, angry, or depressed from time to time about your illness, but bear in mind that your doctors have probably felt similar emotions because they cannot make you well. In this, you are truly partners.

Taking PART

One source of unclear communication can be the lack of time. This is an obstacle to a good patient-doctor relationship. If you or your doctor had a wish for your relationship, it would probably be for you to have more face-to-face time. When time is short, the resulting anxiety can bring about rushed communication. 'You' messages and misunderstandings are common.

Most healthcare professionals are on very tight schedules. They try to stay on schedule, but things happen. This becomes painfully clear when you have had to wait in the GP's surgery because of an emergency or a late patient. Delays like this sometimes cause both patients and doctors to feel rushed. A good strategy to get the most from your visit is to take PART (Prepare, Ask, Repeat, Take action).

Prepare

Before visiting or calling your GP, prepare. What are the reasons for your visit? What do you expect from your doctor? Make a written list of your concerns or questions. After you've walked out of the GP's surgery, have you ever thought to yourself, 'Why didn't I ask about … ?' or 'I forgot to mention …' Making a list beforehand helps ensure that your main concerns get addressed. Be realistic. If you have 13 different problems, your doctor probably cannot deal with all of them in one visit. Star or highlight your two or three most important questions or items.

Give the list to your doctor at the beginning of the visit and explain that you have starred your most important concerns. Be silent a few minutes to give your doctor a moment to review the list. By giving your doctor the list, you let the doctor know which items are the most important to you. Your doctor can also see everything in case there is something medically important that is not starred. If you wait until the end of your appointment to bring up concerns, there will not be time to discuss them.

Here is an example. The GP asks, 'What brings you in today?' and you might say something like 'I have a lot of things I want to discuss'

Take PART

Prepare
Ask
Repeat
Take action

(the doctor looks at the clock, thinks of all the people in the waiting room, and immediately begins to feel tense), 'but I know that we have limited time. The things that most concern me are my shoulder pain, my dizziness, and the side effects from one of the medications I'm taking. The most important thing for me to find out today is if I can go on holiday.' (The GP feels relieved because your concerns are focused and potentially manageable within the appointment time available.)

In addition to your starred list, think about any vitamins and over-the-counter medications and supplements you are taking and make sure that your doctor knows about these. You don't have to list your prescribed medications as your GP will be able to see your previous prescriptions on the surgery's electronic medical records system.

The final thing you need to prepare is your story. Your appointment time is short. When the doctor asks how you are feeling, some people go on for several minutes about this and that symptom. It is better to say, 'I think that overall my anxiety is less, but now I have more trouble sleeping.' You should be prepared to describe your symptoms.

The following are the things your doctor needs to know about your symptoms:

■ when they started

■ how long they last

■ where they are located

■ what makes them better or worse

■ whether you have had similar problems before

- whether you have changed your diet, exercise, or medications in a way that might contribute to the symptoms

- what worries you most about the symptoms

- what you think might be causing the symptoms

If you started a new medication or treatment since your last visit, be ready to report how it went. If you have had any tests in the past 6 months your GP should be able to see the results of these on your medical records.

When you tell your story, talk about trends. Are you getting better or worse, or are you the same? Also mention if your symptoms are more or less frequent or intense. For example, 'In general, I am slowly getting better, but today I don't feel good.'

Be open and share your thoughts, feelings, and fears. Remember, your doctor is not a mind reader. If you are worried, explain why: 'I am worried that I won't be able to work', or 'My father had similar symptoms before he died.' The more open you are, the more likely it is that your doctor can help. If you have a problem, don't wait for the doctor to 'discover' it. State your concern immediately. For example, 'I am worried about this mole on my chest.' Share your hunches or guesses about what might be causing your symptoms, because they often provide vital clues to an accurate diagnosis. Even if it turns out that your guesses are not correct, it gives your doctor the opportunity to reassure you or address your hidden concerns.

The more specific you are (without adding unnecessary details), the clearer the picture you give the doctor of your problem. If you share specific information, you waste less of the doctor's time and less of your own time.

Ask

Your most powerful tool as a self-manager is the question. Asking questions can fill in important missing pieces and close critical gaps in communication. And asking questions shows that you are an active participant in your care. This is critical to restoring your health. Getting answers and information is a cornerstone of self-management.

Be prepared to ask questions about diagnosis, tests, treatments, and follow-up. The following are some guidelines for asking questions:

- **Diagnosis.** Ask what's wrong, what caused it, if it is contagious, and what the outlook (prognosis) is. What can be done to prevent it or manage it?

- **Tests.** If the doctor wants to do tests, ask how the results are likely to affect treatment and what will happen if you are not tested. If you decide to have a test, find out how to prepare for the test and what the test will be like. Ask how and when you will see test results.

- **Treatments.** Ask if there are any choices in treatments and the advantages and disadvantages of each. Ask what will happen if you have no treatment (see Chapter 13, *Managing Your Treatment Decisions and Medications*).

- **Follow-up.** Find out if and when you should call or return for a follow-up visit. What symptoms should you watch for in between visits, and what should you do if they occur?

Repeat

One way to check that you have understood everything that comes up in your appointment is to briefly report back key points. For example, 'You want me to take these three times a day.' Repeating gives the doctor a chance to quickly correct any misunderstandings.

If you don't understand or remember something the doctor said, say that you need to go over it again. For example, you might say, 'I'm pretty sure you told me some of this before, but I'm still confused about it.' Don't be afraid to ask what you think might be a stupid question. Such questions are important and may prevent misunderstanding.

Sometimes it is hard to remember everything. You may want to take notes or bring another person to important visits. You can even record the visit on your phone if you prefer (while it would be polite to ask if it's OK, patients do not need their doctor's permission to record a consultation, because they are only processing their own personal information and are therefore exempt from data protection principles).

Take action

At the end of a visit, you need to understand what to do next. What action do you need to take? This includes treatments, tests, and when to return. You should also know any danger signs and what you should do if they occur. If necessary, ask your doctor to write down instructions, or recommend reading material or online resources.

If for some reason you can't or won't follow the doctor's advice, say so. For example, you might say, 'I didn't take the aspirin. It gives me stomach problems' or 'I've tried to exercise, but I can't seem to keep it up.' If your doctor knows why you can't or won't follow advice, they may be able to make other suggestions. If you don't share the reasons why you are unable to take actions, it's difficult for healthcare professionals to help.

Asking for a Second Opinion

Sometimes you may want to see another doctor or a specialist for a second opinion. Asking for a second opinion can be hard. This is especially true if you and your doctor have had a long relationship. You may worry that asking for another opinion will anger your doctor. Maybe your doctor will take your request the wrong way. If you disagree with your doctor's decision, you can ask them to refer you to another healthcare professional for a second opinion. Although you do not have a legal right to a second opinion, a healthcare professional will rarely refuse to refer you for one. If your condition is complicated or difficult, the doctor may have already consulted with another professional (or more than one). This is often done informally. Asking for a second opinion is perfectly acceptable, and doctors are taught to expect such requests. However, asking for third, fourth, and fifth opinions maybe unproductive.

Ask for a second opinion by using a non-threatening 'I' message such as the following:

'I'm still feeling confused and uncomfortable about this treatment. I feel that another

opinion might reassure me. Can you refer me to someone else I could see?'

Express your own feelings without suggesting that the doctor is at fault. Also confirm your confidence in your doctor by asking for a recommendation. You are not bound by your doctor's suggestion, though. For more information about asking for a second opinion check out the Citizens Advice website (see 'Useful Websites' section at the end of this chapter).

Giving Providers Positive Feedback

When you are pleased with your care, let your healthcare professionals know. Everyone appreciates compliments and positive feedback, especially members of your healthcare team. They are human, and your praise can help nourish and console these busy, hardworking people. Letting them know that you appreciate their efforts is one of the best ways to improve your relationship with them – plus it makes them feel good! Likewise, if you do not like the way you have been treated by any of the members of your healthcare team, let them know that.

Your Role in Medical Decisions

Many medical decisions are not clear-cut. Often there is more than one option. The best decisions, except in life-threatening emergencies, depend on your values and preferences. The decision should not be left solely to your doctor. For example, if you have high blood pressure, you might say, 'I'm very conservative about taking medications. What's a reasonable period for me to try exercise, diet, and relaxation before I start taking the medication?'

No one can tell you which choice is right for you. But to make an informed choice, you need information about the treatment options. Informed choice, not merely informed consent, is essential to quality medical care. The best medical care for you combines your doctor's medical expertise with your own knowledge, skills, and values. Becoming an active self-manager will enable you to develop your health literacy skills. Health literacy is commonly defined as the ability to obtain, read, understand, and use healthcare information in order to make appropriate health decisions and follow instructions for treatment. The more health literacy skills you have, the more you will be able to participate in an effective partnership with your healthcare professionals.

To make an informed choice about any treatment, you need to know the risks of the treatment. This includes the likelihood of possible complications, such as medication reactions, bleeding, infection, injury, or death. It also includes the personal costs such as absences from work. You should also know the risks of doing nothing. You also need to understand how likely it is that the proposed treatments will benefit you in terms of relieving your symptoms, improving your ability to function, or prolonging your life.

Sometimes the best choice may be to delay a decision about treatment in favour of 'watchful waiting'.

Making decisions about treatments can be difficult. Read more about making decisions on pages 27–28 in Chapter 2, *Becoming an Active Self-Manager*. See Chapter 13, *Managing Your Treatment Decisions and Medications*, for advice on evaluating new treatments.

Working with the Healthcare System

If you are unhappy with the care or service you have received, don't suffer in silence. Do something about it. These are the ways in which the NHS in England recommends that you let them know what you think (please note that there are different procedures in each of the four nations of the UK; see the 'Useful Websites' section at the end of this chapter for more information).

■ **Give feedback.** You can give good or bad feedback by telling the NHS organisation or service about it. For example, you can do this through the *Friends and Family Test* or you can speak to a member of staff. Other ways to give feedback should be clearly displayed at the service you visit. If you are unhappy with an NHS service, it is worthwhile discussing your concerns early on with the service, as they may be able to sort the issue out quickly.

■ **Make a complaint.** When making a complaint, you can choose to complain to the organisation where you received the NHS service (for example, your hospital, GP surgery, or dental surgery), or to the commissioner (the organisation that pays for the service or care you received – this will vary depending on the NHS service you are complaining about). You can complain in writing, by e-mail, or by speaking to someone in the organisation. Anyone can complain, including young people, a family member, carer, friend, or your local Member of Parliament (MP – who can complain on your behalf with your permission). You should make your complaint within 12 months of the incident or within 12 months of the matter coming to your attention. This time limit can sometimes be extended if it is still possible to investigate your complaint. If you would like help to make your complaint, contact an NHS Complaints Advocate, who is independent of the NHS and may help you write a letter, attend a meeting with you, or explain the options available to you. This service is free to anyone making a complaint about their NHS treatment or care.

You can find much more information about how to give feedback, make a complaint about NHS England services and how to find an NHS Complaints Advocate at https://www.england.nhs.uk/contact-us/complaint/ or see the 'Useful Websites' section at the end of this chapter.

The following are some common issues that come up when people have to use the NHS. We offer a few hints for addressing these issues and working with NHS services. Not all problems and suggestions will apply to all services, but most do.

■ **'I hate the phone system.'** Often when you call for an appointment or information, you reach an automated system. This is frustrating. Unfortunately, you cannot change this. However, phone systems do not change often. If you memorise the numbers or keys to press, you can move more quickly through the menu of options. Once you do get through, ask if there is a way to contact the clinic/service/person directly. Many systems now let you make appointments online. This often saves time and prevents frustration.

■ **'It takes too long to get a GP appointment.'** Delay in getting a GP appointment is one of the issues most frequently complained about. However, did you know that since April 2015 you don't have to wait on the phone to speak to your GP surgery? You can make a GP appointment on a computer, a tablet or a smartphone using your surgery's website, or the NHS App (see the 'Useful Websites' section at the end of this chapter for further information). Contact your GP surgery and they will help you register for online services. Once registered, you can go online to book and cancel appointments, order repeat prescriptions, and look at part of your GP records (including test results and any medications that have been prescribed to you in the past). In some surgeries, you may also be able to have a video consultation or speak over the phone with your GP: this has becoming increasingly likely since the coronavirus pandemic (ask the reception staff at your GP surgery for more information about online and phone consultations). You can now also see a GP or nurse on a weekday evenings between 6.30 P.M. and 8 P.M. and on Saturdays and Sundays (however, this appointment might not be at your usual surgery). Call your GP surgery if you need an urgent

appointment. If your surgery is closed, a recorded message will tell you who to contact. Before you make an appointment to see your GP, think about what other services might be able to help. Go to a pharmacy for advice and treatment for minor conditions that do not need a prescription. Call NHS 111 if you have an urgent medical problem, but you're not sure what to do. Visit the NHS website at https://111.nhs.uk for urgent medical advice for people aged 5 and over.

If you think your problem is life-threatening, do not waste time going online or trying to contact your doctor directly. Call 999 or go to A&E.

■ **'I see so many doctors and nurses, and I do not know which one to ask.'** It is usually your GP who is the 'gatekeeper' or coordinator of your care. It may be a good idea to let your GP know if another healthcare professional you have seen orders a test or new medication.

■ **'What is a Summary Care Record anyway?'** There are a number of different types of health record. If you are registered with a GP surgery, you'll have a Summary Care Record (unless you've chosen not to have one). Summary Care Records include information about your medications and any reactions you've had to medicines in the past, allergies, vaccinations, previous illnesses, test results, hospital discharge summaries, appointment letters, and referral letters. This information can also be accessed by those administering emergency treatment. Accessing your Summary Care

Record is free, and healthcare professionals have a legal requirement to allow you to see it. If you'd like to see your Summary Care Record, speak to your GP.

■ **'I can never get an appointment with my regular doctor.'** In an effort to manage the flow of demand for services, GP practices are increasingly working with bigger teams of healthcare professionals so that they can offer more support to patients closer to their home. Healthcare professionals such as pharmacists, physiotherapists, paramedics, physician associates, and social prescribing link workers will be working with GPs and nurses so that patients can get a convenient appointment with the right person for their needs. This means that the receptionist at your GP surgery might make you an appointment with a healthcare professional other than your GP, depending on what you tell them you need the appointment for. If you would like to see a particular doctor for personal reasons, then make sure to let the receptionist know when you make the appointment.

■ **'I have to wait too long in the waiting room or the examination room.'** Delays caused by emergencies happen. Or when every patient before you takes an extra 5 minutes, those extra minutes mean a delay for you and everyone after you. There are two ways you can help prevent this problem. First, use your time with the healthcare professional wisely. Be prepared for your visit. Try hard not to take extra time. If every patient takes 5 extra minutes, it means 2 or 3 extra hours of work for the healthcare professional and extra waiting time for the patients whose appointments are later in the day. Second, if you do not need all your time, do not chitchat. When you have what you need, thank the doctor, say you have gotten what you needed and that you are going to give your extra 5 minutes to the next patient. This is a very big gift and will be appreciated and long remembered.

■ **'I don't have enough time with my doctor.'** This may be a booking system problem, since someone other than your healthcare professional often decides how many patients to schedule and for how long. The decision is sometimes based on what you tell the receptionist. If you say you need a blood pressure check, you will be given a short visit. If you say you are very depressed and cannot function, you may be given a longer appointment. You can also ask for the last appointment in the day. You may have to wait awhile, but at least your doctor will not rush your visit to get to other waiting patients.

The following are a few parting words of advice for dealing with the NHS:

■ **If something is not working, ask how you can help make it work better.** Very often, if you learn how to navigate the service, you can solve or at least partially solve your problems.

■ **Be nice – or at least as nice as possible.** If the service or your healthcare professional sees you as a difficult patient, life will become more difficult.

Many people think that things should not be this way. It is not fair to place this burden on the patient. The NHS should be responsive and patient-friendly. The NHS is striving to provide a better service to people living with long-term conditions. In the meantime, use the suggestions in this chapter to help you deal with difficult situations.

Useful Websites

Citizens Advice (NHS patient's rights): https://www.citizensadvice.org.uk/

mygov.scot (Scotland): https://www.mygov.scot/nhs-complaints/

NHS (Friends and family Test): https://www.nhs.uk/using-the-nhs/about-the-nhs/friends-and-family-test-fft/

NHS (Getting started with GP online services): https://www.england.nhs.uk/wp-content/uploads/2016/11/pat-guid-getting-started-gp-online.pdf

NHS (GP appointments and bookings): https://www.nhs.uk/using-the-nhs/nhs-services/gps/gp-appointments-and-bookings/

NHS App: https://www.nhs.uk/using-the-nhs/nhs-services/the-nhs-app/

NHS England (How to make a complaint): https://

NHS Wales (How to make a complaint): https://

Northern Ireland (How to make a complaint): https://www.nidirect.gov.uk/articles/raising-concern-or-making-complaint-about-health-services

thebmj My patient wants to record our appointment – what should I do?): https://www.bmj.com/content/364/bmj.l1101

Wikipedia (Health literacy): https://en.wikipedia.org/wiki/Health_literacy

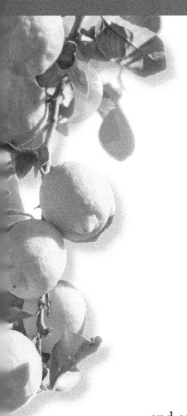

CHAPTER 12

Enjoying Sex and Intimacy

L OVING RELATIONSHIPS THAT INCLUDE INTIMACY and physical pleasure are an important part of healthy living. Sex and other physical intimacies – including touching, holding hands, hugging, cuddling, and kissing – promote emotional connections that strengthen relationships. Intimacy helps you to build trust, feel valued, and manage life better. Sometimes intimacy involves the physical pleasure of sex with your partner, but mostly it is about creating relationships and making connections with the people you love. These connections in turn positively affect your physical, mental, and emotional health. Intimacy also improves your outlook on life.

Over the years, studies have shown that sex and physical intimacy have physical and mental health benefits, including the following:

- **Improved heart health.** Sex is a less intense form of endurance exercise. Depending on the individual, sex can provide benefits like those gained by taking a short, moderately intense walk. It helps strengthen muscles, burn calories, lower blood pressure, and reduce your risk of heart disease, stroke, and hypertension. Studies also show that people with active sex lives tend to exercise more and eat healthier, which adds to their overall physical fitness, health, and well-being.

- **Stronger immunity.** Sex can increase important antibodies that help you fight off infection and protect you from getting sick. Sex also improves circulation and helps maintain fluid balance, which leads to less bloating and better resistance to minor health problems.

- **Stress reduction and relaxation.** Like any form of physical activity, sex can help reduce levels of the stress hormone cortisol, which can cause anxiety. Sex and other physical intimacies can also relieve muscular tension, which promotes both physical and mental relaxation.

- **Better quality of sleep.** During sexual activity, the body produces beneficial hormones, especially during orgasm. These hormones can act like sedatives, calming your nerves and helping to centre the mind. This can help you to fall asleep and stay asleep during the night.

- **Increased sense of well-being and improved mood.** Sex, like exercise, causes the body to release endorphins that make you feel happier and more energetic.

Despite these benefits, many individuals and couples with long-term physical or mental health problems find it challenging to maintain this important part of their lives. Emotions, including fear of worsening symptoms, being unable to perform, or causing a health emergency, can create frustration and decrease desire in one or both partners.

Common Concerns About Sex

For many people with long-term conditions, intercourse is difficult because of the physical demands it makes on your body. Intercourse increases your heart rate and breathing and can tax someone with pain, limited energy, or with breathing or circulatory problems. It may be helpful to start by spending more time on sensuality or foreplay rather than intercourse. Working on ways to arouse yourself and your partner and give pleasure comfortably will increase intimacy and satisfaction. Sharing pleasure through physical intimacies such as caresses and kisses can also be gratifying. Using the mind – either by refocusing thoughts, engaging in visualisation or fantasy, or concentrating on the pleasurable feelings instead of the physical discomfort – can also enhance your experience.

Fear or other difficult emotions can also affect intimate relationships. For example, after people have had a heart attack or a stroke, they often fear that sexual activity will bring on another attack, so they avoid sex. People with breathing difficulties worry that sex is too strenuous and will trigger coughing, wheezing, or worse. Their partners may fear this as well and feel that they would be responsible if something bad happened. Some long-term conditions, such as diabetes, can make erections difficult or cause vaginal dryness that makes intercourse uncomfortable or embarrassing. All these worries can affect a physical relationship.

Loss of self-esteem and a changed self-image can be subtle and devastating sexual barriers as well. Many people with long-term conditions believe that they are physically unattractive. This may be due to paralysis, shortness of breath, weight gain from medications, the changing shape of their joints, or the loss of a breast or other body part. Mental health problems also damage people's sense of self. This can make them avoid sexual situations; they 'try not to think about it'.

Ignoring the sexual part of a relationship or physically and emotionally distancing oneself from a partner can contribute to feeling depressed, which in turn leads to lack of interest in sex and more depression – a vicious cycle. Depression can be treated, and you can feel better. Please refer to Chapter 5, *Understanding and Managing Common Symptoms and Emotions*, to learn more about depression. Sometimes self-management techniques are not enough, so do talk to your GP or a counsellor, or contact an organisation like Mind if depression is a concern for you.

When you avoid sex and intimacy, you have a difficult problem. Not only are you denying yourself an important, pleasurable part of life, but you probably also feel guilty about disappointing your partner. Also, your partner may feel more fearful and guilty than you do – afraid that he or she might hurt you during sex and guilty for feeling resentful about it. This dynamic can cause serious relationship problems. But as an active self-manager, you do not have to allow this to happen. After all, sex and other types of intimacy are supposed to be fun and pleasurable, not scary or uncomfortable!

Fortunately, for humans, intimacy is less about having sex or reaching orgasm and more about sharing ourselves emotionally with our partner or others who are close to us. Remember, making changes enables you to continue doing the things you enjoy. Making changes is one of the tasks discussed in Chapter 2, *Becoming an Active Self-Manager*. So, if sex and intimacy are a priority in your relationship, strive for open communication with your partner. Discuss with your partner the possibility of exploring and experimenting with different types of physical and mental stimulation to experience more sensuality and intimacy, as well as to manage any fears you may have about sex.

Managing Fear During Sex

For successful intimate and sexual relationships, the most important thing is communication. The best way to address the fears of one or both partners is to confront them. Once the fears are out in the open, then you can find ways to talk about them and use problem solving to address them. Without good communication, learning new positions and ways to increase

Misconceptions About Sex

Many sexual attitudes and beliefs are learned – they are not automatic or instinctual. You begin learning these from family, friends, older children, and other adults when you are young. The jokes you hear and the things you read and watch such as magazines, TV, films, and the Internet also influence you. Unfortunately, much of what many people learn about sex are the 'shoulds' and 'should nots', which reflect our society's inhibitions and misconceptions.

To explore their sexuality and maximise enjoyment, people often need to break down these inhibitions and misconceptions. Some of the following are common beliefs about sexuality that simply aren't true:

- Older people can't enjoy sex.
- Sex is for people with beautiful bodies.
- A 'real man' is always ready for sex.
- A 'real woman' should be sexually available whenever her partner is interested.
- Lovemaking must involve sexual intercourse.
- Sex must lead to orgasm.
- Orgasm should occur simultaneously in both partners.
- Kissing and touching should only be done when they lead to sexual intercourse.

sensuality are not going to be enough. This is particularly important for people who worry about how their health problem makes them look physically to others. Often they find that their partner is far less concerned about their looks than they are.

When you and your partner are comfortable with talking about sex, you can then find solutions to the issues you may have. Often, people start by sharing what kinds of physical stimulation they prefer and which positions they find most comfortable. Then, they might share the fantasies they find most arousing. It's difficult to dwell on fears when your mind is occupied with a fantasy.

To get this process started, you and your partner may find some help with the communication skills discussed in Chapter 11, *Communicating with Family, Friends, and Healthcare Professionals*, and the problem-solving techniques outlined in Chapter 2, *Becoming an Active Self Manager*. Remember, if your self-management tools are new, give them a chance before deciding they don't work or giving up. As with any new skill, it takes time, practice, and patience to learn to use them well.

Sensual Sex

In our society, sexual attraction has become almost solely dependent on the visual experience. This leads to an emphasis on our physical image. Sight, however, is only one of your five senses. When you think about being sensual, appreciate the seductive qualities of your partner's voice, scent, taste, and touch. Sensual sex is about connecting with your partner through all the senses, making love not only with the eyes but with your ears, nose, mouth, and hands as well.

Sensual touch is particularly important because the largest sensual organ of our bodies is the skin, which is rich with sensory nerves. The right touch on almost any area of our skin can be very erotic. Fortunately, sexual stimulation through touch can be done in just about any position and can be enhanced with the use of oils, flavoured lotions, scents, feathers, fur gloves – whatever the imagination desires. Sensitive areas include the mouth, earlobes, neck, breasts and nipples, navel area, hands (fingertips if you are giving pleasure, palms if you are receiving pleasure), wrists, small of the back, buttocks, toes, and insides of the thighs and arms. Experiment with different types of touch. Some people find a light touch arousing; others prefer a firm touch. Many people also become very aroused when touched with the nose, lips, and tongue, or even with sex toys.

Fantasy and Sensuality

What goes on in your mind can be extremely arousing. Most people engage in sexual fantasy at some time or another. There are probably as many sexual fantasies as there are people. It is OK to mentally indulge in fantasy. If you discover a fantasy that you and your partner share, you can play it out in bed, even if it is as simple as an expression you or your partner like to hear during sex.

Engaging the mind during sexual activity can be every bit as arousing as the physical stimulation. It is also useful when symptoms during sex interfere with your enjoyment. But be careful – sometimes fantasy leads to unrealistic expectations. Your real partner might not compare favourably to your dream lover. You may find decreased sexual satisfaction if you regularly fire up your imagination with explicit photos or view online videos of young, hard bodies.

Overcoming Symptoms During Sex

Some people are unable to find a sexual position that is completely comfortable. Others find that pain, shortness of breath, fatigue, or even negative thoughts (self-talk) during sex are so distracting that they interfere with the enjoyment of sex or the ability to have an orgasm. This can pose some special problems. If you are unable to orgasm, you may feel resentful of your partner. If he or she is unable to orgasm, you may feel guilty about it. If you avoid sex because you are frustrated, your partner may become resentful and you may feel guilty. Your self-esteem may suffer. Your relationship with your partner may suffer. Everything suffers.

One thing you can do to help deal with this situation is to time the taking of pain medication so that it is at peak effectiveness when you are ready to have sex. Of course, this involves planning. The type of medication may be important, too. If you take a narcotic-type pain reliever, for example, or one containing muscle relaxants or tranquilisers, you may find that your sensory nerves are dulled along with your pain. Obviously, it is counterproductive to dull the nerves that also give you pleasure. Your thinking may be muddled due to medication, making it more difficult to focus. Some medications can make it difficult to achieve an erection; others can help with an erection. Ask your GP or pharmacist about options relating to the timing of your medication and other alternatives if this is a problem for you.

Another way to deal with uncomfortable symptoms is to become an expert at fantasy. This involves practice and training. Develop one or more sexual fantasies that you can indulge in when needed, making them vivid in your mind. Then, during sex, you can call up your fantasy and concentrate on it. You can keep your mind distracted with erotic thoughts rather than on your symptoms or negative thoughts.

If you have not had experience in visualisation and imagery techniques such as those in Chapter 6, *Using Your Mind to Manage Symptoms*, you need to practice several times a week to learn them well. Your practice, though, does not need to be devoted only to your chosen sexual fantasy. You can start with any guided-imagery CD or script such as the ones in Chapter 6. Work on making the imagery more vivid each time you practice. Start with just picturing the images. When you get good at that, add and dwell on colours. After that, look down to your feet in your mind as you walk. As you become more skilled at this, try listening to the sounds around you. Next concentrate on the smells and tastes in the image and feel your skin being touched by a breeze or mist. Finally, feel yourself touch things in the image.

Work on each one of your senses at a time. Become good at one sense before going on to another. Once you are good at using imagery, you can invent your own sexual fantasy and picture it, hear it, smell it, and feel it. You might even begin your fantasy by picturing yourself setting your symptoms aside. The possibilities are limited only by your imagination.

Learning these concentration skills can also help you focus on the moment. Focusing on your physical and emotional sensations during sex can be powerfully erotic. If your mind wanders (which is normal), gently bring it back to the here and now. *IMPORTANT: Do not try to overcome chest pain or sudden weakness on one side of the body in this way. These symptoms should not be ignored, and you should seek medical help right away.*

If you decide that you wish to abstain from sexual activity because of your long-term condition, or if it is not an important part of your life, that's OK. However, it is important that your partner understands and agrees with your decision. Good communication skills are essential. You may benefit from discussing the situation with a professional counsellor. Someone trained to deal with important interpersonal situations can help facilitate the discussion. Don't be embarrassed to be open with counsellors; remember that they have heard it all.

Sexual Positions

Finding a comfortable sexual position can minimise symptoms during sex. This can also reduce your fear of pain or injury. Experimentation may be the best way to find the right positions for you and your partner. Everybody is different. No single position is good for everyone. We encourage you to experiment with different positions, possibly before you and your partner are too aroused. Experiment with the use and placement of pillows or with a sitting position on a chair. You may find that experimentation itself can be erotic.

No matter which position you try, it is often helpful to do some warm-up exercises before sex. Consider some of the stretching exercises in Chapter 8, *Exercising to Make Life Easier*.

Exercise can help your sex life in many ways. Becoming more fit is an excellent way to increase your comfort and endurance during sex. Walking, swimming, cycling, and other activities can benefit you in bed as well as elsewhere by reducing shortness of breath, fatigue, and pain. Exercises also help you learn your limits and how to pace yourself.

During sexual activity, it may help to change positions once in a while. This is especially true if your symptoms come on or increase when you stay in one position too long. Changing positions can be done in a playful fashion so it becomes fun for both of you. During sex, as during any exercise, stopping to rest is OK.

Sex and Intimacy: Special Considerations

People with certain health conditions have specific concerns about sex and intimacy. In this section of the chapter, we address some of these special considerations.

People who are recovering from a heart attack or stroke are often afraid to resume sexual relations for fear of not being able to perform or of bringing on another attack or even death. This fear is even more common for their partners. Fortunately, there is no basis for this fear, and sexual relations can be resumed as soon as you feel ready to do so. Studies show that the risk of sexual activity contributing to a heart attack is less than 1%. And this risk is even lower in individuals who do regular physical

exercise. After a stroke, any remaining paralysis or weakness may require that you pay a little more attention to finding the best positions for support and comfort. You may also need to devote attention to identifying the most sensitive areas of the body to caress. There may also be concerns about bowel and bladder control. The British Heart Foundation and The Stroke Association both have information on their websites about sex after a heart attack or stroke (see the section 'Useful Websites' at the end of this chapter).

People with diabetes sometimes report problems with sexual function. Men may have difficulty achieving or maintaining an erection. This can be the result of medication side effects or other medical conditions associated with diabetes. Women and men can have reduced feeling in the genital area. The most common complaint from women is not enough vaginal lubrication. If you have diabetes, the best ways to prevent or lessen these problems are to maintain good control of your blood glucose, exercise, keep a positive outlook, and generally take care of yourself. Lubricants can help with sensitivity for both men and women. If you are using condoms, be sure to use a water-based lubricant. Petroleum-based lubricants destroy latex. The use of a vibrator can be very helpful for individuals with reduced feeling in the genital area. Concentrating on the most sensual parts of the body for stimulation may lead to more pleasurable sex. There are also new therapies for men with erectile problems. The Diabetes UK website has detailed information about sex while living with diabetes (see the section 'Useful Websites' at the end of this chapter).

Long-term or recurring pain can decrease sexual interest. It can be difficult to feel sexy when you are hurting or are afraid that sex will make you hurt. Pain is often the main symptom of arthritis, migraine headaches, bowel disease, and many other long-term conditions. People who live with these conditions have the challenge of overcoming pain to become sexually aroused or to have an orgasm. Concentration and focus, as discussed earlier in this chapter and in Chapter 6, *Using Your Mind to Manage Symptoms*, are helpful skills. Learning to focus on the moment or on a sexual fantasy can

distract you from the pain and allow you to concentrate on your partner. Time your pain medication so that you receive its maximum effect during sex, find a comfortable position, take it slow and easy, relax, and enjoy foreplay.

People who are missing a breast, testicle, or another body part because of their treatment for cancer or some other medical condition may also have fears about sex and intimacy. This is also true for people with surgical scars or swollen or disfigured joints from arthritis. In these cases, you may worry about what your partner thinks. Will your partner or potential partner find you undesirable? Although this may happen, it happens less often than you think. Usually when you fall in love with someone, you fall in love with who the person is, not that person's breast, testicle, or other body part. Here again, good communication and sharing your concerns and fears with your partner can help. If this is difficult to do, perhaps a couples counsellor or therapist can help. Often the things you worry about do not become serious problems.

Fatigue is another symptom that can kill sexual desire. Chapter 5, *Understanding and Managing Common Symptoms and Emotions*, discusses how to deal with fatigue. Here is one additional hint: plan your sexual activities around your fatigue. That is, try to engage in sex during the times of day and night when you are less tired. This might mean that mornings are better than evenings.

Many mental health conditions and the medications used to treat their symptoms can also interfere with sexual function and desire.

It is important to talk with your GP about these side effects so that together you can find alternatives. Sometimes the doctor can find another medication, change the dosage and timing of the medication, or refer you to a counsellor or therapist to help you and your partner learn other coping strategies to decrease or eliminate symptoms. Individual or couples counselling or therapy can help in dealing with other personal relationship, intimacy, and sexual problems that are not related to your medications.

No matter what your long-term health issue, your GP is your first consultant for sexual problems that might be related to it. Don't be shy or afraid to mention intimate topics. It's unlikely that your problem is unique. Your doctor has probably heard about it many times before and may have some solutions. Remember, sexual considerations are just another issue associated with your long-term condition, just like fatigue, pain, and physical limitations. These are the kinds of problems that a self-manager can learn to solve. Long-term conditions don't have to mean the end of sex or intimacy. Through good communication, planning, and problem solving, you can enjoy satisfying sex and deeper intimacy. By being creative and willing to experiment, both your sex life and your relationship may improve.

Useful Websites

British Heart Foundation(Sex when you have a heart condition): https://www.bhf.org.uk
/informationsupport/heart-matters-magazine/wellbeing/sex-when-you-have-a-heart-condition

Diabetes UK (Sex and diabetes): https://www.diabetes.org.uk/guide-to-diabetes/life-with-diabetes
/sex-and-diabetes

Mind: https://www.mind.org.uk/

Stroke Association (Sex after stroke): https://www.stroke.org.uk/sites/default/files/sex_after_stroke.pdf

Versus Arthritis (Sex relationships and arthritis): https://www.versusarthritis.org/about-arthritis
/living-with-arthritis/sex-relationships-and-arthritis/

Many of the patient organisations supporting people living with your long-term condition will have information and advice on sexual relationships. The treasure hunt begins here!

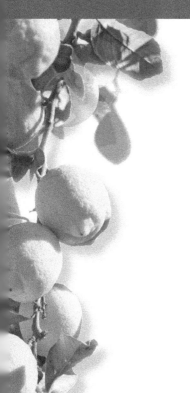

CHAPTER 13

Managing Your Treatment Decisions and Medications

I N THE UK ADVERTISING FOR PRESCRIPTION MEDICINES is closely regulated, so we are protected to some degree from being pressurised about new medication treatments. Nevertheless, we still hear about new over-the-counter medications, nutritional supplements, and alternative treatments on a regular basis. Hardly a week goes by without a new treatment or research of some kind being reported in the news. Pharmaceutical companies spend thousands of pounds advertising and marketing to doctors and patients. Imagine if such marketing power was behind promoting self-management skills. There might be far fewer long-term conditions and less need for medications, surgery, herbs, supplements, and the myriad of alternative medicine offerings.

For the UK edition, special thanks to Rachael Thornton, BPharm(Hons), PGClinDip, MRPharmS, IP, MFRPSII, for contributions to this chapter.

What can you believe? How can you decide what might be worth a try? Managing your own care involves being able to evaluate these claims. You must make an informed decision before trying something new. This chapter provides information on how you can make informed decisions and manage your treatment and medications effectively.

Evaluating Medical and Health Claims

To make informed decisions, you need to learn about any treatment, whether it is a mainstream medical option or an alternative treatment. When evaluating medical and health claims, start with the following questions:

Where did you learn about the treatment?

Was it reported in a scientific journal, in the supermarket, online, in print, a television advert, a website, or a flyer you picked up somewhere? Did a friend, neighbour, or family member suggest it? Did your GP recommend it?

The source of the information is important. Results that are reported in a respected scientific journal are more believable than those you might see in a magazine at a newsagent's or in an advert. Results reported in scientific journals are usually from research studies. Scientists carefully review these studies before publication. Although bias, errors, and fraud can still occur in mainstream scientific publications, they are much less likely and there are ways to correct errors. Many alternative treatments and nutritional supplements have not been studied scientifically. Testimonials, anecdotes, unsupported claims, and opinions aren't the same as objective, evidence-based information. If it sounds too good to be true, it probably is.

Consider this example. A woman returns from a stay at a spa. She reports that her arthritis improved. She credits the special diet, herbs, and supplements. But could it be that the warm weather, relaxation, and pampering caused her improvement? This example shows that it is important to look at everything that has changed since someone started a treatment. It is common to take up a generally healthier lifestyle when starting a new treatment – could that be playing a part in the improvement?

Does the treatment involve extreme diet changes or stopping other medications or treatments?

Is a magic food or supplement being promoted? If you change your eating habits, be sure that you don't sacrifice important nutrients. According to the US National Center for Complementary and Integrative Health, 'alternative care' is used *in place of* conventional medicine, while 'complementary care' is used *along with* conventional medicine. When you use complementary care, you may be getting treatment from your doctor while you are also using additional therapies to manage the same condition. For example, you may be taking medication for arthritis and doing yoga. If, on the other hand, an alternative treatment requires you to stop other medical treatments, be cautious. Talk with your healthcare professional before stopping any treatment or making a change.

Is the treatment safe and effective?

All treatments have side effects and possible risks. Only you can decide if the potential problems are worth the possible benefit.

Many people think that if something is 'natural' or 'organic', it must be good for them. This may not be true. When something is strong enough to have an effect, it's also strong enough to have side effects. 'Natural' isn't necessarily better or safer than a manufactured product just because it comes from a plant or animal. The heart medication digoxin (*Lanoxin*) comes from a plant, but it can be deadly if the dose is not right. Some treatments, herbs, or even vitamin supplements may be safe in small doses but dangerous in larger doses.

Just because many people use a product or practice, or it has been used for many years, doesn't mean that it's safe or effective. Some practices, such as meditation, have proven health benefits and little or no risk. Other traditional methods may not be safe for certain people to use. And others simply don't work or haven't yet been proven.

Nutritional supplements and traditional herbal medicines are regulated in the UK according to whether they are classified as food or medicine. If they are classified as food, they are regulated by the Food Standards Agency and enforced through local Trading Standards Offices. Food supplements are regulated under food law, which is based on the principle that products must be safe for consumption and not misleadingly labelled. Food law does not permit any food to make any claim, or imply that it can treat, prevent, or cure any disease or adverse medical condition. If they are classified as medicine, they are regulated by the Medicines and Healthcare Regulatory Agency (MHRA). Herbal supplements and vitamins do not have to meet the same standards for safety, effectiveness, and manufacturing that over-the-counter and prescription medications must meet. Tests of some supplements have found striking differences between what's listed on the label and what's in the bottle. Do some research about the company selling the product before you try it.

What is the 'cost' of the new treatment?

Is this treatment currently available in your area? Would you be able to attend clinics regularly for treatment? Is your health strong enough to maintain this new regime for the time it will take to produce an improvement? Will you be able to handle it emotionally? Will it put a strain on your ability to function at home or at work?

Learning More About Treatments

You may be wondering where you can get more information about treatments to help you make good decisions about them. The Internet can provide information about new treatments and can be a resource for up-to-date information. But be cautious – especially when you are on sites that are selling products or services. Not every piece of information on the internet is correct or even safe. Seek out the most reliable sources by noting the author or sponsor of the site and the site's internet address (also called its URL). Addresses ending in .edu, .org, and .gov are generally more objective and reliable; they originate from universities, not-for-profit organisations, and government agencies, respectively. Some .com sites can also be good, but because they are maintained by commercial or for-profit organisations, their information may be biased in favour of their own products. Review Chapter 3, *Finding Resources*, to learn more about how to find reliable sources of information. The following are some sites to explore (contact details are provided under the 'Useful Websites' section at the end of this chapter.)

- **NHS website.** As ever, the NHS website is a good place to start. You can find pages on medicines information (which provides a detailed overview of every medicine listed), how the medicines become available and the difference between branded medications and generics. The generic versions will be the same as the branded medicine because they contain the same active ingredients. They are used more often by the NHS because they're just as effective but cost far less. It's similar to buying branded goods or a supermarket's own label – the supermarket's version is usually cheaper. There is a comprehensive database of medicines (A–Z of medicines) and a page on complementary and alternative medicines (CAMs) with information about treatments that fall outside of mainstream healthcare (including among others, acupuncture; homeopathy; aromatherapy; meditation and colonic irrigation). To understand whether a treatment is safe and effective, the NHS website provides a summary of the evi-

dence for particular CAMs and an index for a list of all conditions and treatments covered by the NHS. The availability of CAMs on the NHS is limited and in most cases the NHS will not offer such treatments. The National Institute for Health and Care Excellence (NICE) provides guidance to the NHS on effective treatments that are value for money. NICE has recommended the use of CAMs in a limited number of circumstances – for example, the Alexander technique for Parkinson's disease.

- **Osteopathy and chiropractic** are regulated in the same way as conventional medicine by laws that ensure that practitioners are properly qualified and adhere to certain standards or codes of practice. This is called statutory professional regulation. All osteopaths must be registered with the General Osteopathic Council and all chiropractors must be registered with the General Chiropractic Council. You can use the General Osteopathic Council and General Chiropractic Council websites to find a registered practitioners near you.

- **Professional associations and accredited registers for CAMs.** Apart from osteopathy and chiropractic, there is no professional statutory regulation of complementary and alternative treatments in the UK. If you decide to use a CAM, it's up to you to find a practitioner who will carry out the treatment in a way that's acceptable to you. Professional associations and accredited registers can help you do this. Many CAMs have voluntary registers (some of which are accredited by the Professional Standards Authority for Health and Social Care, known as the PSA) or professional associations that practitioners can join if they choose.

■ **The Complementary and Natural Healthcare Council (CNHC)** is the independent UK regulator for complementary healthcare practitioners of therapies or healthcare approaches that are used in addition to, or alongside, conventional care. These therapies are commonly used by people living with long-term conditions. Such treatments include among others, the Alexander technique; aromatherapy; healing; hypnotherapy; massage therapy; shiatsu and yoga therapy.

■ **Herbal medicines** are defined by the NHS as those with active ingredients made from plant parts, such as leaves, roots or flowers. But being 'natural' doesn't necessarily mean they're safe for you to take. If you want to try a herbal medicine, look out for a traditional herbal registration (THR) marking on the product packaging. This means that the medicine complies with quality standards relating to safety and manufacturing, and it provides information about how and when to use it. You can find a list of banned and restricted herbal ingredients on the GOV.UK website.

■ **National Centre for Integrative Medicine** offers a variety of holistic services and well-being courses from a team of holistic doctors and associate therapists. These services are not provided by the NHS and are therefore not free.

Just because something is commonly done doesn't mean that it is always the best thing to do.

Making decisions about new treatments can be difficult. A good self-manager uses the questions presented in this chapter and the decision-making steps in Chapter 2, *Becoming an Active Self-Manager*, to achieve the best results. If you ask yourself all these questions and decide to try a new treatment on your own, it is very important to inform your healthcare professionals about it.

You and your healthcare professional are partners, and you need to keep your partner informed on your progress during the time you are taking the treatment.

A Few General Words About Medications

In the UK the classification of medicines determines how they can be obtained. There are three major classifications: Prescription Only Medications (POM), which are prescribed by a qualified medical practitioner and dispensed by a qualified pharmacist; Pharmacy Medicines (P), which can be sold over-the-counter by a qualified pharmacist; and General Sales List (GSL) medicines, which are available over-the-counter and do not require a trained pharmacist to sell them. The advertising of POMs in the UK is strictly controlled by the Medicines and Healthcare Products Regulatory Agency (MHRA).

But your body is often its own healer, and given time, many common symptoms and conditions will improve. The prescriptions filled by the body's own 'internal pharmacy' are frequently the safest and most effective treatments. Patience, careful self-observation, and monitoring are often excellent choices.

It is also true that medications can be a very important part of managing a long-term condition. Although most medications do not cure long-term conditions, they can:

- **Relieve symptoms.** For example, an inhaler delivers medications that help expand the bronchial tubes and make it easier to breathe. A nitroglycerine tablet expands the blood vessels to relieve chest pain. Paracetamol may relieve pain.

- **Prevent further problems.** For example, medications that thin the blood help prevent blood clots, which cause strokes and heart and lung problems.

- **Improve or slow the progress of the disease.** For example, nonsteroidal anti-inflammatory medications (NSAIDS) quiet the inflammatory process of arthritis. Antihypertensive medications can lower blood pressure. Sometimes even if medications do not stop symptoms, they help by slowing the underlying condition or illness.

- **Replace substances that the body is no longer producing adequately.** This is why people with diabetes take insulin and why thyroid medication is prescribed for underactive thyroid.

As these examples show, most medications for long-term conditions lessen the consequences of illness or slow the disease. When you take medications like these, you may not feel anything. You may think that the medication isn't working. But it may be preventing complications or keeping you from getting worse. For this reason, it is important to continue taking your medications and discuss medication use with your doctor when you have questions.

Medications can be very helpful. But we pay a price for having such powerful tools. Besides being helpful, all medications can have undesirable side effects. Some of these effects are predictable and minor, and some are unexpected and life-threatening. Adverse medication reactions account for a significant number of hospital admissions in the UK every year (at the same time, not taking medications as prescribed is also a cause of hospitalisation). The Yellow Card Scheme is the UK system for collecting and monitoring information on suspected safety concerns or incidents involving medicines and medical devices. The Yellow Card Scheme allows people to report the side effects of their medications, amongst other things. You can find details of the Yellow Card Scheme website at the end of this chapter.

Using Mind Power: Expecting the Best

Medication affects your body in two ways. The first is determined by the chemical nature of the medication. The second is triggered by your beliefs and expectations. Your beliefs can change your body chemistry and your symptoms. Your beliefs can even enhance how *any* medication or treatment works. Placebos do not contain an active substance meant to affect health. The phrase 'placebo effect' refers to what happens when people take a so-called sugar pill and their symptoms improve. It is an example of how closely the mind and body are connected.

Many studies have shown the power of the placebo – the power of mind over body. When people are given a placebo, some of them improve anyway. *Every time you take a medication, you are swallowing your expectations and beliefs as well as the pill.* You can learn to take advantage of your powerful internal pharmacy along with taking medications. *Expect the best!*

Consider the following ways to do that.

■ **Examine your beliefs about the treatment.** If you tell yourself 'I'm not a pill taker' or 'medications always give me bad side effects', how do you think your body is likely to respond? If you don't think the prescribed treatment is likely to help your symptoms or condition, your negative beliefs will undermine the ability of the pill to help you. You can change these negative images into more positive ones. (Reviewing the discussion of positive thinking in Chapter 6, *Using Your Mind to Manage Symptoms*, can help with this.)

■ **Think of your medications the way you think of vitamins.** Many people associate healthy images with vitamins – more so than with medications. Taking a vitamin makes you think that you are doing something positive to prevent disease and promote health. If you regard your medications as health restoring and health promoting, like vitamins, you may get more benefits.

■ **Imagine how the medicine is helping you.** Develop a mental image of how the medication is doing its job inside you. For example, think of taking thyroid hormone replacement as filling a missing link in your body's chemical chains to help balance and regulate your metabolism. Or think of an antibiotic as a broom sweeping germs out of your body. For some people, forming such a vivid mental image is helpful. Don't worry if your image of what's happening chemically inside of you is not medically accurate. Your belief in a clear, positive image is what counts.

■ **Keep in mind why you are taking the medication.** You are not taking your medication just because your doctor told you to. You are taking your medication to help you live your life. It is important to understand and remind yourself how the medicine is helping you. You can use this information to help the medicine do its job. For example, suppose a woman with cancer is given chemotherapy. She has been told that it will make her feel like she has the flu, she will vomit, and her hair will fall out. This knowledge may worsen her side effects. But suppose she is also told that the symptoms will last only a few days and that her hair falling out is a good sign because it means that cells that grow fast (cancer and hair) are being destroyed. Her hair will recover but not the cancer cells. The presence of side effects can sometimes be proof that the medicine is working.

Taking Multiple Medications

People with several conditions often take many medications. For example, a person might take a medication to lower blood pressure, a medication to help arthritis, a medication for diabetes, and an antacid for heartburn. They might also take vitamins, herbs, and over-the-counter remedies. The more medications you are taking, the greater the risk of side effects. Not all medicines react well together. When they are taken together, they sometimes cause problems. Fortunately, it is often possible to take fewer medications and lower the risks. However, you should not do this without the help of your doctor or pharmacist. Most people would not change the ingredients in a recipe or throw out a few parts when fixing a car. It is not that these things can't be done. It is just that if you want the best and safest results, you may need expert help.

How you respond to any medication depends on your age, daily activity, the ups and downs of symptoms, long-term conditions, genetics, and frame of mind. To get the most from your medications, your doctor depends on you. Report what effect, if any, the medications you take have on your symptoms and if there are any side effects. Based on this information, your doctor continues, increases, discontinues, or changes your medication. In a good doctor-patient partnership, continuing information flows in *both* directions.

Unfortunately, this interchange often does not happen. Studies indicate that often patients getting new prescriptions don't ask any questions about them. Doctors tend to think that if their patients are silent, it means that they understand and will take the medications properly. Problems often result when patients do not get enough information about medications or do not understand how to take them. In addition, people often do not follow instructions. Safe, effective medications use depends on your doctor's expertise and equally on your understanding of when and how to take the medicine. You must ask questions to get the information you need. (See 'Communicating with Members of Your Healthcare Team' in Chapter 11, *Communicating with Family, Friends, and Healthcare Professionals.*)

Some people are afraid to ask their doctor questions. They are afraid that they will seem foolish or stupid or that the doctor will think they are difficult. But asking questions is not an annoyance – it's a necessary part of a healthy doctor-patient relationship.

The goal of treatment is to get the most benefits with the fewest risks. This means taking the fewest medications, in the lowest effective doses, for the shortest period. (Note that some medications need to be taken for life.) Whether the medications are helpful or harmful often depends on how much you know about your medications, how well you communicate with your doctor, and taking them as directed. Another important way to be informed is to read the leaflet that always comes with the medication. This gives you a comprehensive summary of practically all you need to know about the medicine that has been prescribed for you.

Things You Need to Tell Your Doctor Before You Get Any Test, Treatment, or Procedure (Even If Your Doctor Doesn't Ask!)

As we noted previously in this chapter and in Chapter 11, *Communicating with Family, Friends, and Healthcare Professionals*, communication is key. Your doctor needs to know the answer to the following questions even if he or she doesn't ask them:

Are you taking other medications?

Your GP will be able to see on their electronic patient medical records system what medications you have been prescribed in the past, but you do need to let your doctor know about any non-prescription medications you are taking. Report to your dentist all the prescription and non-prescription medications you are taking. An easy way to do this is to carry a list of all medications and the amounts you take (dosage). You can look at your GP records (including a list of the medications you have been prescribed) on a computer, a tablet, or a smartphone by registering with your GP surgery or the NHS App (See Chapter 11, *Communicating with Family, Friends, and Healthcare Professionals*, to learn more about accessing your medical records online.) Saying that you are taking 'the little green pills' isn't very helpful.

If you are seeing a hospital consultant or a healthcare professional outside your GP surgery, then each one may not know what the others have prescribed. Unless you know that all your healthcare professionals are using the same medical records system, you should always bring a list of your medications and supplements. This is necessary for correct diagnosis and treatment. For example, if you have symptoms such as nausea or diarrhoea, sleeplessness or drowsiness, dizziness or memory loss, or impotence or fatigue, a medication side effect rather than an illness or ailment may be the cause. If your doctors do not know all your medications, they cannot protect you from medication interactions.

Have you had allergic or unusual reactions to any medications?

Describe any symptoms or unusual reactions caused by medications, anaesthetics, or X-ray contrast materials (substances introduced into the body prior to an imaging examination). Be specific: describe which medication you took and exactly what type of reaction you had. A rash, fever, or wheezing that develops after taking a medication is often a true allergic reaction. If any of these develop, call your GP at once. Nausea, diarrhoea, ringing in the ears, light headedness, sleeplessness, and frequent urination are likely to be side effects rather than true medication allergies.

What are your long-term conditions and other medical conditions?

Some conditions can make a medication less effective or increase the risks of side effects. Your kidneys or liver can control how the body uses and breaks down a medication. Your doctor may also avoid certain medications if you have ever had high blood pressure, peptic ulcer disease, asthma, heart disease, diabetes, or prostate problems. Be sure to let your doctor know if you have a history of bleeding or are possibly pregnant or are breastfeeding. Many medications are not safe in those situations.

What medications or treatments were tried in the past to treat your illness?

It is a good idea to keep your own records. What medications or treatments were used in the past and what were the effects? You can also usually find some of this information by accessing your medical records online. But also be sure to record self-care, self-prescribed, over-the-counter, and alternative treatments, herbs, and supplements. Knowing what has been tried and how you reacted informs the recommendation of any new medications or treatments. However, the fact that a medication did not work in the past does not necessarily mean that it can't be tried again. Long-term conditions change, and a medication that did not work the first time may work the second time.

Asking Questions Before You Get Tests, Treatments, Procedures, or Take New Medications

Ideally, you should ask the following questions before any test, treatment, surgical procedure, or before you take a new medication. Realistically, you probably want to save the time and effort and ask these only before more significant or risky interventions. Remember, except for in extreme emergencies, when a doctor 'orders' something, this 'order' is really just a recommendation for you. *You* make the final decisions. (See Chapter 11, *Communicating with Family, Friends, and Healthcare Professionals*)

Do I really need this test, treatment, procedure, or medication?

Some doctors prescribe medications or order tests not because the tests are necessary but because they think patients want and expect them to do so. Doctors often feel pressure to do *something* for the patient, so they prescribe a new medication. Don't pressurise your doctor. If your doctor doesn't prescribe a medication, consider that good news.

Instead of asking for new medications, ask about non-medication alternatives. In some cases, you should consider lifestyle changes such as exercise, diet, and stress management. When any treatment is recommended, ask what may happen if you postpone treatment. Would your condition likely get worse or perhaps better with time? Sometimes the best medicine is none. Sometimes the best option is taking a powerful medication early to avoid permanent damage or complications.

When it comes to medical tests, ask, 'What happens if the result is not normal?' and 'What happens if the result is normal?' If the answers are the same, then you probably do not need the test. If you have already had a similar test or medication, providing that information can sometimes prevent unnecessary treatment and risk.

What are the risks and benefits of this test, treatment, procedure, or medication?

No test, no procedure, no medication is without risk. Weighing the possible risks and benefits can be difficult, but it is very important. You are the one who will live with the results. Side effects and complications may range from minor, common, and reversible to major, rare, and permanent. Reading about all the possible side effects on patient information leaflets can be scary. Talk with your doctor or pharmacist to help sort out your risks. *Remember, there are also risks associated with not taking a medication that is necessary and helpful.*

Your doctor may have to try several medications before finding the one that is best for you. You need to know what symptoms to look for and what action to take if they develop. Should you seek immediate medical care, discontinue the medication, or call your doctor? Though the doctor cannot be expected to tell you every possible side effect, the most common and important ones should be discussed. So it may be up to you to ask your doctor or pharmacist if there are any likely adverse reactions. The Patients Association website has a page to help you understand your medicines and how to manage them, including suggested questions to ask about side effects (see the 'Useful Websites' section at the end of this chapter).

Even medical tests carry a risk of inaccuracies or errors. A 'false positive' result incorrectly reports that you are sick. A 'false negative' is a result that fails to identify that you are sick. Such inaccuracies can lead to anxiety, delayed diagnosis, and further risky testing.

Being aware of and avoiding unnecessary risks is important, but there is another side to this story. Some tests such as mammograms, vaginal examinations, prostate examinations, and colonoscopies (examination of the rectum and colon), are somewhat unpleasant and can be embarrassing. Some medications, such as chemotherapy, have side effects. However, these are not reasons to avoid these tests or medications. They can be lifesaving. As a self-manager, you must weigh the risks and benefits. Your doctor can help.

What can I expect from this test, treatment, procedure, or medication?

If you are prescribed a new medication, you should know its name, how much to take, how you should take it, and for how long.

Is the medication intended to prolong your life, completely or partially relieve your symptoms, or help you function better? Some medications help prevent problems in the future and other medications treat acute problems today. For example, if you are given a medicine for high blood pressure, the medication is usually given to prevent later complications (such as stroke or heart disease) rather than to stop a headache. On the other hand, if you are given a pain reliever such as ibuprofen (*Nurofen*), the purpose is to help ease a headache.

You should also know how soon you should expect results. Medications that treat infections or inflammation may take several days to a week to produce improvement. Antidepressant medications and some arthritis medications typically take several weeks or even months to start providing relief.

Taking medication properly is vital. If you are not sure about your prescription, contact your pharmacist or doctor. For example, does 'every 6 hours' mean every 6 hours while awake or every 6 hours around the clock? Should the medication be taken before meals, with meals, or between meals? What should you do if you accidentally miss a dose? Should you skip it, take a double dose next time, or take it as soon as you remember? Should you refill and continue taking the medication until you have fewer symptoms or until you finish the current medication? Some medications are prescribed on an as-needed ('PRN') basis. Others need to be taken regularly. Some medications need blood tests to check for side effects. If you are taking one of these medications, work with your doctor to make sure you are getting the necessary blood tests.

If a surgical procedure is recommended, it is important that you discuss the options for anaesthesia and how to prepare for the operation. For example, should you continue taking medications? Stop eating and drinking? When? Can you drive to the procedure? Discuss how long recovery is likely to take and when you can resume normal activities. You will probably be given medications to relieve pain, but also ask about some of the nonmedication pain-relief tools we talked about in Chapter 6, *Using Your Mind to Manage Symptoms.*

Can a less expensive alternative or generic medication be prescribed?

Most medication has at least two names: a generic name and a brand name. The generic name is the medication's scientific name. The brand name is the name given to the medication by its developer. When a pharmaceutical company develops a new medication in the UK, it is granted exclusive rights to produce that medication for 20 years. Sometimes the licence can be extended. After this 20-year period, other companies may market chemically identical versions of that brand-name medication. These generic medications are as safe and effective as the original brand-name medication but usually cost much less. In some cases, your medicine may be prescribed by brand as this will be the safest way for you to have your medicine prescribed (for example, insulin).

What foods, drinks, and other medications or activities should I avoid while I am taking medication?

Food in your stomach may help protect it from some medications but may render another medication ineffective. For example, milk products or antacids block the absorption of the antibiotic tetracycline. This medication is best taken on an empty stomach. It is very important to ask questions. For example, will the prescribed medication interfere with driving safely? Will drinking alcohol lessen or amplify the effects of the medication? The greater the number of medications you are taking, the greater the chance of an undesirable interaction between the medications. So ask your doctor or pharmacist about possible drug-drug and food-drug interactions. Take great care to know exactly which tablet is which and follow the instructions on how to take it. Using a tablet organiser box can help to make sure you get the right tablets and the right dose at the right time and on the right day.

Are there any tests necessary to monitor the use of my medication?

Most medications are monitored according to the improvement or worsening of symptoms. However, some medications can disrupt body chemistry before any noticeable symptoms develop. Some medications require routine blood monitoring to ensure they are still safe for you to take or are having the desired effect. In addition, with a few medications your blood level needs to be measured on a regular basis to make sure you are getting the right amounts.

Ask your doctor if the medication being prescribed has any of these special requirements.

Is there any written or online information about the test, treatment, procedure, or medication?

Your doctor may not have time to answer all your questions. You may not remember everything you heard. Fortunately, there are many other good sources of information. Don't forget pharmacists! All pharmacists train for 5 years in the use of medicines. They are also trained in managing minor illnesses and providing health and well-being advice. Pharmacists can answer your questions on prescription and over-the-counter medicines, and can help you understand the correct dose and how often you need to take it. The New Medicine Service is available at some pharmacies to give you extra help and advice if you're just starting certain new medicines. This service is for people living with asthma, chronic obstructive pulmonary disease (COPD), type 2 diabetes, and high blood pressure, and those who have been given a new blood-thinning medicine. You can make an appointment with a community pharmacist for a more detailed consultation called a Medicines Use Review. This is especially useful if you regularly take several prescription medicines. You can talk about what you're taking, when you should be taking it, and any side effects that you might be concerned about. As a self-manager, you can also consult nurses, information leaflets that come with your medications, pamphlets, books, and websites. Review Chapter 3, *Finding Resources* and the 'Useful Websites' section at the end of this chapter.

Managing Your Medications

Medicine won't work if you don't take it! That sounds obvious. Yet nearly half of all medicines are not taken as prescribed. Some people refer to this as 'the other medication problem'. There are many reasons why people don't take their prescribed medication: forgetfulness, lack of clear instructions, complicated dosing schedules, side effects, and sometimes the cost of prescriptions. Whatever the reason, if you are having trouble taking your medications as prescribed, discuss this issue with your doctor. Often simple changes can make it easier. For example, if you are taking many different medications, sometimes one or more can be stopped. If you are taking one medication three times a day and another four times a day, your doctor may be able to prescribe medications you only need to take once or twice a day.

If you are having trouble taking your medications, read the following questions and discuss the answers that concern you with your doctor or pharmacist.

- Do you tend to be forgetful?

- Are you confused about the instructions for how and when to use the medications?

- Is the schedule for taking your medications too complicated?

- Do your medications have bothersome side effects?

- Is your medicine too expensive? Certainly, those who need to take several medications and are not eligible for free prescriptions can find that the costs mount up alarmingly.

- Do you feel that your condition is not serious enough to need regular medications? (With some conditions such as high blood pressure, high cholesterol, or early diabetes, you may not have any symptoms.)

- Do you feel that the treatment is unlikely to help?

- Are you denying that you have a condition that needs treatment?

- Have you had a bad experience with the medicine you are supposed to be taking or another medication?

- Do you know someone who had a bad experience with the medication, and are you afraid that something similar will happen to you?

A Word About Pharmacists

Pharmacists are an underused resource. They have gone to university for many years to learn about medications, how they act in your body, and how they interact with each other. Your pharmacist is an expert on medications who will readily answer questions face-to-face, over the phone, or even via e-mail. Pharmacists can be based in, or near your local GP surgery, local chemist, and hospital. As a self-manager, don't forget to seek the advice of your local pharmacist, especially if you need help understanding the instructions on your prescription label

- Are you afraid of the medication's effects or becoming addicted to it?

- Are you embarrassed about taking the medication? Do you view taking it as a sign of weakness or failure, or fear you'll be judged negatively if people know about it?

- What are the benefits you might get if you take the medication as prescribed?

Reading a Prescription Label

Prescription labels can be a great source of information on name, dose, appearance, how to take, precautions, and more. The label will repeat the verbal instructions for using the medication that your doctor will have given you. The label will provide all the information you need to ensure you take the medication safely.

Remembering to Take Your Medicines

If forgetting to take your medications is a problem, here are some suggestions to help you remember:

- **Make it obvious.** Place the medication or a reminder next to your toothbrush, on the breakfast table, in your lunch box, or some other place where you're likely to 'stumble over' it. Be careful where you put the medication if children are around. Or put a reminder note on the bathroom mirror, toothbrush, fridge door, coffee machine, television, or some other obvious place. If you link taking the medication with some well-established habit such as mealtimes, brushing your teeth, or watching your favourite television show, you'll be more likely to remember.

- **Use a checklist or an organiser.** Make a medication chart listing each medication you are taking and the time when you take it. Check off each medication on a calendar as you take it. You might also buy a medication organiser at the pharmacy. This container separates pills according to the time of day they should be taken. You can fill the organiser once a week so that all your pills are ready to take at the proper time. A quick glance at the organiser lets you know if you have missed any doses and prevents double dosing. Some pharmacy services are now able to sort and pre-package medications for each day in 'blister' packs. There are also websites that have charts you can print to help you track your medications.

- **Use an electronic reminder.** Get a watch or mobile phone that you can set to beep at pill-taking time. There are also electronic medication containers that beep at pre-set times to remind you. If you have a smartphone, you can download apps that remind you to take your medication at the right times.

- **Have others remind you.** Ask members of your household to remind you to take your medications at the right times.

- **Don't run out.** Don't let yourself run out of your medicines. When you get a new prescription, add a reminder to your calendar on the date one week before your medications will run out. This will remind you to order a repeat prescription. Don't wait until you take the last pill to order more. Most prescriptions are now electronic, which means you do not have to go into your GP surgery to get a repeat prescription. You can order your medicine online and get it delivered to you or collect it from a pharmacy (see the 'Useful Websites' section at the end of this chapter for more information about how to order repeat prescriptions online.)

- **Plan before you travel.** There are a number of things you need to be aware of if you plan to travel (some relating to short trips others to much longer ones).

  ▸ Talk to your GP at least 2 months ahead of your trip so you will be aware of any special arrangements you need to make.

  ▸ Check the rules for taking your medication out of the UK and into the country you are travelling to.

  ▸ Be aware that some over-the-counter medicines that you may have bought in the UK may be controlled in other countries and vice versa.

  ▸ Always carry your medication in a correctly labelled container.

  ▸ Carry your medication in your hand luggage but also take spare medication in your luggage in case one or the other is lost.

  ▸ It's a good idea to carry a copy of your prescription with you and a letter from your GP explaining the details of your medicine and the condition(s) for which you are taking them.

  ▸ Check the NHS website for guides to healthcare in other countries inside and outside the European Union (see the 'Useful Websites' section at the end of this chapter).

  ▸ Make sure you have the correct travel insurance and especially the cover relating to pre-existing medical conditions. This will be even more important from 1 January 2021, when the Brexit transition period comes to an end. The GOV.UK website has a comprehensive guide to foreign travel insurance which you can access at https://www.gov.uk/guidance/foreign-travel-insurance.

Taking Non-Prescription or Over-the-Counter Medications

You may take non-prescription or over-the-counter (OTC) medications or herbs. Many OTC medications are highly effective and may even be recommended by your doctor. But if you take non-prescription medicines and supplements, you should know what you are taking, why you are taking it, and how to use these products wisely.

The main message of medication advertising is that for every symptom, every ache and pain, and every problem, there is an OTC solution. Although many OTC products are effective, they may keep you from managing your condition in other less medication-centred ways. They may also interfere or interact with your prescription medications.

Whether you are taking prescribed medications or using OTC medications or herbs, here are some helpful suggestions:

- **If you are pregnant or breastfeeding, have a long-term condition, or are already tak-**

ing multiple medications, consult your GP or pharmacist before self-medicating.

■ **Always read medication labels and follow directions carefully.** Reading the label and reviewing the individual ingredients may prevent you from taking medications that have caused problems for you in the past. If you don't understand the information on a product's label, ask a pharmacist or your GP before buying or using the product.

■ **Do not take more than the recommended dose or take it for longer than recommended** unless you have discussed this plan with your doctor.

■ **Be careful if you are taking other medications.** OTC and prescription medications can interact, either cancelling or exaggerating the effects of one or all medications. Ask your doctor or pharmacist before mixing medicines.

■ **Try to select medications with a single active ingredient rather than combination ('all-in-one') products.** If you use a product with multiple ingredients, you are likely to get medications for symptoms you don't even have. Why risk the side effects for medications you don't need? Single-ingredient products also allow you to adjust the dosage of each medication separately for the best symptom relief with the fewest side effects.

■ **Learn the generic names for active ingredients and look for generic products.** Generics contain the same active ingredient as the brand-name product, usually at a lower cost.

■ **Never take a medication from an unlabelled container or a container that** has a label you cannot read. Keep your medications in their original labelled containers or transfer them to a labelled medication organiser or pill dispenser. Do not mix different medications in the same bottle.

■ **Do not take medications that were prescribed for someone else,** even if you have similar symptoms.

■ **Do not share your medications.** The largest source of prescription opioid misuse is medications that are borrowed or stolen from family or friends.

■ **Drink at least a half glass of liquid with your pills** and remain standing or sitting upright for a short while after swallowing. This can prevent the pills from getting stuck.

■ **Store your medications where children or young people cannot find them.** Poisoning from medications is a common and preventable problem. Despite its name, the bathroom medicine cabinet is not usually an appropriate place to store medications. A locked cabinet is far safer.

■ **Make sure you read the instructions on how to store your medications.** For example, in a cool place away from sunlight.

■ **Every medication will have an expiry date. Check this before you take your medicine.** All out-of-date medicines should be taken to your pharmacy for disposal – do not put them in domestic waste or down the toilet.

Medications can help or harm. What often makes the difference is the care you exercise when taking them and the partnership you develop with your doctor when talking about them.

Prescriptions and Prescription Charges

The prescription charges quoted here are correct as of June 2020 and apply to England only (prescriptions are free of charge in Northern Ireland, Wales, and Scotland).

- The current prescription charge is £9.15 per item.

- You can save money by purchasing a Prescription Prepayment Certificate (PPC) for an unlimited number of prescriptions. The charge is £29.65 for 3 months or £105.90 for 12 months (or 10 Direct Debit instalments of £10.59). This means if you're going to buy 4 or more prescriptions in 3 months, or 12 or more prescriptions in 12 months, it may be cheaper to buy a PPC.

- Wigs and fabric supports are available on the NHS, but you will be charged for them unless you qualify for help with charges (see the 'Useful Websites' section at the end of this chapter for more information).

- You may be eligible for free prescriptions, if at the time the prescription is dispensed you:
  - are 60 or over
  - are under 16
  - are aged16 to 18 and in full-time education

  - are pregnant or have had a baby in the previous 12 months and have a valid Maternity Exemption Certificate (MatEx)
  - have a specified medical condition and have a valid Medical Exemption Certificate (MedEx)
  - have a continuing physical disability that prevents you going out without help from another person and have a valid Medical Exemption Certificate (MedEx)
  - hold a valid War Pension Exemption Certificate and the prescription is for your accepted disability
  - are an NHS inpatient
  - are receiving, or your partner is receiving, certain means tested benefits or you're under the age of 20 and the dependant of someone receiving them
  - are entitled to or named on a valid NHS Tax Credit Exemption Certificate
  - are entitled to or named on a valid NHS certificate for full help with health costs (HC2)

There's a simple way to find out if you're eligible for free NHS prescriptions and any help with other NHS costs by using the eligibility checker on the NHS website:

https://www.nhs.uk/using-the-nhs/help-with-health-costs/get-help-with-prescription-costs.get-help-with-prescription-costs.

Using Alcohol and Recreational Drugs

The use of alcohol and recreational drugs (illegal or prescription medications used for nonmedicinal purposes) has been increasing in recent years. These drugs, whether legal or illegal, can cause problems. They can interact with prescription medications, making them less effective or even causing harm. They can fog judgment and cause problems with balance. This can in turn cause accidents and result in injury both to you and others.

In some cases, alcohol or recreational drugs can make existing long-term conditions worse. Alcohol use is associated with higher risk of hypertension, diabetes, gastrointestinal bleeding, sleep disorders, depression, erectile dysfunction, breast and other cancers, and injury. The NHS advises men and women not to drink more than 14 units per week on a regular basis. This is equivalent to drinking no more than 6 pints of average-strength beer (4% ABV) or 7 medium-sized glasses of wine (175ml, 12% ABV) a week. To keep health risks from alcohol at a low level, spread your drinking over 3 or more days if you regularly drink as much as 14 units a week, and if you want to cut down try to have several drink-free days each week. Regularly drinking more than 14 units of alcohol a week risks damaging your health. Avoiding alcohol altogether may be best, depending upon your medical conditions, history, and how you react to alcohol.

According to the NHS, the previously held position that some level of alcohol was good for the heart has been revised. It's now thought that the evidence of a protective effect from moderate drinking is less strong than previously thought. If you drink less than 14 units a week, this is considered low risk drinking. It's called 'low risk' rather than 'safe' because there's no safe drinking

level. To keep health risks from alcohol at 'low risk' follow the guidance set out above.

If you are drinking above the 'low risk' level or are regularly using recreational drugs, seriously consider cutting down or stopping their use. Talk to your doctor. Doctors are often hesitant to raise the issue because they don't want to embarrass you. So it is up to you to bring up the subject. Doctors will be very willing to talk about it. They have heard it all, and they will not think less of you. An honest conversation may save your life.

Using Medical Cannabis

'Medical cannabis' is a broad term used by the NHS for any sort of cannabis-based medicine used to relieve symptoms.

Very few people in England are likely to get a prescription for medical cannabis. You cannot get cannabis-based medicine from a GP; it can only be prescribed by a specialist hospital doctor. As of June 2020 it is only likely to be prescribed for children and adults with rare, severe forms of epilepsy, adults with vomiting or nausea caused by chemotherapy, and people with muscle stiffness and spasms caused by multiple sclerosis (MS). It will only be considered when other treatments were not suitable or had not helped. There is some evidence that medical cannabis can help certain types of pain, though this evidence is not yet strong enough to recommend it for pain relief.

You can find out much more about medical cannabis and cannabis oils by visiting the NHS website, https://www.nhs.uk/conditions/medical-cannabis/.

Useful Websites

Complementary and Natural Healthcare Council: https://www.cnhc.org.uk/

General Chiropractic Council: https://www.gcc-uk.org/

General Osteopathic Council: https://www.osteopathy.org.uk/home/

GOV.UK (Foreign travel insurance): https://www.gov.uk/guidance/foreign-travel-insurance

GOV.UK (Banned and restricted herbal ingredients): https://www.gov.uk/government
/publications/list-of-banned-or-restricted-herbal-ingredients-for-medicinal-use/banned-and
-restricted-herbal-ingredients

Medicines and Healthcare Products Regulatory Authority: www.gov.uk/mhra

National Centre for Integrative Medicine: https://ncim.org.uk/treatments/holistic-doctor

NHS (Am I entitled to free prescriptions?): https://www.nhs.uk/using-the-nhs/help-with-health
-costs/get-help-with-prescription-costs

NHS (Complementary and alternative medicine): https://www.nhs.uk/conditions
/complementary-and-alternative-medicine/

NHS (Herbal medicines): https://www.nhs.uk/conditions/herbal-medicines/

NHS (How to order repeat prescriptions online): https://www.nhs.uk/using-the-nhs/nhs-services
/pharmacies/how-to-order-repeat-prescriptions-online/

NHS (Medical cannabis and cannabis oils): https://www.nhs.uk/conditions/medical-cannabis/

NHS (Medicines A-Z): https://www.nhs.uk/medicines/

NHS (Medicines information): https://www.nhs.uk/conditions/medicines-information/

NHS (The risks of drinking too much): https://www.nhs.uk/live-well/alcohol-support/the-risks
-of-drinking-too-much/

NHS (Travelling and living abroad): https://www.nhs.uk/using-the-nhs/healthcare-abroad
/healthcare-when-travelling-abroad/

NHS (What to expect from your pharmacy team): https://www.nhs.uk/using-the-nhs/nhs-services
/pharmacies/what-to-expect-from-your-pharmacy-team/

NHS (Wigs and fabric supports on the NHS): https://www.nhs.uk/using-the-nhs/help-with
-health-costs/wigs-and-fabric-supports-on-the-nhs/

Patients Association (Understanding your medicines): https://www.patients-association.org.uk
/understanding-your-medicines

Professionals Standards Authority for Health and Social Care: https://www.professionalstandards
.org.uk/what-we-do/accredited-registers/find-a-register

Yellow Card Scheme: https://yellowcard.mhra.gov.uk/the-yellow-card-scheme/

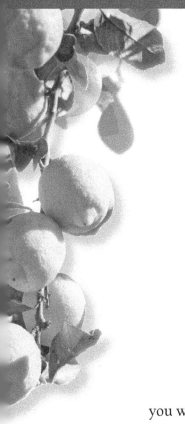

Managing Diabetes

LIVING WELL WITH DIABETES REQUIRES both good medical care and active day-to-day self-management. In this chapter, you will learn about diabetes and tools you need for diabetes self-management.

What Is Diabetes?

There are multiple forms of diabetes – type 1, type 2, and gestational diabetes (which sometimes happens during pregnancy) are the most common. Diabetes occurs when your body cannot properly use the carbohydrate content of the food you eat for energy.

Special thanks to Ann Constance, MA, RDN, CDE, FAADE, Robin Edelman, MS, RDN, CDE, and Yvonne Mullan, MSc, RD, CDE, for contributions to this chapter. For the UK edition special thanks to Catherine Washbrook-Davies BSc (Hons) RD (All Wales Dietetic Lead for Diabetes – Adult), for contributions to this chapter.

Carbohydrates are found in grains, fruits, vegetables, and dairy products. To understand diabetes, it is helpful to know a little about the digestive process, how insulin is made in the pancreas, and how insulin is used by the body's cells (see Figure 14.1).

During digestion, your body breaks down the carbohydrates that you eat or drink into a simple sugar called glucose. Glucose is absorbed into the bloodstream from your stomach and intestines, causing the level of glucose in your blood to rise. The glucose in your blood is also known as blood sugar. For the cells of your body to use the glucose in your blood as fuel, your body needs insulin. Insulin is a hormone. A hormone is a kind of chemical messenger in your body. The pancreas, a small gland located below and behind your stomach, makes insulin. Insulin helps the blood glucose get from the bloodstream into the cells. Once glucose is inside the cells, the cells use the glucose as their energy source.

Glucose in the body can be compared to petrol in a car. Like petrol, glucose is a fuel and a source of energy. Petrol alone, however, is not enough to make the car move. We also need a key to start the car engine, which converts the petrol into energy. Like a car, our bodies also need a key. Insulin is the key that enables us to use glucose as energy. Insulin allows the glucose to pass from the bloodstream into the cells, where it produces energy for the body.

In the bodies of people with diabetes, insulin is not able to carry out this function for one of two reasons:

1. The pancreas makes little or no insulin. This occurs in type 1 diabetes, which must be treated with insulin.

2. The body makes insulin but has trouble using the insulin. This occurs in type 2 diabetes.

In either case, the amount of glucose in the bloodstream remains high (see Table 14.1).

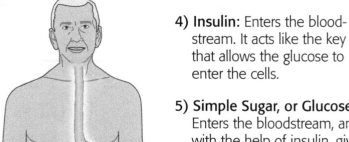

1) **The Mouth:** Starts the process of food intake. Chews and breaks up the food so it can be passed down to the stomach.

2) **The Stomach and Intestines:** Break down the food into simpler substances that the body can absorb, including the simple sugar called glucose.

3) **The Pancreas:** Produces hormones and substances that help with digestion. One of these hormones is insulin.

4) **Insulin:** Enters the bloodstream. It acts like the key that allows the glucose to enter the cells.

5) **Simple Sugar, or Glucose:** Enters the bloodstream, and, with the help of insulin, gives nutrients to the cells, producing energy.

Figure 14.1 **The Digestion Process**

Table 14.1 **Overview of Type 1 and Type 2 Diabetes**

Characteristics	Type 1 Diabetes (insulin dependent)	Type 2 Diabetes (may or may not need insulin and may need other medications)
Age	Usually occurs before age 20, but can occur in adults	Most commonly occurs in adults but can occur at any age
Insulin	Little or no insulin is produced by the pancreas	The cells cannot use insulin normally because they are resistant to its effect. This is called insulin resistance
Onset	Sudden	Slow
Heredity	Some hereditary tendency	Strong hereditary tendency
Weight	Prior to diagnosis, majority experience weight loss and are thin	Carrying extra weight is a risk factor of developing type 2 diabetes
Ketones	Ketones found in the urine	Usually there are no ketones found in the urine
Treatment	Insulin, diet, exercise, and self-management	Diet, exercise, self-management, and, when necessary, medication(s) that may include insulin

When the kidneys filter the blood of people with diabetes, that extra glucose is removed and ends up in the urine. Raised blood glucose levels can lead to a number of symptoms such as frequent urination due to large amounts of glucose sugar in the urine, thirst, and tiredness.

The exact cause of diabetes is not known. Type 1 diabetes usually starts in childhood. It is an autoimmune disease, meaning that for people with type 1 diabetes, the body's immune system doesn't work right and damages the cells in the pancreas that make insulin. Type 2 diabetes, in contrast, does not seem to be an autoimmune disease. It tends to run in families and may result from other factors. These include being overweight, lack of physical activity, and other lifestyle habits. Type 2 diabetes used to be called adult-onset diabetes. However, in recent years more and more teens and even children are developing type 2 diabetes.

Type 2 diabetes is more common among people who are overweight. Excess body fat does not allow the body to properly use insulin. When people have type 2 diabetes, there is an overproduction of insulin due to the body having trouble using the insulin; their bodies are 'resistant' to insulin. This resistance prevents the body from moving the glucose from the blood into the cells, where it can be used as energy. Glucose builds up in the blood because the body cannot use it. Fortunately, we know some ways to manage this type of diabetes, which we discuss later in this chapter.

The key difference between the two types of diabetes is that type 1 requires the person to use insulin every day, whereas most people with type 2 may not initially need insulin to control their diabetes. However, if blood glucose levels cannot be controlled with diet, exercise, and non-insulin medications, using insulin can be tremendously helpful in type 2 diabetes.

Diagnosing Diabetes

Healthcare professionals usually diagnose diabetes when a person has elevated blood glucose levels. Doctors will also diagnose diabetes using the haemoglobin A1C blood test, which is commonly known in the UK as the HbA1c test. The HbA1c test measures average blood glucose over the past 2 to 3 months. The HbA1c test will also be used to find out how well your treatment programme is working. In 2011 the system for expressing the results of HbA1c was changed in the UK. It was previously given as a percentage but is now given as millimoles of HbA1c per mol of haemoglobin. For example, 6% is now expressed as 42 mmol/mol, as you can see from Table 14.2.

Diabetes UK recommends that people with diabetes should have a HbA1c level of 48 mmol/mol (6.5%) or below. However, they also acknowledge that everyone is different and that people should talk to their healthcare team about setting an individual target level that is

Table 14.2 **Measuring HbA1c Blood Glucose Levels**

(%)	(mmol/mol)
6.0	42
6.5	48
7.0	53
7.5	58
8.0	64
9.0	75

right for you. In the UK, HbA1c levels between 42 and 47 mmol/mol (6.0% and 6.4%) are considered prediabetes. (For more on prediabetes, see pages 331–332.) For people with diabetes, the usual aim is to keep HbA1c at or below 48 mmol/mol (6.5%). Some doctors recommend a slightly higher goal for certain people, especially for those who are over 65 years old and have other health conditions. Most people with diabetes will have the HbA1c test every 3 to 6 months. It is recommended that you have the HbA1c test at least once per year. Your healthcare team will arrange this for you, but chase it up with your GP if you haven't had one for a few

Symptoms of Diabetes

Some people with diabetes have no symptoms, while others have some or all of the following symptoms:

- extreme tiredness
- extreme thirst
- frequent urination, especially at night
- blurry vision or a change in vision
- increased hunger

- unintentional weight loss
- sores or cuts that heal slowly
- numbness or tingling in the feet
- frequent infections of skin, gums, bladder, or vagina (yeast infections)

Table 14.3 **HbA1c as an Indicator of Diabetes Control**

HbA1c	mmol/mol	%
Normal	Below 42 mmol/mol	Below 6.0%
Prediabetes	42 to 47 mmol/mol	6.0% to 6.4%
Diabetes	48 mmol/mol or over	6.5% or over

months. You may need one more often if you're planning for a baby, if you are adjusting to your treatment plan, or you're having problems managing your blood glucose levels. People with prediabetes should be checked for diabetes at least once a year. Other adults should get checked for diabetes and prediabetes at least every 3 years, starting at age 45. Many GP practices are now screening adults aged 45 to 75 years old who are overweight and have one or more diabetes risk factors for diabetes/prediabetes.

Preventing Type 2 Diabetes

Type 2 diabetes is a growing epidemic. Like most long-term conditions, diabetes does not happen overnight. Instead it happens slowly over time. Many people have a condition known as prediabetes. People are usually diagnosed with prediabetes if their HbA1c results are 42 to 47 mmol/mol (6.0% to 6.4%). This means that their blood glucose levels are higher than normal but not high enough to be diagnosed as having diabetes.

Prediabetes is an early warning sign. However, maintaining a healthy weight and being physically active can often reverse prediabetes and delay or prevent the development of type 2 diabetes. If you have prediabetes, the single most important thing you can do is prevent diabetes by using self-management tools. If you are overweight, losing 5% of your weight can help

prevent diabetes. This is a 10-pound (4.5kg) loss for a 14-stone (90kg) person. Along with the weight loss, being physically active for 150 minutes a week has been shown to drastically lower your risk of developing type 2 diabetes. The self-management advice for prediabetes and diabetes is very similar. One difference is that self-monitoring blood glucose is not necessary for those with prediabetes.

You are at risk for prediabetes and type 2 diabetes if you:

- are overweight or obese, especially if you are large around the middle

- are over age 40, or over 25 if you are African-Caribbean, Black African, or South Asian

- have a parent, brother, sister, or child with type 2 diabetes

- are a member of a higher-risk population group (African-Caribbean, Black African, or South Asian)

- have a history of heart disease or stroke

- have ever had high blood pressure (140/90 or above) or are taking medication for high blood pressure

- have blood glucose levels that are 5.5 to 6.9 mmol/L or HbA1c equal to 42 to 47 mmol/mol. (This is a prediabetes level that indicates need for checking for diabetes.)

- have an HDL cholesterol (good cholesterol) level less than 1 mmol/L and/or a triglyceride (a combination of fatty acids and glycerol used by the body for energy)' level greater than 2.3 mmol/L.

- are a woman with polycystic ovary syndrome or previous gestational diabetes (diabetes that started during pregnancy) or a large baby (weighing 9 pounds or more)

- are not physically active

- have acanthosis nigricans (thick, velvety skin around neck or armpits)

- drink alcohol beyond the recommended guidelines

- are a smoker

If you think you are at risk for diabetes, talk

In the UK, the standard unit of measure for blood glucose, cholesterol, and triglycerides is millimoles per litre (mmol/L).

with your GP. Knowing early about prediabetes can help prevent type 2 diabetes. Even if you do not have prediabetes, you can reduce your risk factors by lowering your blood pressure; losing weight; eating fewer processed foods and more whole grains, nuts, fruits, vegetables, and beans and pulses; and becoming more physically active. Depression can increase your risk for diabetes. More information about recognising and treating depression is available on pages 117–122. Not smoking is also important, as smoking has been linked to developing diabetes. You can find more advice on pages 109–113 in Chapter 5, *Understanding and Managing Common Symptoms and Emotions*.

Diabetes Self-Management

Successful diabetes management involves maintaining blood glucose levels in a safe range, detecting early problems, and taking action to prevent complications. You need to work closely with your doctor and healthcare team and practice effective self-management. The tools in your self-management toolbox, such as problem solving, decision making, and action planning, can be very important in helping you manage your diabetes. Recall from Chapter 2 that these are the tools that help you to decide which other tools work best for you, as well as when and how to use your tools successfully. You can add to your toolbox with additional

skills and strategies to manage diabetes, including the following:

- Observe symptoms, monitor your blood glucose (where appropriate), and know how to respond to changes.

- Prevent dehydration.

- Follow a healthy eating plan.

- Be physically active.

- Manage stress and emotions.

- Manage sick days, infections, and other illnesses.

- Use prescribed medications in a safe and effective way to control blood glucose, blood pressure, and cholesterol, and to prevent complications.

▪ Get necessary tests, examinations, and immunisations.

▪ Wear an emergency alert necklace or bracelet.

Note the last item. It is recommended that people with diabetes who take certain diabetes medications wear an emergency alert necklace or bracelet or carry an emergency card in their wallet (or both). The emergency card should list information about the medications you are taking, your GP's contact information, and an emergency contact person's name and telephone number. The MedicAlert Foundation UK provides a range of medical ID services (see the 'Useful Websites' section at the end of this chapter for more details.) Also, if you use insulin or a medication that can cause low blood glucose, always carry a 'hypo treatment' or 'remedy food' or fast-acting carbohydrate source (see page 334) with you to quickly manage low blood glucose.

In this chapter, we address all of these in detail.

Observing Symptoms, Monitoring Your Blood Glucose Level, and Taking Action

The goal of diabetes management is to keep blood glucose levels in a target range. The target level differs for different people. Ask your doctor what range is best for you. Sometimes blood glucose levels get too high. This is called hyperglycaemia. Sometimes levels are too low. This is called hypoglycaemia.

Hyperglycaemia and Hypoglycaemia

The causes of hyperglycaemia and hypoglycaemia include the following:

Hyperglycaemia:

▪ too little medication, including insulin

▪ too much carbohydrate

▪ too little physical activity

▪ illness, infection, or surgery

▪ emotional stress

Hypoglycaemia:

▪ too much medication

▪ missing or skipping meals (if you take medication to manage your diabetes)

▪ too little food, especially carbohydrates

▪ unplanned activity over and above your usual amount

▪ drinking alcohol on an empty stomach (if you take medication to manage your diabetes)

As you can see in Table 14.4 on pages 334 –335, the symptoms of high and low blood glucose are often the same. It is critically important that you learn to recognise the symptoms, take action, and know when and how to seek medical assistance.

Table 14.4 **Hyperglycaemia and Hypoglycaemia***

	Hyperglycaemia (blood glucose too high)	Hypoglycaemia (blood glucose too low)
Symptoms	Extreme tiredness Extreme thirst Blurry vision or a change in vision Increased hunger Increased need to urinate	Feeling sweaty, shaky, or dizzy Hard, fast heartbeat Headache Confusion, irritability, or sudden change in mood Tingling around your mouth, tongue, or lips or in your fingers
What to do if you suspect this condition**	If your blood glucose is greater than 7.0 mmol/L when fasting or above 9.0 mmol/L 2 hours after a meal, or if you cannot check your blood glucose and think you have high blood glucose, take the following actions immediately: Drink water or other sugar-free liquids to prevent dehydration. Consider what may have caused the rise (refer to the causes of hyperglycaemia listed on page 333). If possible, continue to check your blood glucose every 2 to 4 hours. If you have type 1 diabetes, check blood or urine for ketones. Contact your GP surgery or NHS 111 right away if you have moderate to high ketone levels and don't know what to do. Seek immediate medical attention if you develop any of the symptoms described below.	If you feel symptoms of low blood glucose, check your blood glucose immediately. If your blood glucose is below 4 mmol/L† or if you cannot test your blood glucose and think you have low blood glucose, take the following actions: Eat or drink a 'remedy food' that contains 15 grams to 20 grams of fast-acting carbohydrate – or example, 3 glucose tablets, 5 jelly babies, a small carton of pure fruit juice, or 150ml of full-glucose fizzy drink (NOT DIET OR SUGAR FREE). Avoid using foods that contain fat (such as a chocolate bar) or protein (such as milk) to treat low blood glucose. Wait 15 minutes, note your symptoms, and, if possible, check your blood glucose again. After 15 minutes, if your blood glucose level is still less than 4 mmol/L, eat another remedy food and wait 15 minutes.

*Depending on your condition and history, your doctor may provide you with slightly different instructions for managing high or low blood glucose .

**Those with type 1 diabetes and hyperglycaemia will also want to check for ketones and contact a healthcare professional immediately if the ketones are moderate to high. For those with type 1 diabetes and hypoglycaemia, it is important to know about how and when to use glucagon. (A glucagon injection kit is used to treat episodes of severe hypoglycaemia, where a patient is either unable to treat themselves or treatment by mouth has not been successful).

†Some people who have overall high blood glucose (over 10 mmol/L) experience symptoms of hypoglycaemia with blood glucose slightly higher than 4 mmol/L. This is another reason why it is important for you to check your blood glucose, know your body, and learn how you feel at different levels.

Table 14.4 **Hyperglycaemia and Hypoglycaemia** (*continued*)

	Hyperglycaemia (blood glucose too high)	**Hypoglycaemia (blood glucose too low)**
What to do if you suspect this condition (continued)	See page 334.	If your blood glucose doesn't go above 4 mmol/L despite repeated treatments, someone should call 999. Do not wait – it is critical to get immediate medical help. If your blood glucose is above 4 mmol/L and your next meal is more than 1 hour away, or if you are going to be active, eat a meal or a snack such as half a sandwich, a few crackers, bowl of cereal, glass of milk, or a piece of fruit. If you know or think you have hypoglycaemia, do not start driving until you have treated yourself, retested, and your blood glucose is at least 5 mmol/L. Wait at least 40 minutes before driving.
When to call your GP or seek immediate medical help	If you feel confused, disoriented, agitated, or weak If you are unable to eat or drink any carbohydrate-containing food or fluids, go directly to A&E. You cannot safely treat this at home! If you have symptoms of dehydration, such as extreme thirst, dry mouth, and cracked lips, or have not urinated for 8 hours If you have stomach pain and nausea that doesn't go away If you are running a fever If you vomit 2 times or more in a 12-hour period If you have diarrhoea that does not stop or is getting worse If you have a cold, infection, or flu that is getting worse If you have a strong, fruity breath odour (that smells like nail polish or acetone) If your breathing is rapid and deep If your blood glucose level is over 16.6 mmol/L for 8 hours or is much higher than usual	If you have slurred speech, poor coordination, or clumsy movements If you have seizures or loss of consciousness If you are confused or disoriented If your symptoms are not better after repeating the 'what to do' steps If you have low glucose (less than 3.3 mmol/L) twice in one day If your blood glucose is repeatedly lower than usual without cause

Although it is important to learn to recognise how you feel when your blood glucose is very low or high, feelings are not a reliable way to manage diabetes. Many people do not have symptoms until their blood glucose is very high or low. Some people with diabetes are not aware of symptoms or may not link the symptoms to their blood glucose levels. This makes it very difficult to stay within their appropriate blood glucose range. If you don't know your actual blood glucose level, you don't know if your levels are too low or too high, so you won't know what to do. The only way for you to know your blood glucose level is to monitor it.

Blood Glucose Monitoring

Management of diabetes involves keeping blood glucose in a safe range. If you are on certain diabetes medications you will have been provided with a blood glucose monitor, and this can be used to tell if your blood glucose level is in a safe range. Monitoring is not a treatment. It is a tool to find out how you are doing. If you know your levels, you can make any needed day-to-day changes in diet and exercise, as well as changes in your medications, as recommended by your healthcare team.

Depending on your medications, your type of diabetes, and what you want to know, blood glucose monitoring can be done in different ways. Be sure to get instructions on how to monitor your blood glucose levels and what equipment you will need. This will ensure accurate results. Get specific instructions from your GP, practice nurse, or diabetes nurse.

These are the ways to monitor blood glucose levels:

- **Home blood glucose monitoring.** This is done by obtaining a small drop of blood (usually from a prick of a fingertip), placing the drop on a blood glucose strip, and putting the strip in a glucose meter to assess the glucose level. This self-check is easy to do at home or almost anywhere. It may be done a few times a week, once a day, or from 4 to 6 times per day, depending on how your diabetes is being managed. A glucose meter is about half the size of a mobile phone, or even smaller. You can carry one with you wherever you go.

- **Continuous glucose monitoring and flash glucose monitoring for people using insulin and insulin pumps.** In this type of monitoring, a glucose sensor under the skin provides ongoing glucose measurements. These sensors generally need to be replaced every 7 to 14 days. How often you replace your sensor depends on the type you are using. Some monitors have a separate reader, and others let you check your glucose using your mobile phone. Some let you avoid finger sticks. It is especially helpful to have your GP, a nurse, pharmacist, or diabetes nurse observe your technique and give you tips. There is also a system that works with an insulin pump to help you control your blood glucose. Stay in contact with your healthcare team, as there are constantly changes and improvements in this area.

■ **HbA1c blood test.** Your healthcare professional orders this test. The test is done at your GP surgery. The results show your average blood glucose levels over approximately 3 months. For people with diabetes, a reasonable HbA1c goal may be 48mmol/mol to 52mmol/mol. For people with a history of low blood glucose, people with several long-term conditions, and some older people, a higher HbA1c target may be appropriate. Talk with your GP about the best target for you.

Most home blood glucose meters and continuous glucose monitors allow you to upload the results to a computer and can give you multiple displays of your glucose information in special reports. You and your healthcare professional can use this feature to help you better manage your diabetes. If you use insulin, home glucose monitoring, or a continuous or flash glucose monitor, these reports contain valuable feedback for adjusting your insulin timing and dosage.

Blood glucose monitoring is a useful tool to help you manage your diabetes. It can help you learn more about the following:

■ if you think you might have low or high blood glucose

■ if you want to know how diabetes medication or insulin changes affect your blood glucose

■ if you want to know how eating, exercise, and emotions affect your blood glucose

■ if you are sick and not sure what is happening with your blood glucose

■ if you want to know how you are doing day to day

How often should I monitor?

How often you check your blood glucose depends on how you and your healthcare team are going to use the information. Remember, monitoring is not a treatment. Monitoring gives you information so that you can make changes if you need to do so. You may want to monitor several times a day or perhaps once a week. If you use insulin more than once a day or are using an insulin pump, you may have been recommended to monitor more frequently, for example, at least four times per day. Monitor any time you want to know how you are doing with your self-management plan. There are a few times when it is especially important to monitor, including these:

■ when you start a new medication

■ when you change the dose of a medication

■ any time you think you might have low or high blood glucose

■ when you are sick

The important thing about monitoring is that the information is for you. Blood glucose levels change often throughout the day and night. Monitoring shows you how your eating, exercise, medications, stress, illness, and infections affect your blood glucose. Checking your own blood glucose gives you and your healthcare professionals more flexibility when you are making decisions about how to control your blood glucose levels. Checking your blood glucose also helps you evaluate and take action if the levels are too high or too low (see pages 334–335).

You may also be instructed by your GP or diabetes nurse on how to check your urine at home for ketones if your blood glucose tends to be high. Ketones in the urine are a sign that your body is using fat for energy instead of using glucose because you do not have enough insulin to use glucose for energy. This is especially important for people with type 1 diabetes, as high ketones may be serious and life threatening.

Blood glucose targets

When you monitor your own blood glucose, it is important to know your targets for various times of the day. Talk with your GP about your personal targets. For many people, blood glucose targets are as follows:

- before a meal, including in the morning after fasting: 4.4 to 7.2 mmol/L.

- two hours after a meal: less than 10 mmol/L.

If these are your targets, the goal is to have as many blood glucose values between 4.4 to 10 mmol/L as possible.

Remember that your GP may recommend slightly different targets for you.

Blood glucose naturally rises and falls during the day. It is usually highest an hour or two after you eat. Your target range is likely from a low of about 4.4 mmol/L (first thing in the morning) to a high of 10 mmol/L after meals. Do not be concerned if your blood glucose fluctuates within this target range.

Experimenting to learn more and improve self-management

One way to learn more about your blood glucose is to do an experiment. If you have a blood glucose meter, you may want to do the following:

On two days – one weekday and one weekend day – monitor your blood glucose five times. Take measurements at the following times:

- first thing in the morning before eating

- before a meal

- 2 hours after a meal

- before exercising

- after exercising

- before going to bed

We know that this is a lot of finger pricking! However, if you do this only a couple of days, you and your healthcare professionals will learn a lot. Plot your blood glucose levels on the 'Your Blood Glucose Profile' chart on page 340 (or make copies of the chart to use). If there are things about these numbers that you do not understand, or if you want help to figure out what these numbers mean, talk with your GP, nurse or dietician.

Again, do not be concerned if your blood glucose fluctuates within your target range. The important thing is that your numbers be about the same each day in relationship to the same activities (for example, your numbers should be about the same both days an hour or two after meals or after exercising).

The dawn effect

If you have been managing your diabetes (eating well, exercising, and taking your medication) and your early morning blood glucose is almost always high, talk to your GP. Some people go to bed with blood glucose in their target range but then find that the levels are much higher in the morning. This is known as the 'dawn effect' or 'dawn phenomenon'. Blood glucose levels may rise a few hours before getting up in the morning in response to the release of hormones and extra glucose from the liver. If you think you have the 'dawn effect', you are not a self-management failure. This is just the way the body sometimes works. To prevent or correct high blood glucose levels in the morning, your GP may adjust your dosage of medication or insulin or switch you to a different medication. This adjustment will be based on the results of blood testing throughout the night.

Preventing Dehydration

Dehydration (not having enough fluid in your body) can be a special problem for people with diabetes. Common symptoms of dehydration include the following:

- Infrequent urination. If you have not urinated over a period of 8 hours you may be dehydrated. However, know that because your body is trying to get rid of excess glucose, you can be dehydrated and still be urinating.
- Dry mouth.
- Dizziness when you move or change positions, particularly when you stand.
- Nausea. (This can also be a sign of infection, ketosis, or a more serious problem.)

To prevent dehydration, drink water and other non-sugary fluids frequently throughout the day. Coffee and tea (with or without caffeine) may also be used to help prevent dehydration. See the recommendations to check the colour of your urine on page 250 to help you know if you are drinking enough.

Healthy Eating

Healthy eating is the core of diabetes self-management. You are the only one who can manage your blood glucose levels. The good news is that this is not as hard as it might seem. Small changes in your eating can help improve your blood glucose levels and how you feel. If you have diabetes, you may need to be more careful than other people about what you eat. However, you do not have to go hungry. You do not need to eat special foods. You can still eat the foods you like. Healthy eating for diabetes is also healthy eating for your whole family. In Chapter 10, *Healthy Eating*, you will find information about healthy foods and eating habits.

There are three basics to healthy eating while managing diabetes:

- what you eat
- how much you eat
- when you eat

Your Blood Glucose Profile

Use the following table to plot your blood glucose profile.
Then ask yourself the questions below it.

My Daily Blood Glucose Results

Day 1

When Tested	Time of Day	Blood Glucose Level (mmol/L)
First thing in the morning (before eating or taking medicine)		
Before a meal		
2 hours after lunch or dinner		
Before exercising		
After exercising		

Day 2

When Tested	Time of Day	Blood Glucose Level (mmol/L)
First thing in the morning (before eating or taking medicine)		
Before a meal		
2 hours after lunch or dinner		
Before exercising		
After exercising		

Questions to Ask Yourself

- Are your blood glucose levels within the recommended range?

- Are any of your numbers under or over your recommended target?

- Do you notice any daily pattern(s)?

- Are there specific times during the day that your blood glucose is lower than your target range?

- Are there specific times during the day that your blood glucose is higher than your target range?

- Can you think of any reasons why your blood glucose levels change as they do?

What to Eat if You Have Diabetes

All the food you eat affects your blood glucose levels. However, carbohydrate (carbs) is the nutrient that determines your blood glucose levels the most. (You can read more about carbohydrates in Chapter 10, *Healthy Eating*, on pages 246–247.) Your job is to monitor your carbs, especially refined carbohydrates such as sugar, foods made with white flour, and fizzy drinks and juices that are not made with reduced sugar or calories. During processing, refined grains lose healthy, naturally occurring nutrients. Sugar and other refined carbs are often added to processed foods to give them flavour and texture, so it is good to eat fewer of these foods.

To learn more about managing your eating plan, spend some time with a member of your diabetes healthcare team. These healthcare professionals have been specially trained to teach diabetes management. A dietitian is a qualified health professional who, as well as providing general health advice, can also work with people with special dietary needs (due to health conditions) tailor their eating plan to their lifestyle and develop individualised meal plans to help meet their goals. You can ask to be referred to a registered dietitian in your local area by contacting your local hospital or GP surgery. Some dietetic departments also accept self-referrals. The title 'dietitian' is protected by law. This means that you're not allowed to call yourself a dietitian unless you're properly qualified and registered with the Health and Care Professions Council (HCPC) (see the 'Useful Websites' section at the end of this chapter for more details).

Vegetables, fruits, and whole grains provide you with essential nutrients such as fibre and healthy fats and are lower in energy compared to many processed foods. Limit refined carbohydrates and high-carbohydrate snacks, such as chocolate, cakes, biscuits, regular (non-diet) fizzy drinks, and ice cream. These raise blood glucose levels and add calories without providing healthy nutrients. Moderation is the key to successful management of blood glucose. We are not saying you can't ever have these foods if you like them, but it is helpful to limit them in your diet. If you do eat cake or another high-carb food at a meal, consider limiting other carbs at that meal. Review the content on carbohydrates and nutrition labels in Chapter 10, *Healthy Eating*, on pages 241–242. Knowing how to read a food label and the ingredients list will help you know the difference between high- and low-carb foods. A good starting place for people with diabetes is to keep the total grams of carbohydrates per meal between 45 and 60. Your age and activity levels will affect the amount of carbohydrate you need. Some people with repeated high blood glucose levels successfully manage their levels by eating fewer carbohydrates.

Planning meals when you have diabetes may sound complicated, but here's a simple tip for healthy eating. Use the Eatwell Guide developed by the Food Standards Agency (Figure 14.2) to plan your meals. As the Diabetes UK website explains, the Eatwell Guide aims to make it easier for you to identify foods you should try to eat more of, foods you should aim to eat less of, and how much of what you eat overall should come from which food group. Following the guidelines can help with effective diabetes management, encouraging you to make healthier choices for your body. When using the Eatwell Guide try to choose a variety of different

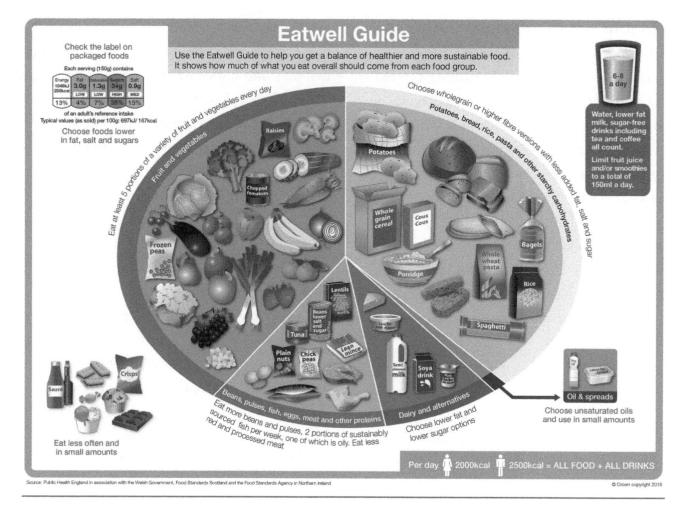

Figure 14.2 **The Eatwell Guide**

foods from each of the five main food groups to help you get the wide range of nutrients your body needs to stay healthy. Remember that, as a person living with diabetes, you might want to check with your healthcare team, or with a registered dietitian, on how to adapt the Eatwell Guide to meet your own individual needs.

The Mediterranean and DASH (Dietary Approaches to Stop Hypertension) diet plans also help you choose healthier carbohydrates: whole grains, fruits, vegetables, and healthy choices of protein. These diet plans have been shown to help people with diabetes. The Diabetes UK website has information about the Mediterranean plan and a selection of meal plans for people living with diabetes. Please see the 'Useful Websites' section at the end of this chapter to find out more about diet plans, including the Mediterranean and DASH plans.

How Much to Eat if You Have Diabetes

What you eat is just part of the picture. You may choose healthy foods but still not be eating healthfully. Many of us eat too much. To control how much you eat, be aware of the portions of the foods you eat. Understanding what a recommended portion size is for each food group in the Eatwell Guide can help you to achieve a well-balanced diet. See Figure 10.2 in Chapter 10, *Healthy Eating*, on page 239 for a handy guide to getting portion sizes right.

A serving is how much you actually eat. If you eat a small bowl of ice cream, that is your serving. However, if you eat a half carton of ice cream, that is also your serving (and a likely cause of extra weight gain).

You need to be aware that sometimes the terms 'portion' and 'serving' are used the other way around, (especially in information originating from the United States). So on some food labels 'portions' are called 'servings'. This can all be very confusing!

So, a portion is the amount of food that appears on a food list, meal plan, or nutrition label. Many people eat more than a single portion of food. If you are like most people, you may benefit from eating smaller servings. You can learn more about portions and serving sizes in the discussion 'The Importance of Food Labels' in Chapter 10, *Healthy Eating*, on pages 239–241.

Choose to put the recommended portion size on your plate. The portion size is different for every food. A good starting place for people with diabetes is to keep your total grams of carbohydrates per meal in the range of 45 to 60; some may find that lower carb meals help with blood glucose control. A registered dietitian can help you set personalised carbohydrate targets for meals and snacks.

To learn more about the portions you are eating, try an experiment. Measure how much carbohydrate-dense foods (such as cereal, rice, pasta, beans, ice cream, fruit, and milk) you eat or drink each time you sit down to enjoy these foods. Measure your serving using a food scale or measuring cup and compare the amount you eat to the portion size on the package. How many carbohydrates are you eating?

Being aware of portion size is also important when you are trying to lose weight. Just as you can check out the number of carbohydrates in your servings, you can also check out the number of calories. The number of calories in a standard portion (not serving) is listed on the nutrition label. If you are eating several portions, you are eating more calories. And the more calories you eat, the less likely you are to lose weight. In fact, when you eat more calories than your body needs you gain weight. By cutting back on your portion and serving sizes, you are also cutting your calories. The British Nutrition Foundation has produced a guide to help people *Get Portion Wise*. The guide contains a useful reference for understanding and measuring your portions. See the 'Useful Websites' section at the end of this chapter for more information.

When to Eat If You Have Diabetes

Some people with diabetes find it helpful to eat smaller meals every 4 to 5 hours. Be sure not to skip breakfast. This is when your body most needs fuel, as you have not eaten for a long time. Eating smaller meals more frequently is an easy way to spread your carbs throughout the day and to make sure that you do not get too hungry.

Some Special Considerations About Healthy Eating and Diabetes

Here are some additional suggestions for people with diabetes:

- Unfortunately, diabetes, cardiovascular disease, and stroke often go together. For this reason, it is very important that people with diabetes eat a heart-healthy diet. Using the Eatwell Guide (page 342) can help with effective diabetes management. The Mediterranean and DASH diet plans (page 342) are also heart-healthy. Learn more in the section 'Heart Disease and Stroke and Healthy Eating' in Chapter 10, *Healthy Eating*, pages 263–264.

- The salt recommendations for people with diabetes are the same as for everyone else: a maximum of 6 grams (that's around 1 teaspoon) a day.

- Sweeteners with few or no calories have not been shown to help with blood glucose control. However, substituting sugar with these sweeteners can help lower the carbohydrate content of many different foods and drinks. Sugar alcohols or polyols (for example, sorbitol), contain about 50% of the calories contained in sugar. Polyols are usually used in products marketed as 'diabetic' or 'suitable for diabetics' and, as these products can be as high in fat and calories as standard products, Diabetes

UK and the European Commission Regulations don't recommend them. Consuming large amounts of polyols can have a laxative effect, causing bloating, flatulence, and diarrhoea. Most other sugar substitutes contain very few calories. Diabetes UK suggest that if you do decide to use sweeteners, but you're unsure, speak to your diabetes healthcare team for individual advice, and check nutrition labels and ingredients on food packaging, as this can help you to make informed choices.

- Diabetes UK encourages drinking water to quench one's thirst (make water your beverage of choice). They also recommend that you stay hydrated by drinking milk, tea, herbal teas, coffee, chai, and hot chocolate (cut back on sugar and use semi-skimmed or skimmed milk). However, if you have been drinking fizzy sugary drinks, replacing these with sugar-free alternatives may help lower how many calories and how much carbohydrate you are taking in.

- Moderate alcohol use has the same effects on people with diabetes as it has on the general population. The NHS advises men and women not to drink more than 14 units per week on a regular basis. This is equivalent to drinking no more than 6 pints of average-strength beer (4% ABV) or 7 medium-sized glasses of wine (175ml, 12% ABV) a week. To keep health risks from alcohol at a low level, spread your drinking over 3 or more days if you regularly drink as much as 14 units a week and if you want to cut down, try to have several drink-free days each week. Alcohol can lead to hypoglycaemia, especially for those who use insulin or medications like sulfonylureas; low blood glucose can occur several hours after drinking alcohol. Alcohol also adds calories that can lead to weight gain. If you do drink, make sure you eat food when you have a drink to help avoid a low blood glucose reaction. Check your blood glucose to see how alcohol affects you.

■ Vitamins and mineral supplements have not been shown to improve diabetes outcomes for people who do not have vitamin deficiencies. People who take metformin should be checked once a year for B_{12} deficiencies. People in some circumstances such as planning a pregnancy, treating a new condition, or following an eating plan that restricts specific food groups can ask their health providers whether a multivitamin supplement is recommended.

Being Physically Active

Exercise helps people with type 2 diabetes in several ways. Mild to moderate aerobic exercise decreases your need for insulin and helps control your blood glucose levels. It does this by increasing the sensitivity of your body cells to insulin and lowering your blood glucose levels both during and after exercise. Regular exercise is also essential for weight management and reducing cardiovascular risk factors, such as high levels of blood lipids (cholesterol and triglycerides) and high blood pressure. However, exercise alone does not improve blood glucose control for people who manage their diabetes with insulin; they need to learn how to adjust their carbohydrate portions or their insulin when they are going to be active. Speak to your healthcare team before starting a new exercise routine. Experts agree that exercise is important in achieving overall health goals for people with any type of diabetes.

The exercise programme recommended for people with diabetes is generally the same as the endurance exercise programme described in Chapter 7, *Being Physically Active*. In Chapter 7, we discussed how there are four major types of exercise: endurance, flexibility, strength, and balance (see pages 166–167). Adults should do moderate endurance (aerobic) exercise for at least 150 minutes (2.5 hours) each week or vigorous intensity activity for at least 75 minutes each week. Try not go more than 2 days without exercising. In addition, you should take part in strength training (exercises with weight or weight machines or resistance training) 2 or more days a week. Do not do strength training 2 days in a row. If you would like to do more vigorous exercise – for example, if you wish to run a marathon – check with your healthcare team, as you may need to adjust your eating or medications (or both). Balance and flexibility training are also recommended for people with diabetes, especially for older people. You can find much more information and suggested exercises in

Chapter 7, *Being Physically Active*, and Chapter 8, *Exercising to Make Life Easier*.

Additional considerations for people with diabetes include the following:

- Keep in touch with your healthcare professional or diabetes nurse to make changes to your medication and eating plan if needed.

- Coordinate eating, medication, and exercise to avoid hypoglycaemia (low blood glucose).

- If you are able, check your blood glucose levels before and after exercise so that you develop a sense of how your body responds to exercise.

- If you take a medication that can cause low blood glucose, plan to be active within an hour after eating your meals or snacks to prevent low blood glucose. You may need to reduce your insulin dose on days that you are exercising. Speak to your healthcare professional or diabetes nurse to learn more

about the best option for you. Carry a 'hypo treatment remedy food' when you exercise (see page 334).

- If you take insulin and your blood glucose is less than 5.6 mmol/L before exercising, eat 15 to 20 grams of carbohydrate for every 30 minutes of moderate to intense activity unless advised otherwise by your healthcare team.

- Stop exercising right away if you are dizzy, have shortness of breath, feel nauseous, or are in pain.

- Drink extra fluids before, during, and after exercise.

- If you have problems with sensation in your feet or poor circulation, check your feet regularly and protect yourself from blisters and abrasions. Inspect your feet and practice good skin and nail care regularly. Shoe inserts can be tailored to help protect the soles of the feet.

Managing Stress and Emotions

After learning that you have diabetes, or if you develop diabetes-related complications, you may be feeling angry, scared, or depressed. These feelings are normal, understandable, and manageable. If you have diabetes, stress and emotions such as anger, fear, frustration, and depression can raise your blood glucose levels. For this reason, it is important to learn effective ways to deal with these feelings. You can

find tools for dealing with stress and negative emotions in Chapter 5, *Understanding and Managing Common Symptoms and Emotions*, and Chapter 6, *Using Your Mind to Manage Symptoms*. If negative thoughts and emotions about diabetes are interfering with your life, you may want to get help from a trained counsellor. Ask your healthcare professional or diabetes nurse for a referral.

Managing Sick Days, Infections, and Other Illnesses

People with diabetes, like all people, sometimes get sick. When you get an infection, a cold, or the flu, your blood glucose levels tend to go up due to your body's response to fighting the infection. For this reason, it is important to know what to do to keep your blood glucose levels as close to target as possible. Some people will know these as *sick day rules*.

Handling Sick Days: Planning Ahead

The following points should be included in your action plan for sick days:

■ Let a family member or friend know how you're feeling. Ask a family member or friend to check on you. This person can help you with home care, call your GP, or get you to A&E if necessary.

■ Have plenty of both sweetened and unsweetened or sugarless (or sugar-free) liquids available unless you have been told to limit fluids.

■ Have a thermometer at home and know how to use it.

■ Have your emergency medical information available and put it in an obvious place in your home (including your GP's phone number and a list of your medications and dosages).

■ Be sure to ask your diabetes team under what circumstances you should call them.

Some general guidelines on managing sick days as recommended by Diabetes UK and diabetes nurses across the UK are provided in the following section.

What to Do When You Are Sick

When you do get sick, follow these 10 steps to manage your situation:

1. **Don't panic.** Contact your diabetes team, who will help you if you have any questions or if you are unsure what to do.

2. **Rest.** Avoid strenuous exercise.

3. **Treat symptoms such as a high temperature or a cough with basic over-the-counter medicines such as painkillers and cough syrups.** These do not have to be sugar-free varieties, as they contain very little glucose and are taken in small quantities. Ask your pharmacist for advice.

4. **Contact your GP if you think you have an infection.** You may need antibiotics.

5. **Keep taking your diabetes medication – even if you don't feel like eating.** If you are taking insulin, you might need to adjust your insulin doses while you are sick – particularly if you are not eating or have high or low blood glucose levels. There are some medications that you shouldn't take as much of or stop taking altogether. Make sure you talk to your diabetes team as soon as you're feeling ill so they can give you the right advice.

6. **If you check your blood glucose at home you'll probably need to do it more**

often – at least every 4 hours, including during the night. If you don't test your blood glucose levels at home, be aware of the signs of hyperglycaemia. See pages 334–335.

7. **Stay hydrated.** When you are sick, fluids are more important than food. They can help prevent dehydration. Have plenty of sugar-free drinks and sip them gently throughout the day (at least 2.5 to 3.5 litres or 4 to 6 pints over 24 hours).

8. **Keep eating or drinking.** If you can't keep food down, try snacks or drinks with carbohydrates in them to give you energy. Try to sip on sugary drinks (such as fruit juice or non-diet cola or lemonade) or suck on glucose tablets or sweets like jelly babies. Letting fizzy drinks go flat may help keep them down. If you're vomiting, or not able to keep fluids down, get medical help as soon as possible.

9. **If you have type 1 diabetes, it's important to check for ketones.** You usually check when your blood glucose level is 15mmol/l or more, or 13mmol/l if you use an insulin pump. However, your diabetes team may have given you different targets, so regardless of what your blood glucose levels are saying – test for ketones. If you find ketones, contact your diabetes team.

10. **If you take a certain type of diabetes tablet called *SGLT2i* and become unwell – stop taking them.** You need to check your ketones and your blood glucose (if you have been told to do this and have the kit) and speak to your healthcare team. There are different types of SGLT2i tablets (you can check the Diabetes UK website for brand names at https://www.diabetes.org.uk/guide-to-diabetes/managing-your-diabetes/treating-your-diabetes/tablets-and-medication/sglt2-inhibitors). Taking these tablets when you are not very well can increase your risk of developing diabetic ketosis (DKA – a serious condition that happens when there is severe lack of insulin in the body). Make sure you know the symptoms of DKA, which you can find on the Diabetes UK website. See the 'Useful Websites' section at the end of this chapter.

Preventing Diabetes Complications

High blood glucose levels that last over months and years can have serious complications. For most people, the higher the blood glucose level, the higher the chance of complications. However, the most common complications of diabetes are related to damaged blood vessels and nerves.

Most diabetes complications are also related to high blood pressure, so you can often delay and sometimes avoid complications by maintaining good blood pressure along with blood glucose control. If you do not have cardiovascular problems, your blood pressure target is less

SEEK MEDICAL HELP IF:

- your readings remain higher than usual, you feel unwell, and you are not sure what to do

- you are unable to take in liquids or solids or to keep them down

- you have diarrhoea or are vomiting for more than 6 hours

- your temperature is 38.3 C (101 degrees F) or more

- you have stomach pains that do not go away

When you call your doctor or NHS 111, have the following ready and be prepared to tell them:

- your type of diabetes

- your blood glucose level (if you know it)

- your urine ketone level (if you have type 1 diabetes and if you know it)

- your temperature

- a list of your symptoms

- the medications you are taking

- what you have done to treat your symptoms

Ask your GP or diabetes nurse if you do not know how to adjust medications when you are sick. Tell your GP or diabetes nurse if you are having ongoing problems with:

- frequent urination

- extreme thirst

- weakness

- difficulty breathing

than 140/90. If you have cardiovascular risks or problems, the target is less than 130/80, if it can be achieved safely.

Blood pressure changes day to day and over the day. For this reason, measure it frequently, not just when you visit your GP or diabetes team. You can monitor your blood pressure at home. Ask your GP or diabetes nurse about the most accurate monitors and have them teach you how to use them. It is not too hard, and you can learn to do it. If you cannot, or if you do not wish to monitor your blood pressure at home, go to your GP surgery or pharmacy. When you monitor your blood pressure, write down the date, what you

were doing, and your blood pressure measurement. Take your readings with you when you visit your GP. If you ever feel that your blood pressure tends to be too high or too low, talk to your doctor. You can be healthier and avoid complications if you monitor and manage your blood pressure.

The following is a list of common complications that may affect people with diabetes:

- **Heart disease and stroke.** High blood glucose levels and high blood pressure over time cause problems that harden and block the arteries in the heart and brain. There are many things you can do to help reduce these potential problems. For more information on heart disease, high blood pressure, and stroke, see Chapter 4, *Understanding and Managing Common Conditions.*

- **Nerve damage.** High blood glucose levels can cause damage to nerves (neuropathy), resulting in a burning or tingling sensation, numbness, or severe pain, especially in the feet and hands. Nerve damage can also lead to sexual problems such as erection problems in men and vaginal dryness in women. It can also cause problems with digestion and urination. The nerves that help control your heart rate and your blood pressure can also be damaged.

- **Kidney damage.** High blood glucose levels can damage the blood vessels in the kidneys, especially when blood pressure is high. In the long term this can cause kidney failure. The first signs of kidney damage may be detected by testing for small amounts of protein in the urine.

- **Vision problems.** Blurred vision can occur when high blood glucose levels temporarily cause the lens in the eye to swell. More serious and permanent damage to the blood vessels in the retina in the back of the eye (retinopathy) can lead to poor vision or even blindness.

- **Infections.** Diabetes can decrease immune function and reduce blood flow, which can lead to slower healing and more frequent infections of the skin, feet, lungs, and other parts of the body.

- **Gum disease.** Gum (periodontal) disease and infection are often more serious and

may be more common in people with diabetes. It is important to discuss your diabetes with your dentist and to get regular dental checkups. Follow the dental health tips on pages 134–135.

The following checklist helps you make sure you are doing the things and getting the care that will help significantly prevent or delay complications of diabetes. These tips may even save your life!

- **Maintain blood glucose levels within the recommended range.** Eating a healthy diet, getting regular exercise, maintaining a healthy weight, learning to manage your stress, and (if needed) taking medications are the keys to controlling blood glucose levels and preventing complications. For people with diabetes, a reasonable HbA1c goal is 48 mmol/mol to 53 mmol/mol.

- **Control your blood pressure.** If you do not have cardiovascular problems, your blood pressure target is less than 140/90. If you have cardiovascular risks or problems, the target is less than 130/80, if it can be achieved safely. Lower blood pressure means less stress on your heart and blood vessels, eyes, and kidneys. To prevent complications of diabetes, controlling blood pressure can be as important as controlling blood glucose levels.

- **Control your blood cholesterol.** LDL ('bad') cholesterol, rather than total cholesterol, is the measure that is usually monitored for people with diabetes. The target LDL level for people with diabetes is below 2.0 mmol/L (check with your GP what is right for you). You may have been prescribed statins. These are medicines that decrease inflammation and lower cholesterol, reducing the chance of a heart attack or stroke.

■ **Protect your kidneys.** Keeping blood glucose and blood pressure under control can help keep your kidneys healthy. Regular tests that check for protein in the urine can detect problems early. Along with regular testing, taking an ACE inhibitor or angiotensin receptor blocker (ARB) if you have high blood pressure and kidney disease may help protect your kidneys and help your heart health too.

■ **Check your feet.** When you have diabetes, your feet need extra care and attention. Diabetes can damage the nerve endings and blood vessels in your feet, making you less likely to notice when your feet are injured. Diabetes also limits your body's ability to fight infection and get blood to areas that need it. If you get a minor foot injury, it could become an ulcer or a serious infection.

▸ Examine your feet every day. You or someone else should look between the toes and on the tops and bottoms of the feet for cuts, cracks, sores, corns, calluses, blisters, ingrown toenails, extreme dryness, bruises, redness, swelling, or pus. Using a mirror with a handle makes this easier to do. Also check for warm spots on the feet – this can mean there is an infection.

▸ Wash your feet every day. Use warm (not hot) water and mild soap. Check the water temperature with your wrist or another part of your body, not your feet,

and dry thoroughly, especially between the toes. Do not soak your feet, as this causes drying.

▸ Cut your toenails straight across, not too short, and file any sharp edges. If you can't safely trim your toenails yourself, ask a family member to do it or get professional help from a nurse or podiatrist. Also, do not clean under your toenails or remove skin with sharp objects.

▸ After you dry your feet, apply a mild lotion (except between your toes). Avoid lotions that contain alcohol or other ingredients that end in *-ol*, as these tend to dry out the skin.

▸ If your feet sweat, sprinkle on a non-medicated powder before putting on your socks.

▸ Wear clean socks. White socks allow you to notice drainage or bleeding if you have a sore or cut. Avoid socks with tight elastic tops.

▸ Never go barefoot except when bathing, swimming, or in bed.

▸ Wear comfortable shoes. Your shoes should support, protect, and cover your feet. It is best to have at least two pairs of shoes and wear a different pair every other day or so. This helps prevent rubbing at the same place every day.

▸ Before putting on shoes, check inside for rough places or any sharp objects such as drawing pins or nails on the sole of the shoe. Break in new shoes gradually.

- Do not wear the same shoes 2 days in a row. If you have any problems with your feet, change your shoes in the middle of the day.

- Get a member of your diabetes team or a podiatrist to check your feet at each review. As a reminder, take off your shoes and socks.

- Get early treatment for foot problems. A minor irritation can lead to a major problem.

■ **Take these additional precautions.**

- Be sure to tell your healthcare professional if you are taking aspirin (75 to 162 mg/day) to lessen your risk of heart attacks and stroke.

- Do not smoke regular or E-cigarettes, or if you do smoke, take steps to quit. If you smoke, see pages 109–113 on how to become a non-smoker.

- In general, moderate alcohol use (no more than 14 units per week) does not seem to have any negative long-term effects on blood glucose levels. However, alcohol can cause a sudden and drastic drop in blood glucose for people with diabetes. Alcohol also adds calories that can lead to weight gain. If you do drink, make sure you eat food when you have a drink to help avoid a low blood glucose reaction. Check your blood glucose to see how alcohol affects your blood glucose. In addition, people with high triglycerides should avoid drinking alcohol.

- Protect your skin. Don't get sunburned and keep your skin clean.

- Wear an emergency alert necklace or bracelet and carry a list of all your medications with you. Share with your healthcare team what over-the-counter medications, herbs, and vitamins you take – some of these may affect your diabetes or interact with other medications you take.

- At every visit relating to your health and if you are ever hospitalised or go to A&E, remind the doctor and nurse that you have diabetes.

Using Medications:
Controlling Blood Glucose and Preventing Complications

People with type 2 diabetes may be prescribed a variety of medications. Medications help keep blood glucose, blood pressure, and cholesterol levels in your target ranges. Although they can be helpful, many people do not like taking medications. There are many lifestyle changes that can have a positive impact on blood pressure, blood glucose, and cholesterol levels. You might want to manage your conditions naturally. Sometimes it is possible to manage without medications. However, many people with type 2 diabetes may need to take one or more medications or insulin to maintain blood glucose control and prevent diabetes complications. Taking medications (including insulin) does not mean that you have failed in your efforts to maintain healthier habits.

Diet and exercise changes continue to be important when you take medications. Medications can help prevent such complications as heart attack, stroke, and kidney disease, and early death. Unfortunately, you cannot wait to see what happens before you decide to take medications. Once you have diabetes complications, they cannot usually be reversed.

Blood Glucose Medications

Your doctor recommends medications based on your type of diabetes, how well your blood glucose is controlled, and your other medical conditions. Medication options differ for people with type 1 and type 2 diabetes as described here:

- **Insulin for type 1 diabetes.** Insulin is required from the time of diagnosis and for the rest of your life because your body is no longer able to make its own insulin.

- **Medications for type 2 diabetes.** There are several types of glucose-lowering medications, including a variety of pills and medications you inject. These medications can be used separately or in combination to help control your blood glucose levels.

- **Insulin for type 2 diabetes.** Over time, your pancreas doesn't produce enough insulin. When this happens, you will need to start insulin to lower your blood glucose levels into the target range. Injected insulin is a safe and effective choice for many people with type 2 diabetes.

Getting Necessary Tests, Examinations, and Vaccinations

If you have diabetes, get regular checkups, examinations, and vaccinations. Use the following list to make sure you are actively managing your condition:

- Have an HbA1c test at least every 6 months if your diabetes is well controlled or at least 3-month intervals if it is not well controlled.

- Get kidney function tests at least once a year (or more if you have kidney disease).

- Have your blood cholesterol and lipid levels tested at least once a year or as indicated by your healthcare professional. More frequent testing may be necessary for people taking cholesterol medications.

- Have a dilated eye examination (eye drops are used) by an optician every 1 to 2 years (or as recommended by your doctor). Report any changes in vision to your doctor. The retinal examination is different than the test to check your vision to see if you need glasses.

- Remind your healthcare professional to check your feet and legs at each visit or at least once a year. One way to do this is to always take off your shoes and socks in the examining room. (See the list on pages 351–352 for more tips about foot care.)

- Have your blood pressure checked at every visit (or as recommended by your

A Word About Driving

If you are diagnosed with diabetes and treated with insulin you must, by law, inform the DVLA. If your diabetes is treated by tablets or non-insulin injections you will need to check with your diabetes team if you need to inform DVLA. You can be fined up to £1,000 if you don't tell DVLA about a medical condition that affects your driving. You may be prosecuted if you're involved in an accident as a result. For more information, visit https://www.gov.uk/diabetes-driving.

healthcare professional) and keep track of the numbers.

- Get your free yearly flu jabs and ask your healthcare professional about when to get pneumonia vaccinations. In addition, have all the other vaccinations appropriate for your age.

- Have a dental examination once a year or as recommended by your healthcare professional. Brush your teeth twice a day and use a 'TePe' or floss daily. (See pages 134–135 in Chapter 5, *Understanding and Managing Common Symptoms and Emotions*, for more tips on managing your dental health.)

Diabetes UK has produced a useful ticklist of 15 free essential checks, tests, and services that you are entitled to if you live with diabetes (see the 'Useful Websites' section at the end of this chapter), so in addition to this list talk to your GP about the following:

- advice on diet
- emotional and psychological support
- group self-management education
- care from diabetes specialists
- good care if you are in hospital
- support with any sexual problems
- help to stop smoking
- specialist care if you are planning to have a baby

Self-Management and Diabetes: Your Role Is Important

To be a good diabetes self-manager, you must learn a lot. Putting all this information into action is sometimes difficult. Set personal goals to control your diabetes, review them regularly, and revise them as needed. Be sure to talk to your doctor or diabetes team about your questions, problems, and concerns. Find other information and resources in your community. Attend a diabetes education programme. Consider joining a

diabetes support group either in your community or online (see the 'Useful Websites' section at the end of this chapter).

Most complications of diabetes can be prevented, delayed, and treated. You have an important role in this. Maintain your blood glucose, blood pressure, blood cholesterol, and lipid levels within the recommended ranges. Be aware of your body and symptoms. Report changes early.

Time is important. Recall the important tools you have as a self-manager:

- Observe symptoms, monitor your blood glucose, and know how to respond to changes.

- Prevent dehydration.

- Follow a healthy eating plan.

- Be physically active.

- Manage stress and emotions.

- Manage sick days, infections, and other illnesses.

- Use prescribed medications in a safe and effective way to control blood glucose, blood pressure, and blood cholesterol to help prevent complications. Take medications as prescribed. If you have problems with your medications, work with your GP to find solutions.

- Get necessary tests, examinations, and vaccinations.

- Wear an emergency alert necklace or bracelet.

Useful Websites

British Nutrition Foundation (*Get Portion Wise*): https://www.nutrition.org.uk/healthyliving/find-your-balance.html

Diabetes Chat (Scheduled chats with healthcare professionals or just the chance to talk to others): https://www.diabetes.co.uk/diabetes-chat/index.html

Diabetes UK (15 healthcare essentials): https://diabetes-resources-production.s3-eu-west-1.amazonaws.com/diabetes-storage/migration/pdf/15-healthcare-essentials-2016.pdf

Diabetes UK (Collection of blogs on work and diabetes, food, eyes, and more): https://blogs.diabetes.org.uk/

Diabetes UK (Diabetic ketoacidosis): https://admin.diabetes.org.uk/guide-to-diabetes/complications/diabetic_ketoacidosis

Diabetes UK (Diabetes and blood pressure): https://www.diabetes.org.uk/guide-to-diabetes/managing-your-diabetes/blood-pressure

Diabetes UK (Diabetes health guidelines): https://www.diabetes.co.uk/diabetes-health-guidelines.html#:~:text=Charity%20Diabetes%20UK%20lists%20the,1.2%20mmol%2Fl%20(women)

Diabetes UK (Diabetes Support Forum – discussions about living with and managing diabetes): https://www.diabetes.org.uk/how_we_help/community/diabetes-support-forum

Diabetes UK (Mediterranean meal plan): https://www.diabetes.org.uk/guide-to-diabetes/enjoy-food/eating-with-diabetes/meal-plans-/mediterranean

Diabetes UK (Mediterranean and DASH plans): https://www.diabetes.co.uk/diet/mediterranean-diet.html

Diabetes UK (Sugar, sweeteners, and diabetes): https://www.diabetes.org.uk/guide-to-diabetes
/enjoy-food/carbohydrates-and-diabetes/sugar-sweeteners-and-diabetes

Diabetes UK (The Eatwell Guide): https://www.diabetes.org.uk/guide-to-diabetes/enjoy-food/
eating-with-diabetes/the-eatwell-guide

Diabetes UK (What to drink when you have diabetes): https://www.diabetes.org.uk/guide-to
-diabetes/enjoy-food/what-to-drink-with-diabetes

DVLA (Diabetes and driving): https://www.gov.uk/diabetes-driving

Food Standards Agency (Nutrition labelling): https://www.food.gov.uk/business-guidance
/nutrition-labelling#front-of-pack-nutritional-labelling

Freelance Dieticians: https://freelancedietitians.org/

Health & Care Professions Council (HCPC): https://www.hcpc-uk.org/standards/standards-of
-proficiency/dietitians/

MedicAlert: https://www.medicalert.org.uk/

NHS (Alcohol units): https://www.nhs.uk/live-well/alcohol-support/calculating-alcohol-units/

NHS (Salt: the facts website guide): https://www.nhs.uk/live-well/eat-well/salt-nutrition/

NHS (The Eatwell Guide): https://www.nhs.uk/live-well/eat-well/the-eatwell-guide/

NHS Apps Library (Apps and tools to help you manage your diabetes): https://www.nhs.uk/apps
-library/

Public Health England (*The Eatwell Guide* booklet): https://www.gov.uk/government/publications
/the-eatwell-guide

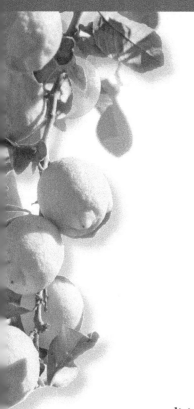

CHAPTER **15**

Working and Living with Long-Term Conditions

MANAGING A LONG-TERM CONDITION can feel like a job all by itself. Yet many working people also have a long-term condition. If you have a job and you have a long-term condition, you have the added challenge of balancing your work and home lives while also taking care of your health.

Work is a large part of many people's lives. If you are working full time, you may spend more time at work than you do at home. In fact, for many people who are working, the only thing that they do more than work is sleep! People work for a variety of different reasons, primarily financial. But many people also work because they receive mental and social health benefits from their jobs. At the same time, a job can also be a source of stress, challenges, and conflict. Because work has both positive and negative effects and makes up a significant part of our life, it is important to think about how work impacts health and health impacts work. Learning to work and live with a long-term condition is another self-management task.

357

Working while managing a long-term condition presents special challenges, including:

- **Physical challenges.** At work, physical challenges include dealing with symptoms such as pain or fatigue, experiencing other symptoms during work time, and being limited in what you can do because of your condition.

- **Missed work.** You may miss work because of your symptoms or because of healthcare appointments.

- **Dealing with what others think.** What your colleagues or managers think about you can affect how you deal with your condition. They may think you must not be that sick if you can work, or they may think you are lazy or not doing a good job. They may not see your symptoms or really know why you miss work, and that can lead to misunderstanding or confusion.

- **Time management.** Everyone who works must balance home and work responsibilities. Having a long-term condition can tip the balance or make finding a balance much more difficult.

Unfortunately, you can't leave your symptoms at home when you to go work every day. Many people with jobs and long-term conditions just put up with their symptoms and don't take care of their own health. This leaves them exhausted. In the long run this can lead to poor health. Poor health leads to poor job performance, poor work attendance, and a decline in the quality of your home life and your life in general. Instead of toughing it out and ignoring your own health, you should focus on taking care of yourself. This improves not only your quality of life but also makes you a better employee.

Managing a condition at work presents unique challenges when dealing with symptoms. This is because many things about your work environment, your work responsibilities, and your work schedule are out of your hands. There are many things at work that you cannot control or change. In most jobs, there are set schedules, responsibilities, and expectations that employees must meet.

Imagine someone with joint pain. For them, sitting and typing at a computer can make their pain worse. However, if sitting and typing is part of that person's job, it may be difficult to avoid. Or consider fatigue. Fatigue can make it difficult to focus and accomplish tasks. And for most people it is not possible to rest or take a nap during work. Despite these difficulties, there are things that you can do and choices that you can make to be a better self-manager. At work, just like at home, you must be a good problem solver, just as we discussed in Chapter 2, *Becoming an Active Self-Manager*.

Finding Work/Life Balance

The relationship between your work life and your home life can be complex. It is more so when you are dealing with a long-term condition. The term 'work/life balance' is misleading because it is probably impossible to achieve a perfect balance. You may not even want this. Your work and home responsibilities both require time and resources that quite often pull you in different directions. It is up to you to find a balance between the two. Working toward work/life balance doesn't mean that work and home should be equally important. It means that both work and home fit into the picture, and taking care of one doesn't mean not taking care of the other.

Work can take on many forms. You may work full time or part time or have a job with flexitime. Although many people you know might still work in what you would typically consider an office environment, there has been an increase in alternative work arrangements in recent years. These arrangements allow some people to work at home or in a shared space near home. And some working people never go to an office. For some, work means driving all day, and for others it means manual labour. All jobs have their own challenges, and all workplaces have different policies and procedures. Just as people's work is diverse, home can also mean many different things to different people. Home can include family, friends, home responsibilities, community involvement, hobbies, and many other non-work activities.

Most people's work and home lives interact in complex ways. Work can affect home, and home can affect work. Having a busy, stressful day at work can make you feel fatigued and more likely to pick up a takeaway on the way home. After work, you may feel physically tired, emotionally run down, and as if there is little left to give at home. Conflict or problems at home can distract people from work and cause things to pile up and make people less productive.

Work/life balance isn't static; it changes day to day and can tilt one way or the other. As a good self-manager, you can work to anticipate the times when your work and life are out of balance and identify ways to get back on track.

Managing Your Time

When your work and life are out of balance, the first step is to identify the problems that are causing the lack of balance. Effective time management is the most important tool for finding balance. The goal is to make time for home, time for work, and a bit of time for yourself.

Start to notice how you are spending your time. Tracking your time (in the same way that you track what you eat or how much you exercise) can help you identify how and where you are currently spending your time. Make a list of how you spend your time each day by breaking the day down into hours. For each hour, use general categories to describe how you spent that time (for example, work, chores, watching TV, exercise, etc.). Make sure to include at least one workday and at least one non-workday. You will find a time management worksheet (Figure 15.1) on pages 360–361. You may find it helpful as you start to track your time.

After a few days, look for patterns. Once you discover your patterns, you may find changes you can make. Think about how you are spending your time. Is this helping you meet your personal or professional goals? Is this a 'good' use of your time?

Building Good Habits

How people use time is similar to other behaviours. People tend to do the same things over and over. Those things become habits.

Figure 15.1 **Time Management Worksheet**

Write down everything you do in hour-long blocks. You may have many tasks in the same hour.

Time	Task	Priority	Use of time
7:00 A.M.		☐ High ☐ Medium ☐ Low	☐ Good ☐ Poor
8:00 A.M.		☐ High ☐ Medium ☐ Low	☐ Good ☐ Poor
9:00 A.M.		☐ High ☐ Medium ☐ Low	☐ Good ☐ Poor
10:00 A.M.		☐ High ☐ Medium ☐ Low	☐ Good ☐ Poor
11:00 A.M.		☐ High ☐ Medium ☐ Low	☐ Good ☐ Poor
12:00 P.M.		☐ High ☐ Medium ☐ Low	☐ Good ☐ Poor
1:00 P.M.		☐ High ☐ Medium ☐ Low	☐ Good ☐ Poor
2:00 P.M.		☐ High ☐ Medium ☐ Low	☐ Good ☐ Poor
3:00 P.M.		☐ High ☐ Medium ☐ Low	☐ Good ☐ Poor
4:00 P.M.		☐ High ☐ Medium ☐ Low	☐ Good ☐ Poor
5:00 P.M.		☐ High ☐ Medium ☐ Low	☐ Good ☐ Poor
6:00 P.M.		☐ High ☐ Medium ☐ Low	☐ Good ☐ Poor

Figure 15.1 **Time Management Worksheet (*continued*)**

Write down everything you do in hour-long blocks. You may have many tasks in the same hour.

Time	Task	Priority	Use of time
7:00 P.M.		☐ High ☐ Medium ☐ Low	☐ Good ☐ Poor
8:00 P.M.		☐ High ☐ Medium ☐ Low	☐ Good ☐ Poor
9:00 P.M.		☐ High ☐ Medium ☐ Low	☐ Good ☐ Poor
10:00 P.M.		☐ High ☐ Medium ☐ Low	☐ Good ☐ Poor
11:00 P.M.		☐ High ☐ Medium ☐ Low	☐ Good ☐ Poor
12:00 A.M.		☐ High ☐ Medium ☐ Low	☐ Good ☐ Poor
1:00 A.M.		☐ High ☐ Medium ☐ Low	☐ Good ☐ Poor
2:00 A.M.		☐ High ☐ Medium ☐ Low	☐ Good ☐ Poor
3:00 A.M.		☐ High ☐ Medium ☐ Low	☐ Good ☐ Poor
4:00 A.M.		☐ High ☐ Medium ☐ Low	☐ Good ☐ Poor
5:00 A.M.		☐ High ☐ Medium ☐ Low	☐ Good ☐ Poor
6:00 A.M.		☐ High ☐ Medium ☐ Low	☐ Good ☐ Poor

It becomes easy to come home, turn on the TV, or surf the web, and before you know it, a great deal of time has passed. There is a place for those activities that help you unwind and relax, such as watching TV, reading, or shopping – but moderation is key. Make sure that those activities are not keeping you from accomplishing your goals. If you find yourself spending more time than you like doing things that don't help you meet your personal or professional goals, consider breaking those time spending habits.

Changing habits can be hard; it takes effort and time. A good first step is to identify one hour of time that you could spend in a more enjoyable or productive way and make an action plan. Review the discussion of action planning in Chapter 2, *Becoming an Active Self-Manager*. Keep a calendar and schedule the things that are important to you and are priorities in your life. Those may include exercise, time for self-care, playing with children or grandchildren, attending a football match or live theatre performance, or anything else.

Managing Stress and Working

Juggling workloads, family responsibilities, and your health often results in high stress. Experiencing high stress over a long period is not good for your body or your mind. Stress can affect your condition as well. Prolonged stress can increase blood pressure, raise blood sugar, make pain and fatigue worse, and cause depression and anxiety to worsen. Stress can also weaken the immune system.

Stress is common; everyone feels stress at some point in their lives. But stressors (the things that cause stress) are very personal. What causes stress for one person may not be stressful for another person. Many times stress is brought about by positive things. For example, beginning a new job or buying a new house can be good things that still cause us stress. Stress is therefore not always bad. Stress can motivate us to accomplish goals and help us make changes. However, long periods of high stress can be very harmful to our health. The good news is

that you can learn what is causing your stress. Once you have done this, stress is much easier to manage.

What Is Stress and What Causes It?

As we discussed in Chapter 5, *Understanding and Managing Common Symptoms and Emotions*, stress is a natural reaction that your body has to a demand or a threat. It is not important if the threat is real. What is important is that you think it is a threat. Stress is the body's way of protecting you. The 'stress response' causes the nervous system to release hormones such as adrenaline and cortisol. These hormones cause your heart to beat faster and your muscles to tighten up. It raises your blood pressure and makes your breathing faster. Stress can sharpen your senses and make your body ready for 'fight or flight'. This was all very useful when our ancestors came into contact with a lion.

In small doses, these changes focus and prepare you to meet challenges. However, the part of your brain that sets off this reaction is not very good at telling the difference between real and imagined threats or between emotional and physical threats. A deadline at work or an unpaid bill can cause the body to react just as strongly as if you were facing a life-or-death situation. So although the 'stress response' is helpful in times of physical danger, over time it becomes a learned behaviour and is more easily activated. The more it is triggered, the harder it becomes to shut off. It is a vicious cycle: stress leads to more stress.

Common causes of stress include both external or outside causes (such as major life changes, work, relationship difficulties, financial problems, and children and family) and internal or inside causes (such as rigid thinking, negative self-talk, and unrealistic expectations). According to the Holmes and Rahe Stress Scale (a questionnaire developed by psychiatrists Thomas Holmes and Richard Rahe in 1967 for identifying major stressful life events), the top ten stressful life events for adults are the following:

1. death of a spouse
2. divorce
3. marriage separation
4. imprisonment
5. death of a close family member
6. injury or illness
7. marriage
8. job loss
9. marriage reconciliation
10. retirement

As you can see, having an illness is the sixth most stressful life event. If you have a long-term condition, you are experiencing one of the top ten stressors! Do any of these others apply to you as well? When you add in trying to balance work and life, knowing how stressful an illness can be helps to explain why finding work/life balance may be so difficult. Work stress adds another dimension to stress management. Common causes of workplace stress include fear of being laid off or losing your job, overtime or overwork, pressure to perform, and lack of control.

Symptoms of Stress

If stress is part of your daily life, it can be easy to not even know when you are stressed. Feeling stressed may be your 'normal'. Here are some warning signs that you are under too much stress:

■ memory problems
■ problems concentrating
■ poor judgement
■ constant negative thinking
■ anxiety or constant worrying thoughts
■ depression
■ moodiness, irritability, or anger
■ feeling overwhelmed, isolated, or lonely
■ aches and pains
■ diarrhoea or constipation
■ nausea or dizziness
■ eating more or less
■ muscle tension or headaches
■ sleeping too much or too little

- withdrawing from others

- nervous habits such as biting your nails or fidgeting

- using alcohol or drugs to relax

- pulling your hair, tapping your foot, or other repetitive habits

- grinding your teeth or clenching your jaw

- tension in your head, neck, or shoulders

- feeling anxious, nervous, or helpless

- frequent accidents

- fatigue and exhaustion

Stress Management Tools

How much stress is too much? This level is different for everyone. We all have different limits. How much stress you have may depend on your support from family and friends, your sense of control, your attitude, how you manage your emotions, your knowledge of stress, and your preparation to handle stress. There are many tools in this book to help you manage stress. You can find a guide to these problem-solving tools in the material on stress in Chapter 5, *Understanding and Managing Common Symptoms and Emotions*. Getting enough sleep is also key to stress management. It is not just the amount of sleep that matters but the quality of sleep. There are tips for dealing with sleep disruption in Chapter 5. You can also find tools for relaxation in Chapter 6, *Using Your Mind to Manage Symptoms*, exercises that can help with stress reduction in Chapter 8, *Exercising to Make Life Easier*, and information about eating a healthy diet in Chapter 10, *Healthy Eating*.

Another great way to manage stress is to reach out to those around you. You can use the communication skills covered in Chapter 11, *Communicating with Family, Friends, and Healthcare Professionals*, to help someone understand what you are going through. Your friends and family do not necessarily have to 'fix' the problem, but just having someone to listen is helpful! When you are experiencing stress at work, colleagues can be a great source of support because they understand your work environment. If you feel that you have no one you can talk to, it may be time to seek out professional help.

There are things that you cannot change about your job, but by prioritising and organising, you can help regain a sense of control and decrease your stress response at work. The following are useful tips for dealing with workplace stress:

1. Plan regular breaks where you take a walk, chat with a friend, or relax.

2. Establish boundaries. Though it is easy to feel the need to be connected to phones and email 24 hours a day, set up a time to no longer think about work. It may take some practice to break the habit of being available 24/7, but lower stress levels will be your reward.

3. Learn to say no. Don't overcommit to things, avoid scheduling things back to back, and don't be afraid to say no to things that you can't do or things you do not want to do.

4. Prioritise your work tasks and break projects into small steps. Use action plans (see

Chapter 2, *Becoming an Active Self-Manager*) to make and reach your small goals.

5. Delegate work tasks when you can do so and be willing to compromise.

6. Resist the urge to set unrealistic work goals for yourself. Make sure that your goals are achievable.

7. Reduce negative talk and focus on the positive. Find something in your job that you enjoy and focus on that.

8. Take time off!

Finally, if these small tips are not working, you may need to think about speaking with your manager, supervisor, or the human resources (HR) department about your responsibilities and expectations. If you feel like your stress levels are having an impact on your health or your condition, share this with your GP or other healthcare professional.

Communicating and Working

One of the hardest self-management tasks is talking to others about your long-term conditions and how they affect your life. This is even harder when your conditions impact your work. This section includes some suggestions to make this easier or at least not so frightening.

You do not have to tell anyone about your condition unless you want to. It can be scary to talk about your health at work. Many people fear that they will be treated differently or even lose their job. However, if your condition is impacting the way that you do your job, your attendance at work, or your job performance, it may be time to talk with your manager or someone else in the organisation. If you choose not to talk, people may make assumptions or jump to conclusions about your job performance.

When communicating with people at work about your health, it is important to think about:

■ **When you want to disclose.** When is the right time for you to bring it up?

■ **Whom you want to disclose it to.** Should you tell supervisors, colleagues, managers, HR?

■ **What you want to disclose.** Will it help you to share this information?

■ **How much you want to disclose.** Do they need to know all the details, or will something more general be enough?

Remember, it is always your choice to share!

Deciding When to Share

Talking about your long-term conditions can be a very sensitive topic. However, *not* communicating can have consequences as well. You may want to ask yourself the following questions to help you decide:

■ **Do your symptoms interfere with your work duties, assignments, or projects?** Does pain or fatigue cause you to miss deadlines? Does it take longer to accomplish tasks because of your symptoms?

■ **Do you sometimes need time off because of your condition?** Do you have frequent doctor's appointments or symptom flare-ups? Does it happen more than once in a while?

■ **Do you have pain that is so severe it can affect your mood and the ability to deal with customers or colleagues?** Do you feel more stressed and have a shorter temper because you are in pain or are tired?

■ **Does your job impact your symptoms?** Does standing all day make your pain worse? Are you being exposed to something in the work environment that is worsening your condition?

If you answered yes to any of these questions, it may be time to consider saying something to someone at work. People are often afraid of being discriminated against, but without all of the information, your manager or employer may make incorrect assumptions about you or what is impacting your work. Someone who knows what you are dealing with is less likely to make false assumptions about you.

Deciding What to Share and Whom to Tell

Remember, communicating about your health needs is different from disclosing your condition. It is possible to discuss the problems you are facing and how your health is being affected without naming your condition or going into too much detail. How much to share is a very personal decision that you should make based on your circumstances, your job, your managers, and your desired outcomes. If you decide to discuss your condition with a supervisor or manager, give some thought ahead of time as to when, how much, and what you will share. Ask yourself, 'What do *I* want and need from this conversation? How can I make sure this conversation

helps me? When is a good time when both my manager and I can discuss the problem?'

Consider how much you want to share. You may want to disclose only the *symptoms* you experience that are related to your job performance. Keeping the focus on the symptoms and not getting into details about your condition can help protect your privacy. You may want to limit the conversation to how your condition affects you at work. However, depending on the condition, discussing what your condition is may provide more context and allow the other person to understand more about what you are dealing with. Think about your own boundaries – does the idea of sharing make you feel empowered, or would it make you feel exposed? If it makes you feel empowered, then more disclosure may help.

Discussing Your Condition at Work

When it is time to discuss your health with someone at work, it can be helpful if you can control the conversation. Let the person know that you want to discuss something about your health. Explain why you are disclosing this information now (for example, does it explain an absence or justify why you can't do something related to your job?), and keep the focus on the impact of your condition on your work. Here is an example:

I know that I am often late. I have rheumatoid arthritis, and in the mornings, I am stiff and have lots of pain. For me to get going in the morning takes several hours. I am wondering if I might come to work a bit later and leave a bit later.

Set clear boundaries about the spread of information by saying something like, 'I would like this information to stay between you and me.' Have a plan of action for what you would like to see happen as a result of this conversation, such as coming to work later. Do you need your work hours adjusted? Do you need to take more frequent breaks? Is there a system that needs to be worked out to cover your absences? Make sure that what you are sharing always comes back to what you want to happen, as in the following example:

Hello, I'd like a minute of your time to talk about something important to me. I have been dealing with a health concern for some time now. Because of this, I will need to take some time for doctors' appointments, and there may be days when I am unable to come in. I want to be up front with you so that we can discuss how best to handle those days.

Remember, you do not have to share anything with anyone that you do not want to share. Think about what is in your best interest and what will result in a better and healthier work environment for you. In most cases, it is better to be up front and communicate at least the basics than not communicate at all.

By sharing that you have a condition that may affect you at work, you can become an advocate for yourself. Ask for what you need: adjustments to your workspace, changes to work hours, changing the way that you work, and so on. Laws vary between UK nations about workplace responsibilities and accommodations. Know your rights. Check out the laws that apply in your nation. Your company's HR department should also have resources.

The primary legislation used to protect people with long-term conditions at work across England, Scotland, and Wales is the Equality Act of 2010. Under this act it is against the law to discriminate against anyone at work because of their disability. You're disabled under the law if you have a physical or mental impairment that has a 'substantial' (is more than minor or trivial) and 'long-term' (meaning 12 months or more) negative effect on your ability to do normal daily activities. People with progressive conditions (ones that get worse over time) are classed as disabled. An employer has to make 'reasonable adjustments' to avoid you being put at a disadvantage compared to non-disabled people in the workplace. For example, adjusting your working hours or providing you with a special piece of equipment to help you do the job. There are also special rules about recurring or fluctuating conditions such as arthritis.

The Equality Act 2010 protects disabled people in the workplace in relation to the following:

■ application forms
■ interview arrangements
■ aptitude or proficiency tests
■ job offers
■ terms of employment, including pay
■ promotion, transfer, and training opportunities
■ dismissal or redundancy
■ discipline and grievances

The Equality Act 2010 does not apply to Northern Ireland, where people with disabilities share the same general employment rights as other jobseekers and employees. However, there are also special terms for them under the Disability Discrimination Act 1995.

In addition, the UN Convention on disability rights has been agreed by the UK to protect and promote the rights of disabled people.

There are links to government websites in the 'Useful Websites' section at the end of this chapter where you can find more details about employment rights. You can also contact your local Citizens Advice or check out one of the many condition-specific charities across the UK who may also provide employment rights advice.

Finally, in many work environments, colleagues can be supportive. People spend a lot of time at work and sometimes spend more time with colleagues than with family. Getting some support from those around you can help you get through the tough times. If you do ask for support, do it carefully. If you do not want everyone to know your concerns, share only with the people you trust. One benefit of this sharing is that as someone learns more about you, they are also more likely to share something about themselves. This is the basis of trust and friendship.

Communicating About Work at Home

Often work stresses and problems show up at home. You may be quiet, not have the energy to help around the house, or snap at your partner or children. In turn, your home life may not be everything you want it to be. You may think, *'They just don't understand'* or *'They should know I am working as hard as I can and appreciate me more'* or *'There is nothing that can be done.'* The reason people at home do not 'understand' and don't 'know' what you are going through is often poor communication. When work is stressful, communicate with those at home. Find a time to talk with your family about what is going on at work, how they can help, and changes that can be made. When people understand, they are often inventive. Maybe the children can walk the dog, or your partner can prepare lunches for everyone. They might even have ideas that you could try at work. At the same time, you might learn that the children have stresses at school and your partner has his or her own concerns. Anytime you find yourself thinking *'they don't understand'* or *'they should know'*, take this as a clue that more communication is needed.

Being Physically Active and Working

Being active has many physical and mental benefits. Being active can help you be better at your job by improving thinking, improving memory, increasing your mental stamina, and boosting creativity. Exercise can improve your mood and decrease stress. Despite knowing all of this, many of us think of exercise and physical activity as a luxury – something we would like to do if only we had more time.

Staying physically active when you are working can be a challenge. Getting enough physical activity is often hard to do if you spend long hours at work. You may find yourself sitting or standing in one place for most of the workday. Because of job responsibilities, inactivity can be hard to avoid. When you add in your commuting time, you can end up spending a large part of your life sitting. Standing or sitting for a long time without a break can have many negative effects.

Research has found that being active during leisure time is not enough to make up for sitting down all day. To make things worse, you may find yourself exhausted at the end of the day so that you also spend your non-work time in sedentary activities. When you are sitting, your muscles are not working, and when your major muscles (like those in your legs) aren't working, your metabolism slows down, your muscles and joints get stiff, and symptoms such as pain, fatigue, and depression can get worse.

Other studies have shown links between being sedentary and increased risk of heart disease, poor metabolic health, and poor mental health. Being sedentary can be mentally draining and cause fatigue and memory problems. Sitting is not the only problem. Standing is not much better if you are just standing still in place. It all comes back to moving your big muscles (arms and legs) more and limiting the time that you spend being still.

The following are some suggestions for increasing movement at work:

- Stand up every 20 minutes and move your big muscles, even if it is just for a minute or two.
  - ▸ Walk from one side of the room to the other.
  - ▸ Walk down the corridor to talk to a colleague instead of sending an e-mail.
  - ▸ Use the lavatory that is the furthest away from your office or workstation. If possible, take the stairs to the floor above or below.
- Take a 10-minute activity break at a scheduled time every day.
- Regularly, at least once an hour, stand up and stretch.
- Take the stairs instead of the lift.
- If you are able, have standing or walking meetings. If you do this, be sure that everyone who needs to attend is able to take part.
- Wear comfortable shoes that encourage movement.
- Consider creating a walking group, have challenges with colleagues to see who can sit the least, or think up other fitness challenges. One inclusive way to conduct a fitness challenge is for each person to set a weekly goal – say 5,000, 7,000, or 9,000 steps a day – and the winners are the people who hit their goals on the most days. This allows the very fit and the not so fit to both 'win'.

Sedentary (Non-Active) Jobs

Even if you work at a desk, short bouts of physical activity can improve your fitness and cardiovascular health. With some planning, you can get some of these short bouts of aerobic exercise, strengthening exercises, or stretching in between meetings, calls, or other tasks. Though this type of physical activity may not produce dramatic results, it can improve your strength, burn a few extra calories, give you a much needed mental break, and keep your muscles and joints from getting stiff. Many of the exercises in Chapter 8, *Exercising to Make Life Easier*, can be done at your desk or workstation. Again, the key is that more movement is better than less movement.

For more information on general physical activity, developing an exercise routine, and strength and flexibility exercises, see Chapter 7, *Being Physically Active*, and Chapter 8, *Exercising to Make Life Easier*.

Active Jobs

Many people have active jobs. They are moving and lifting most of their workday. Think about canteen workers, nurses, building-site workers, gardeners, and postal workers. When people exercise during their free time, they can take breaks when they get tired. This is not always true for people with physical jobs. They may do the same labour-intensive tasks for hours, with few, if any, breaks. Moderate physical activity can strengthen the heart and the cardiovascular system. However, when people are very active at work and have limited rest breaks, their heart rate and blood pressure may be high over the whole day. This can put strain on the cardiovascular system. If the work is very repetitive, it can cause muscle strain and injury. In addition, people with jobs that are physically demanding may not exercise outside of work. They don't do the types of activities that could be beneficial, because they are too tired or they feel that their activity at work is enough. People with active jobs need to remember to take breaks during their workday. Be sure to make being active outside of work a priority!

Eating Well and Working

Balancing work and home can affect how you eat, not just at work but also at home. There is a relationship between many long-term conditions and nutrition. Healthy eating is a vital part of a healthy lifestyle. What and how you eat can also affect job performance and mental health.

When you eat, your body breaks down that food into glucose. Glucose is used by the brain to function and stay alert. That's why when we are

hungry, we may struggle to stay focused, or when we overeat, we may feel sluggish and tired. Some foods are better at providing sustained energy than others. Unfortunately, it can be difficult to make healthy decisions about eating when we are hungry, stressed, pressed for time, or have limited choices. Less healthy food choices are often cheaper and faster than healthy ones. Think about a fast food burger versus a bowl of beef stew or a chocolate bar versus a piece of fruit. When you don't eat healthily, your conditions may worsen. You may become more fatigued or gain weight. An unhealthy diet can cause fatigue, poor mental health, irritability, increased stress and depression, low energy levels, and decreased ability to think clearly and work effectively. This leaves you with little energy to prepare healthy food or make healthy choices. Good self-management can break this cycle.

The following are some tips for healthy eating when you are working. You can find more about this topic in Chapter 10, *Healthy Eating.*

- **Decide what you are going to eat before you get hungry.** If you wait to decide when you are very hungry, tired, and stressed, you are more likely to make an unhealthy choice.

- **Plan for your meal at work (usually lunch).** Many of us plan for our non-work meal (usually dinner). Doing the same for our work meal can keep us on track.

- **Plan snacks.** Keep healthy snacks such as fruit, cut-up vegetables, nuts, and seeds easily available at work. This will keep your energy levels up and keep you from overeating.

- **Choose fruits and vegetables.** These foods contain nutrients that improve health. Typically, when people eat better, they feel better. High-fat, high-sugar meals can make you tired and cause you to 'crash' a few hours after eating.

Healthier Desk Dining

According to research carried out by BUPA, almost a third of UK workers usually eat lunch at their desk. This can lead to poor food choices, including eating fewer fruits and vegetables, and eating more foods that are processed and higher in sugars, fat, and salt. One of the biggest reasons *not* to eat at your desk is that often people at their desks are distracted by e-mails, phone calls, or other tasks. If you eat at your desk, you are not fully focused on what and how much you are eating. This encourages overeating and a lack of awareness about what you are eating. People who eat at their desks tend to snack more and eat more calories. One final disadvantage to eating at your desk is that you are missing an opportunity for exercise and social interaction.

If you do have to eat at your desk, here are some tips for healthier eating.

- **Schedule your lunch.** Give yourself a break and stop to eat before you get too hungry. Set an alarm or calendar reminder.

- **Focus on your food.** Even if it is only for 10 minutes, stop what you are doing and focus on what and how much you are eating. There are very few tasks that cannot wait for a few minutes.

- **Pay close attention to your portions (how much you eat).** More information on portion and serving sizes can be found on pages 237–239 and 261 in Chapter 10, *Healthy Eating.*

- **Bring your lunch.** Avoid fast food for lunch. Plan ahead and bring healthy meals from home. Include fruits and vegetables as well as whole grains. See below for more information on recommendations for packing lunches.

- **Disinfect your desk.** Your desk or work-station can be covered with bacteria and germs. Wipe down your desk every day.

- **Socialise when you can.** People who socialise at work are more productive than those who don't.

- **Eat somewhere other than your desk.** Sit somewhere else during lunch, such as an outside picnic table or a staff room.

Whether you are eating at your desk due to a lack of time, too many tasks to accomplish, or to make others think that you are working harder, there are ways to make your lunches healthier. Remember, lunch is about more than consuming calories; it is also a break that you should take advantage of!

Packing Your Lunch

It is easy to get into a rut when it comes to bringing lunch. But there are many benefits. Lunches you pack at home are usually healthier than fast food or restaurants and can be much less expensive. If you buy your lunches and spend between £5 and £10 each day, that can add up to £200 a month! Follow these tips to get the most out of packing your lunches:

- Prepare and pack meals on the weekends or the night before work.

- Repackage leftovers. Use leftover chicken to make a wrap or a sandwich.

- Have fun with basic recipes. Use the Eat-well Guide in Chapter 10, *Healthy Eating,* to help you chose healthy foods to include in your lunch box. By dressing up a sandwich or salad, you can keep your meal interesting and simple at the same time.

Buy good-quality bread and substitute low-calorie mustard for high-calorie mayonnaise. Substitute hummus or avocado for luncheon meat. Include things beyond lettuce, tomatoes, and cucumbers in your salads. Add beans, brown rice, nuts, fruit, and small amounts of cheeses. Try out different dressings. Get a rotisserie chicken to eat for dinner and toss the leftovers on top of your salad or put them in your soup.

- Soups can be great lunches. You can cook them in bulk and freeze smaller portions to bring for lunch.

- Search for easy lunch ideas online.

- Choose healthy frozen dinners.

- Keep a plate, bowl, and utensils at the office.

- If your workplace does not have a refrigerator or microwave, ask for one.

Avoiding Temptations at Work

At work, food is often a distraction or temptation. Many people bring food they want to get out of their house to share at work. There are also endless celebrations in large offices, from birthdays to promotions to baby showers. Almost everyone agrees that it is hard to turn down a doughnut. Invitations to lunch can be hard to resist, even if you have brought a healthy lunch. Planning ahead, anticipating these distractions, and communicating with your colleagues can help. Also consider these tips:

- Make a pact with colleagues to bring only healthy items to share.

- Ask for and choose healthier options in vending machines and cafeterias.

- Communicate with your colleagues: '*I really appreciate it when you bring snacks in to share, but I am finding it hard to resist them. Please do not offer me food. I promise to tell you if I want something.*'

- When there is an event where everyone brings food to share, do not expect others to cook to your needs. Rather, be sure to bring something you can eat and enjoy that will also be enjoyed by others.

- Have a regular 'out for lunch' day. Communicate with your colleagues and ask them not to ask you out for lunch on other days.

■ ■ ■

In this chapter, we have discussed some of the challenges of working with a long-term condition. Although there are many things about work and jobs that are out of your hands, there are things you can control and changes you can make. All of these can lead to a better work/life balance. The keys are managing your time, identifying stressors and managing stress, communicating with colleagues and people at home, being physically active, and eating healthily. Throughout this book you will find much more about all of these topics.

Useful Websites

Citizens Advice: https://www.citizensadvice.org.uk/

Disability Rights (Equality Act 2010 and UN Convention): https://www.gov.uk/rights-disabled -person/the-equality-act-2010-and-un-convention

Disability Rights UK (Equality Advisory Support Service – EASS): https://www.disabilityrightsuk.org /how-we-can-help/helplines/equality-advisory-support-service

NI Direct (Disability Discrimination Act 1995): https://www.nidirect.gov.uk/articles/disability -discrimination-law-employment-rights

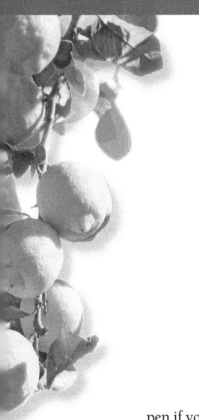

CHAPTER 16

Planning for the Future: Fears and Reality

PEOPLE WITH LONG-TERM CONDITIONS often worry about what will happen in the future. You may wonder what will happen if your condition becomes disabling. You may fear that you will have problems managing your condition and your life. Sometimes you may have this fear not for yourself but for a partner or friend. One way to deal with your fears about the future is to take control and plan for them. You may never need to put your plans into effect. Just the same, you will feel reassured knowing that you have control if the events you fear do happen. In this chapter, we examine some common concerns and offer some suggestions to help you feel more in control. We also provide information about a number of organisations and their contact details can be found in the 'Useful Websites' section at the end of the chapter.

For the UK edition, special thanks to Age UK Thanet and Bassetlaw Action Centre for their contributions to this chapter.

What if I Can't Take Care of Myself Anymore?

Regardless of how healthy you are or feel, most people fear becoming helpless and dependent. This fear is even greater among people with long-term conditions or other health concerns. This fear involves not only how to manage physical challenges, but also financial, social, and emotional ones.

Problem Solving for Physical Day-to-Day Living Concerns

As your health condition changes, you may need to consider changing your living situation. You may consider either paying someone to help you in your home or moving to a place that provides more help. The decision you make depends on your needs and how these can best be met. Most people usually think about only their physical needs, but we all have social and emotional needs. Consider these as well.

Start by evaluating what you can do for yourself. What tasks affect your health, and what activities of daily living (ADLs) require help? ADLs include getting out of bed, bathing, dressing, preparing and eating meals, cleaning the house, shopping, and paying bills. Most people can do these things, even though they may have to do them slowly, with some adjustments, or with some help from devices. In addition to taking care of yourself, you may be responsible for doing these things for someone else. Evaluate which of these tasks you can continue to do and which are becoming too difficult.

Some people find that they can no longer do one or more of these tasks without help.

For example, you may still be able to prepare meals but are no longer able to do the shopping. Or if you have problems with fainting or sudden bouts of unconsciousness, you might need someone around all the time to help. You may find that some activities you enjoyed in the past, such as gardening, are no longer pleasurable.

You can use the problem-solving steps discussed in Chapter 2, *Becoming an Active Self-Manager*, to make a list of potential problems. (This is step 1: Identify the problem. Review the steps of problem solving on page 26.) Once you have this list, you can then solve the problems one at a time. Begin by first writing down your problems and then every possible solution you can think of. (This is step 2: List ideas to solve the problem.) For example:

Can't go shopping

- Ask a family member to shop for me.
- Find a volunteer shopping service.
- Shop at a supermarket that offers a delivery service.
- Ask a neighbour to shop for me.
- Shop on the Internet.
- Get home-delivered meals.

Can't be by myself

- Employ an around-the-clock carer.
- Move in with a relative.
- Get a personal alarm system.

Will my long-term condition affect my ability to drive?

You need to tell DVLA about some medical conditions as they can affect your driving. You can be fined up to £1,000 if you do not tell DVLA about a medical condition that affects your driving. You may be prosecuted if you're involved in an accident as a result. You must give up your driving licence if either your doctor tells you to stop driving for 3 months or more, or you do not meet the required standards for driving because of your medical condition. The GOV.UK website has a handy A to Z list of conditions that you can check to see if you need to report your condition, as well as the relevant form or questionnaire. See the 'Useful Websites' section at the end of this chapter for more information.

■ Move to a retirement community.

■ Move to a residential care or nursing home.

When you have listed your problems and the possible solutions, choose one solution that is workable, acceptable, and within your financial means. (This is step 3 of problem solving.) Your choice will depend on your finances, the family or other resources available to help, and how well the potential solutions will solve your problem.

Sometimes one solution may be the answer to several problems. For instance, if you can't shop and can't be alone, and household chores require help, you might consider a retirement community that offers meals, regular house-cleaning, and transportation for errands and medical appointments.

Even if you are not of retirement age, many facilities accept younger people. Some facilities for the retired take residents who are 50 or younger. If you are a younger person, the local centre for people with disabilities or 'independent living centre' may be able to direct you to a care facility suitable for you. When looking for a retirement community, consider the levels of care that are offered. These usually include the following:

■ **independent living**, where you have your own apartment or small house

■ **assisted living**, where you get some help with daily living activities such as taking medications, chores, and errands

■ **skilled nursing**, which includes help with all ADLs and some medical care

Getting Help with Decision Making

It may help to discuss your wishes, abilities, and limitations with a trusted friend, relative, or social worker. Sometimes this other person can identify things you overlook or would like to ignore. Seeking ideas from others and using other resources are important parts of becoming a good self-manager. (These are also parts of step 6: Use other resources, in the problem-solving process described in Chapter 2.)

As you begin to make changes in your life, go slowly, one step at a time. You don't need to change your whole life to solve one problem. Remember, you can always change your mind.

Just be careful not to make a major change in your life that you cannot reverse. For example, if you are thinking of moving out of your own place to another location (a relative's house, a care home, or elsewhere), don't give up your current home until you are sure you want to stay in your new home.

If you think you need help, hiring help at home is a less drastic solution than moving. If you can't be alone and you live with a family member who is away from home during the day, then going to a community centre may be enough to keep you safe and comfortable while your family member is away. In fact, community centres are ideal places to find new friends, and they often provide activities geared to your abilities.

A social worker at your local community centre, local centre for people with disabilities, hospital, or social services department can help by providing you with information about resources in your community. This person can also give you some ideas about how to deal with your care needs. There are several kinds of professionals who can help.

For example, social prescribing or community link workers are based in GP practices and are able to give people the time to focus on 'what matters to me' while taking a holistic approach to people's health and wellbeing. They also connect people to community groups and statutory services for practical and emotional support.

Social workers are good for helping you decide how to solve financial and living arrangement problems and to locate community resources. Some social workers are also trained in counselling people with disabilities or the elderly to deal with emotional and relationship problems.

Another helpful professional is an occupational therapist (OT). An occupational therapist can assess your daily living needs and suggest assistive devices or changes you can make at home to make life easier. OTs can also help you figure out how to keep doing enjoyable activities.

If you have been hospitalised, you can use the hospital's resources. Most hospitals have discharge coordinators. This person, usually a nurse or social worker, will see you before you go home and check that you and family members know what to do. If necessary, they will help find resources so that when you leave the hospital you are safe and continue to heal. It is very important that you be honest with this person. If you have concerns about your ability to care for yourself, say so. Solutions are almost always available. However, the coordinators can help only if you share your concerns. Many hospitals also have chaplains; they might know about resources within your own religious or spiritual community.

Financial advisers and solicitors are also very useful resources. Financial advisers not only provide advice on investing and managing your money, they can also help you plan for your retirement and discuss your options, including the future need for different types of insurance protection such as disability or long-term care insurance. If you use a financial adviser, make sure you understand how their charges are structured before entering into any agreement with them. Financial advisers come in different guises and aren't always called 'financial advisers'. Sometimes they are named by their speciality, such as 'mortgage adviser', 'investment adviser', or 'pensions adviser'. Sometimes they are known as 'brokers', often when dealing with products such as:

■ mortgages

■ home and car insurance, or

■ investments, including shares

Whatever they might be called (or call themselves), what all financial advisers in the UK do have in common is they are regulated by the Financial Conduct Authority (FCA). This means that there are rules they must follow when dealing with you. The independent Money Advice Service will provide you with detailed advice on finding an independent financial adviser that is right for you.

Solicitors, especially those specialising in adult care, should be on your list of resources. They can help you set your financial affairs in order. They can help you to protect your assets, prepare a proper will, and perhaps execute lasting power of attorney (LPA) for both health care and financial management. (An ordinary power of attorney deals with financial matters, while a lasting power of attorney is for health care or financial matters; this is discussed in detail on pages 394–395.)

If finances are a concern, before you seek paid advice do your research. There are many useful websites and organisations that can inform and support your decision making. You will find more information about these as you read through this chapter. If after that you think you do need to seek paid advice, contact your local Citizens Advice for the names of solicitors and financial advisers who offer low-cost services to older people. Age UK can also help you find the right legal advice. The Focus on Disability website has a list of Law Centres across the UK that can offer free legal advice to people in their local communities. If you are living with a disability, even if you are not a senior citizen, your legal needs are much the same as those of the older person. The sooner you can plan for these in the present, the better prepared and more in control you will feel about the future.

Finding Help at Home

Having a carer come to visit you in your home can make a huge difference to your life, especially if you have difficulty walking or getting around. This type of care is known as homecare or domiciliary care, or sometimes as home help.

Help at home types

The following list describes the various kinds of help you might want and need. The majority of this information has been taken from the NHS website, and you might need to check whether there are different arrangements for people living in Scotland, Wales, and Northern Ireland.

■ **Homecare.** You might need a carer for only an hour a week or for several hours a day. You might need a live-in carer. It can be temporary, for example, for a few weeks while you recover from an illness, or it can be long term. Your local council can arrange homecare for you if you're eligible for it. A carer can visit you at home to help you with all kinds of things including:

- ▸ getting out of bed in the morning
- ▸ washing and dressing
- ▸ brushing your hair
- ▸ using the toilet
- ▸ preparing meals and drinks
- ▸ remembering to take your medicines
- ▸ doing your shopping
- ▸ collecting prescriptions or your pension
- ▸ getting out, for example, to a lunch club
- ▸ getting settled in the evening and ready for bed

If you want your local council to help with homecare, start by asking them for a 'needs assessment'. Your needs assessment will help the council to decide whether you're eligible for care. If you're eligible, the council may recommend help at home from a paid carer. They will arrange the homecare for you and you may get help with the cost from the council. What you will contribute depends on your income and savings. The council will work this out in a financial assessment. If the council is paying for some or all of your homecare, they must give you a care and support plan. This sets out what your needs are, how they will be met, and your personal budget (the amount the council thinks your care should cost).

If you aren't eligible for the council to contribute to your homecare costs, you will have to pay for it yourself. However, the council must still give you free advice about where you can get help in your community. Even if you're intending to make arrangements yourself with an agency or private carer, it's still a good idea to have a needs assessment, as it will help you to explain to the agency or carer what kind of help you need. Check if you're eligible for benefits, as some benefits aren't means tested and they can help you meet the costs of homecare. You can do this at https://www.gov.uk/benefits-calculators.

If you're arranging your own homecare, the two main ways to do this are to use a homecare agency or employ your own carer.

Homecare agencies employ trained carers and arrange for them to visit you in your home. You may not always have the same carer visiting your home, though the agency will try to match you with someone suitable. If you're paying for yourself, the agency should be able to give you a clear price list. They'll send you a monthly bill for your homecare.

There are four main ways to find a local homecare agency:

- Search the NHS website for local homecare services and agencies and a list of national homecare organisations and then contact the ones that interest you.

- Ask your local council's social services department for information on the homecare agencies in your area. They may have a directory of homecare agencies on their website.

- Contact the Care Quality Commission (CQC). All homecare agencies must register with the CQC. It can give you the latest inspection report on an agency.

■ Ask the United Kingdom Homecare Association (UKHCA) for a list of approved homecare agencies in your area.

You have the right to complain if you're not happy about the help at home you're receiving. This might be because the carers arrive late and leave early, they don't give your medication to you properly, they leave your home untidy after visits, or they give you poor care, such as not dressing you properly.

First complain to your local council or, if you're paying for yourself, complain directly to the homecare agency. The council or agency should have a formal complaints procedure on their website. Try to be specific about what happened and include staff names and dates if you can. If you're not happy with the way the council or agency handles your complaint, ask the Local Government & Social Care Ombudsman to investigate further. An ombudsman is an independent person who's been appointed to look into complaints about organisations. You can also tell the Care Quality Commission (CQC), which checks social care services in England.

■ **Personal assistant.** Instead of using an agency, you can hire your own carer, sometimes called a private carer or personal assistant. Choosing to receive your personal budget (the amount of money your local council will pay towards you social care and support) as a direct payment each month gives you the control to employ someone you know to care for you at home rather than using a homecare agency. If

you choose to employ a personal assistant you'll then have the legal responsibilities of an employer, which includes arranging cover for their illness and holidays (check the GOV.UK website for information about your responsibilities when employing someone in your home).

A personal assistant can help you or someone you are caring for by assisting with a variety of tasks:

▸ running errands

▸ driving you or a family member on errands, for social outings, or to medical appointments

▸ grocery shopping

▸ cooking or preparing healthy prepared meals to freeze

▸ performing light housekeeping tasks such as laundry, vacuuming, and kitchen and bathroom cleaning

▸ organising and cleaning wardrobes, drawers, or even the garage

▸ keeping you or another family member company – playing cards or games, helping with hobbies, or just sitting and chatting

■ **Respite care in your home.** Sometimes you might need a break and want a little time for yourself. This is especially true if you yourself are a carer. Having someone come in on a regular basis can be a big help. There are lots of respite care options. They range from getting a relative, friend, or volunteer to sit with you to having homecare.

Your local council or local carers' centre can give you information about local support. Some charities and carers' organisations offer sitting services, where a trained volunteer keeps the person you care for company for a while, usually a few hours at a time. This type of sitting service is often free, or there may be a small charge. Find out about sitting services in your area by contacting your local carers' service, Age UK, or Royal Voluntary Society (RVS).

Local councils will fund respite care only for people that they have assessed as needing it. So, if you want the council to pay for respite care for either yourself as a carer or the person you look after, it's important that you both have an assessment. The carer should have a carer's assessment and the person they are looking after should have a needs assessment in the same way as described for homecare.

- **Live-in care.** Live-in care is when a professional carer lives in their client's home to enable their needs to be met. It is an increasingly popular alternative to moving into a care home. It enables you to stay in your own home and meet your changing needs. For some people, it offers a way of continuing to live as independently as possible at home in their local community.

You can organise live-in care:

- privately, through your own advertising, in which case you would be the employer
- through an introductory agency, where carers are self-employed and you manage and pay for their services directly. Most carers from introductory agencies are responsible for paying their own tax and national insurance (NI) contributions

- via a company that employs its carers and manages the service for you. With this arrangement, the provider employs and trains the carers, finding replacements for cover periods. This service is particularly valuable for people for whom an informal caring network isn't close at hand.

- **Home help.** This is slightly different to homecare and means day-to-day domestic tasks that you may need a helping hand with, such as:
  - cleaning (including putting on clean bed sheets)
  - doing the washing up
  - doing the laundry
  - gardening

You might want some home help instead of or as well as homecare. Most councils don't provide home help. Contact a charity such as the Royal Voluntary Service (RVS), the British Red Cross, or your local Age UK to see whether they can help (the services they provide may not be free).

- Another way to find help that is less expensive is to hire someone *recommended by a friend or through a help wanted advert or posting on a website*. If you choose this option, know that it involves more time – you will be responsible for checking all references and doing all the screening. This person can work for you as an employee, in which case you will have all the legal responsibilities of an employer, so you should make sure you know what these are.

Moving to a New Residence

The time may come when you or your partner needs to move to a new residence. This might be because your health is declining or due to the increased health needs of your partner. This is a difficult decision to make regardless of the reason, and the decision-making tool discussed in Chapter 2, *Becoming an Active Self-Manager*, can help. Once you make that decision, you can then begin to look for the type of community that provides the care you need. The following section outlines some of the options available.

- **Independent living or retirement villages.** If either you or your partner is a 'senior' (usually over age 50), this option is open to you. This type of accommodation may be owned or rented and provides a more protected setting with security and emergency response services. These villages usually offer meals in a dining room and weekly housekeeping. They sometimes also offer laundry service and personal transportation. They often host a variety of activities and outings. This kind of community is an option if you no longer want to cook and clean but do want to be around others every day. The majority of properties in retirement villages are designed for independent living, but some offer care and support for those that need it. This might be in assisted living apartments or on-site care services that can provide home help or personal care. Some schemes have care homes on site, should people require more care in the future. If you're thinking about a retirement village, make sure that it offers the care and support you require and think about your future care needs if possible.

  There are almost always waiting lists for this type of community, often even before they are built and ready for occupancy. If you think such a place would be right for you, get on the waiting list right away, or at least a couple of years before you think you want to move. You can always change your mind or decline if you are not ready when a space is offered. To find these communities in your area, search the Internet for 'independent living for older people' or 'retirement villages' near you. If you have friends living in nearby retirement villages, ask to be invited for a visit and a meal. This will help you to get an insider's view. Some villages even have guest accommodation where you can arrange to stay for a night or two before you commit to a lease or contract.

- **Assisted living facilities.** An Assisted Living Facility (ALF) usually offers all the services that independent living residences do, plus some personal care and help with taking medication. Care offered at assisted living facilities can range between help with basic everyday tasks (like cleaning and shopping) to more advanced care (personal care, medical attention) and caters for a variety of needs and requirements. What is on offer can vary between ALFs. You'll normally have 24-hour on-call assistance and fitted alarms in each property. Care can be administered on a regular basis or one-off, as much or as little as you would like.

- **Sheltered housing.** This can be an ideal option for people who want to retain their independence while having the peace of mind to know that help is on hand if needed. Some common features of sheltered housing include:
  - ▸ help from a scheme manager (warden), or support staff
  - ▸ 24-hour emergency help through an alarm system
  - ▸ communal areas, such as gardens or lounges
  - ▸ social activities for residents

There are various types of sheltered housing ranging from rented accommodation provided by your local authority or by voluntary organisations, to housing that is privately owned and run, which sometimes you can have the option to buy, or rent.

- **Care homes.** A care home may be the best option if you or someone you know is struggling to live alone (even with help from friends, family, or paid carers), has had a needs assessment that suggested a care home is the best choice, or has a complex medical condition that needs specialist attention during the day and night. There are two main types of care home:
  - ▸ **residential homes,** which provide accommodation and personal care, such as help with washing, dressing, taking medications, and going to the toilet
  - ▸ **nursing homes,** which also provide accommodation and personal care, in addition to qualified nurses on duty to provide nursing care. These are sometimes called care homes with nursing. Some nursing homes offer services for people that may need more care and support, for example, for someone who has a colostomy or who is fed through a tube

Some care homes offer both residential and nursing care places. Some care homes also offer activities, such as day trips.

Care homes may be run by private companies, voluntary or charitable organisations, or sometimes by local authorities. The cost of a care home will be different depending on the type of care home you need and where you live. Nursing homes usually cost more than residential homes, as they provide nursing care. Before deciding how to pay for a care home, it's worth asking your local council for a needs assessment. The council can then help you look at all your options. If the local council is paying for your care home, you should be given a care plan by the council, which lets you know your options. The information in your care plan might also help you decide which care home best meets your needs. You can choose which care home you prefer, as long as the council agrees that it meets your needs and is not more expensive than another suitable care home. You may choose to pay for care yourself if you're able to afford it or if you don't want to have your finances assessed. If you are paying for the care home you might have a lot of options. It's important to do some research to make sure it's the right place to meet your needs. Your local authority's adult social care services can give you more information about care homes in your area, and you can speak to organisations like Age UK before you make your decision.

Many people have negative feelings about care homes. You might have read or heard negative stories. Unfortunately, these reports and stories help to create anxiety and fear. Although some of these stories may be true, all the excellent care received in care homes never makes the news. There are organisations that regularly inspect and monitor services provided in care homes, and you may want to look at their reports while conducting your enquiries. The Care Quality Commission (CQC) inspects and rates residential care homes and nursing homes in England. You can download the latest inspection report and information about any care home from their website. In Wales, care home inspections are carried by the Care Inspectorate Wales, whose website also provides a list of things to consider when choosing a care home and a register of service providers. In Scotland, this role is carried out by the Care Inspectorate, and in Northern Ireland the responsibility lies with the Regulation and Quality Improvement Authority.

■ **Continuing care retirement communities (CCRCs).** These have long been a retirement option in the US but have only recently become available in the UK. CCRCs provide a full spectrum of care, from independent living right through to 24-hour care, which is flexible and tailored to individual needs. CCRCs typically comprise a care home and a number of extra care dwellings, where residents can live as independently as possible in the security that care is available on site as and when it is needed. They also provide a range of onsite facilities and opportunities, promoting general health and well-being as well as social interaction.

Whatever options you consider, this step requires a lot of thought and research. It is a big decision. Use the decision-making tools discussed in Chapter 2, *Becoming an Active Self-Manager*, and consider holding a family meeting to discuss this with close family members and friends and get ideas and help from them.

Will I Have Enough Money to Pay for My Long-Term Care?

There are differences in the way that health and social care services are funded across the four nations of the UK.

How is health care funded?

There's more than one NHS in the UK, as responsibility for healthcare has been passed from the UK government to the Scottish Government, Welsh Government, and Northern Irish Assembly. NHS England, NHS Wales (GIG Cymru), and NHS Scotland provide healthcare services in Great Britain. The publicly funded health care service in Northern Ireland isn't officially called the NHS, it's actually called Health and Social Care Services (HSC).

Each NHS organisation and the HSC provide healthcare services free at the point of delivery (that is, free at the point of use). However, there are differences in what is fully funded by government and what services are available across the different UK countries. For example, NHS England asks some people to pay part of the cost of prescriptions, whereas in Wales, Scotland, and Northern Ireland these costs are covered by the government.

Even where people are asked to contribute towards the cost of their healthcare, some people do not have to pay these costs. If this is the case for you, the NHS will ask to see proof of your entitlement. This could be a prescription prepayment certificate (PPC), benefit award notice, or an exemption certificate. It's your responsibility to check whether you're entitled to claim for free treatment or prescriptions.

You can find out what health services are free of charge in each of the UK nations and whether you're entitled to help by following the link to the relevant websites listed in the 'Useful Websites' section at the end of this chapter.

How is social care funded?

If you need support with day-to-day tasks, or you need to move into a care home, your local authority might help with the costs of care. Exactly how much you get will depend on your care needs and how much you can afford to pay.

The NHS website and the government-backed Money Advice Service website offer a range of comprehensive information to help people make decisions about how to fund their long-term social care needs. We have summarised the main points for you:

- **Check if you are eligible for financial support.** You might be eligible for the local

council to pay toward the cost of your care if you have less than £23,250 in savings (correct as of June 2020). Exactly how much your council will pay depends on what care you need and how much you can afford to pay.

- **Check if you are eligible for NHS continuing healthcare.** If you have a disability or complex medical problem, you might qualify for free NHS continuing healthcare (CHC). This is a package of healthcare that's arranged and funded by the NHS. It is provided for you at home, in a care home, nursing home, or hospice. You're more likely to qualify if you have mostly healthcare needs rather than social care needs – in other words, if you need a nurse or medical attention rather than a carer.

- **Ask your local council for a needs assessment.** Your local council (or Health and Social Care Trust in Northern Ireland) may be able to help you with the costs of help at home or a care home. Your local authority or trust can arrange care services for you, or you can choose to receive direct payments and organise things yourself. The first step is for your council to do an assessment to check how much help you need (a needs assessment).

- **Complete a financial assessment.** If the needs assessment shows that you should have care, the council will then do a financial assessment (a means test) to work out what if any, you will have to pay toward the cost of your care.

- **Develop your care and support plan with the local council and have a personal**

budget allocated. If the council is going to pay toward your care, you'll get a personal budget (the amount of money your local council will pay toward any social care and support you need). The amount will be worked out when the council makes a care and support plan with you. You can choose to get your personal budget in three ways:

- ► A direct payment is made into your bank account each month for you to pay for your care.

- ► The council arranges and pays for your care.

- ► A mixed personal budget: the council arranges some of your care and you arrange and pay for the rest with a personal budget.

■ **Work out your finances.** Depending on your circumstances, you might not qualify for funding from the NHS or your local council. Even if you do, the amount you receive might not be enough to completely cover your care costs either at home or in a care home. If this happens, you'll need to think about how you're going to pay your share of the cost, or if you have to pay for it all yourself. It is never too soon or too late to start financial planning for both expected and unexpected future events.

■ **Find out if you are entitled to any benefits.** Even if you have to pay for care, you may still be entitled to claim some benefits. You can contact your local Citizens Advice or Age UK for advice about what help you might receive with your care costs.

Even though the idea of discussing the future may make you and your family feel uncomfortable or uneasy, the sooner you begin this process the better off and more secure you will all feel knowing there is a plan in place. You will also be better prepared if something happens.

I Need Help but Don't Want Help – Now What?

In addition to practical and financial concerns, there are the emotional aspects of needing help. Most people leave childhood wanting and reaching for independence – your driving license, your first job, your first credit card, the first time you go out and don't have to tell anybody where you are going, and so on. In these and many other ways, you demonstrate to yourself and others that you are 'grown up'. You are in charge of your life and able to take care of yourself.

If you realise that you can no longer manage completely on your own, it may feel like a return to childhood. This may seem like a loss of independence. You again find yourself with somebody else in charge of parts of your life. This can be painful and embarrassing.

Some people faced with this situation become depressed and can no longer find any joy in life. Others deny their need for help. They may even place themselves in danger, making life difficult for those who want to be helpful.

Still others give up and expect others to take care of them completely. They may demand attention and support from their children or other family members. If you are having one or more of these reactions, you can help yourself and develop a more positive response.

The idea of 'changing the things you can change, accepting the things you cannot change, and knowing the difference' is key to staying in charge of your life. Take a hard and realistic look at your situation. Identify the activities that require help (such as going shopping and cleaning the house) and those that you can still do yourself (such as getting dressed, paying bills, and cooking easy meals). Another way to look at this is to ask for help from others for the things you least like to do. This gives you time and energy to do the things you like.

Figuring out what kind of help you need means making decisions. And if you are making the decisions, you are in charge. It is important to make decisions and take action while you are still able to do so. Don't let events force someone else to make your decisions. You must be realistic and honest with yourself. Use the decision-making tools on pages 27–28 in Chapter 2, *Becoming an Active Self-Manager*.

Even though you are the decision maker and the manager, you don't need to figure it all out alone. Some people find that talking with a sympathetic listener – either a professional counsellor or a sensible close friend or family member – is comforting and helpful. A thoughtful listener can often point out options you may have overlooked. You may see things in a new light.

Choose your advisers carefully and be cautious when you take advice. Don't take advice from somebody who is selling something. There are many people whose solution to your problem is whatever they are selling – this can include things like health or funeral insurance policies, annuities, special and expensive furniture, 'sunshine cruises', special magazines, or health foods.

When talking with family members or friends, be as open and reasonable as possible. At the same time, try to make them understand that you are the one who decides to accept or not accept help. To gain their cooperation, use 'I' messages. For example, 'Yes, I do need some help with _____, but I still want to do _____ myself.' You can learn more about communicating with 'I' messages and other communication tips in Chapter 11, *Communicating with Family, Friends, and Healthcare Professionals*.

Asking for help does not mean giving up your right to choose. Insist on being asked about all the important decisions that affect you. Early on, lay the ground rules with your helpers. Ask to be presented with options when it is time to make choices. Try hard to weigh good suggestions, and do not dismiss every option that isn't your own idea. If you learn to be a good decision maker, people will see that you can make reasonable decisions and will continue to give you the opportunity to do so.

Be appreciative. Recognise the goodwill and efforts of people who want to help you. When you need help, you maintain your dignity by gracefully accepting help. Getting assistance might be embarrassing, but in the long run getting help can allow you to maintain your independence. If you believe that you are being offered help you don't need, say no with tact and appreciation. For example, 'I appreciate your offer to have Christmas at your house, but I'd like to continue having it here. I could use some help, though. I would like to roast the turkey, but could the rest of you bring the other food and wash up after dinner?'

If you are unable to come to terms with your increasing needs for help from others, talk with a professional. Find a counsellor who has experience with the emotional and social issues of people with long-term health conditions. Ask at your GP surgery for information about free psychological therapy services ('talking therapies') in your area, or get the details of registered counsellors and therapists from the British Association for Counselling and Psychotherapy (BACP). In addition, there may be organisations working for people with your specific long-term condition, such as the MS Society or Parkinson's UK, and they will be able to direct you to local support groups or toward support online.

When you know you cannot do something yourself, reach out to family and friends. Sometimes, people fear rejection and so never ask. Other people try to hide their need for fear that their loved ones will withdraw. Families often complain, 'If we'd only known...'' when they find out that a loved one has needs that were unmet. Like the fear and embarrassment of becoming physically dependent, there is also the fear of being abandoned by family members. Tales of being 'dumped' in a nursing home by children who never come to visit haunt many people. They worry that this may happen to them. A more usual situation is that people who you thought would help don't end up helping. Sometimes this is because they don't know how. You may expect people to 'know what to do'. But often people do in fact not know what to do. Sometimes they are almost as overwhelmed by your situation as you are. Remember from Chapter 11 that you cannot change how others communicate. What you can do is change your communication to be sure you are understood.

If you cannot turn to close family or friends, turn to helpful agencies. Contact your GP surgery and ask for an appointment to see the local link worker or for a referral to your local social prescribing service (or make direct contact with your local social prescribing service). Social prescribing is the way in which GPs and other frontline healthcare professionals refer patients to a link worker to have a conversation about their support options and design their own personalised solutions (that is, helping people 'co-produce' their 'social prescription'), often by connecting them to community services that might be run by the council or a local charity. For example, signposting people who have been diagnosed with dementia to local dementia support groups or signposting to community groups running activities such as volunteering, arts and crafts, group learning, gardening, befriending, cookery, healthy eating advice, and a range of sports.

Social prescribing works for a wide range of people, including people with one or more long-term conditions, who need support with their mental health, who are lonely or isolated and who have complex social needs that affect their well-being.

Grieving: A Normal Reaction to Bad News

When you experience loss – small losses (such as losing a special keepsake) or big losses (such as losing a life partner or facing a disabling or terminal illness) – you go through an emotional process called grieving. This is natural; it helps people to come to terms with the loss.

A person with a long-term disabling health condition experiences a variety of losses. These can include loss of confidence, loss of self-esteem, loss of independence, loss of lifestyle, and perhaps the most painful of all, loss of a positive self-image. This is especially true if your condition has changed your appearance. This can happen with rheumatoid arthritis, Parkinson's disease, paralysis from a stroke, or the loss of a breast due to cancer.

Elizabeth Kübler-Ross, a well-known psychiatrist, described the stages of grief:

- **Shock**, when you feel both a mental and a physical reaction to the initial recognition of the loss.

- **Denial**, when you think, 'No, it can't be true', and proceed to act for a time as if it were not true.

- **Anger**, when you fume 'Why me?' and search for someone or something to blame (if the doctor had diagnosed it earlier, the job caused me too much stress, etc.).

- **Bargaining**, when you promise, 'I'll never smoke again', or 'I'll follow my treatment regime to the letter', or 'I'll go to church every Sunday, if only I can get over this.'

- **Depression**, when awareness sets in, you confront the truth about the situation, and experience deep feelings of sadness and hopelessness.

- **Acceptance**, when you recognise that you must deal with what has happened and make up your mind to do what you must do to move forward.

People do not necessarily pass through these stages one after another. You are more likely to flip-flop between them. Therefore, don't be surprised or discouraged if you find yourself angry or depressed again when you thought you had reached acceptance. This is normal.

Making End-of-Life Decisions

Decisions about the end of life can be very difficult. For all of us, this means dealing with the idea of our own mortality. As you age, you may begin to have fears about death. This is especially true when something happens to bring you face-to-face with the possibility of your own death. Losing someone close, surviving an accident, or learning you have a health condition that may shorten your life usually causes you to think about your own passing.

Attitudes about death are shaped by core attitudes about life. These are the product of your culture, your family, perhaps your religion, and certainly your life experiences. You might wish or pray for yourself or a loved one to be released from suffering, feel guilty about these wishes, or fear dying. Sometimes we have all these feelings. If this is how you feel, you are not alone. These feelings are common. Many people try to avoid these feelings; they do not want to face the future because they are afraid to think about death.

If you are ready to think about your own and your partner's future – about the near or distant prospect that your lives will most certainly end – then the ideas that follow will be useful. If you are not ready to think about this just yet, put this reading aside for now and come back when you are ready.

Taking positive steps to prepare for death is useful and healthy. This means getting your house in order by attending to all the necessary details, large and small. If you avoid dealing with these details, you create problems for yourself and for those who love and care for you. You also may lose your ability to make these important decisions.

Whatever you decide about your future, it is important to tell others. What are your wishes about how and where you want to be during your last days? Do you want to be in a hospital or at home? When do you want to stop procedures that prolong your life? At what point do you want nature to take its course? Who should be with you – only the few people who

are nearest and dearest, or all the people you care about and want to see one last time? What will happen if you can no longer manage your affairs? Most people have very definite ideas about what they would like. Share these ideas and wishes with others.

This kind of end-of-life planning is hard and sometimes frightening. People do not like thinking about all the 'what ifs'. Nevertheless, such planning is necessary for you, your partner, and your family. Good planning will protect you and ensure that your wishes are understood and carried out.

However, if your plans are not written down, and more importantly written into legal documents, your wishes might not be followed. In this next section, we discuss the types of legal documents you should have in place. If you are not sure what you have, or you do not have any of these, do your homework first before consulting a solicitor. Many people worry that going to a solicitor will be very expensive, which it can be! However, some solicitors will offer a fixed-fee initial consultation where you discuss your needs. Use this first meeting to establish the cost of any further advice. Also, solicitors' fees do vary. Shop around to find one whose fees fit best with what you can afford to pay. Contact Citizens Advice, Age UK, your local Law Centre, or your condition-specific charity to see if they can advise you about how to find a solicitor.

Legal Planning

Preparing legal documents should be done now, not later. This is especially true if your mental abilities are affected by your long-term health condition. Solicitors who are consulted about legal end-of-life planning are required by law to determine that a person is 'of sound mind' and able to make these decisions for themselves. You can download a factsheet on obtaining legal and financial advice from the Age UK website.

The Office of the Public Guardian (OPG) helps people in England and Wales to stay in control of decisions about their health and finance and make important decisions for others who cannot decide for themselves. They have a telephone helpline where you can obtain some general advice about planning for the future: 0300 456 0300 (Monday–Friday, 9:30 A.M.–5 P.M.) or you can visit their website, https://www.gov.uk/government/organisations/office-of-the-public-guardian. For contact details of the Office of the Public Guardian (Scotland) and the Office of Care and Protection (Northern Ireland), see the 'Useful Websites' section at the end of this chapter.

First, a disclaimer: the following discussion is not complete. Also, the laws are different for each of the UK nations. These are just the basics to prepare you for a deeper discussion with your partner, family, and solicitor.

Advance Decisions (Living Wills)

Although none of us has control over our own death; our death, like the rest of our life, is something we can help manage. That is, you can have input, make decisions, and probably add quality to your final days. Proper management can make your death easier on family and friends. An advance decision can help you manage some of the medical and legal issues concerning death as well as help you plan for both expected and unexpected end-of-life situations. You and other adult family members should prepare an advance healthcare decision as early as possible. This is true even for people

who do not have any long-term health conditions. Without this decision, your wishes may not be followed.

Advance Decisions (sometimes known as an advance decision to refuse treatment, an ADRT, or a living will) are instructions that tell your doctor what kind of care you would like to receive when you are not able to make medical decisions for yourself (for example, if you are unconscious, in a coma, or mentally incapacitated). If you want to refuse potentially life-sustaining treatment your decision must be in writing, signed, witnessed, and include the statement 'even if life is at risk as a result'.

The treatments you're deciding to refuse must all be named in the advance decision. You may want to refuse a treatment in some situations, but not in others. If this is the case, you need to be clear about all the circumstances in which you want to refuse this treatment. An advance decision is legally binding, which means that those caring for you must follow your instructions. However, it will only be used if you lose the capacity to make or communicate decisions about your treatment.

You should discuss your advance decision with a healthcare professional who knows your medical history and the risks and benefits of refusing certain treatments. You may also want to discuss it with your family and friends so that they understand your wishes. Your GP and medical team must know about your advance decision so they can include it in your medical notes. You should review it regularly and can change it at any time. You must make sure that you clearly communicate and record these changes, being sure to date and sign it.

An advance decision is not something you should make without careful consideration, and it's best to seek advice in the first instance from the Office of the Public Guardian and also, if necessary, to seek legal advice about setting up an advance decision.

Advance Statement

An advance statement is also used when you are unable to communicate your wishes and is a more general statement about how you would like to be looked after. It can cover any aspect of your future health or social care. An advance statement is not legally binding. The aim of an advance statement is to provide a guide to anyone who might have to make decisions in your best interest if you have lost the capacity to make decisions or to communicate them. It also takes into account who you would like to be involved when discussions about you need to be made so that you can have your wishes followed. You can make sure people know about your wishes by talking about them. By writing your advance statement down, you can help to make things clear to your family, carers, and anybody involved in your care.

CPR and a 'Do Not Attempt CPR' decision

Cardiopulmonary resuscitation (CPR) is a treatment that attempts to start breathing and blood flow in people who have stopped breathing (respiratory arrest) or whose heart has stopped beating (cardiac arrest). Everyone has the right to refuse CPR if they wish. You can make it clear to your healthcare professionals that you do not want to have CPR if you stop breathing or your heart stops beating. This is known as a do not attempt cardiopulmonary resuscitation (DNACPR) decision, or DNACPR order. Once a DNACPR decision is made, it's put in your medical records, usually on a special form that healthcare professionals will recognise. It's also helpful to let your family or other carers know about your DNACPR decision so that it does not come as a surprise to them if the situation arises.

Lasting Power of Attorney (LPA) – Health and Welfare

A lasting power of attorney (LPA) is a legal document that lets you (the 'donor') appoint one or more people (known as 'attorneys') to help you make decisions or to make decisions on your behalf. This gives you more control over what happens to you if you have an accident or an illness and cannot make your own decisions (you 'lack mental capacity'). You must be 18 or over and have mental capacity (the ability to make your own decisions) when you make your LPA. There are two types of LPA, one for health and welfare and the other for financial and property affairs. You can choose to have either one or both (see the GOV.UK website for more information).

Under the health and welfare LPA your attorney can make decisions about anything to do with your health and personal welfare. This includes decisions about medical treatment, where you are cared for, the type of care you receive, day-to-day things like your diet, how you dress, and your daily routine. You can list any instructions that your attorney must follow, or any preferences that you'd like them to take into account when making decisions on your behalf. You'll also need to choose whether or not you want your attorney to be able to make decisions about life-sustaining treatment. If you choose not to, then all decisions about life-sustaining treatment will be made by your healthcare team, unless you've made an advance decision (living will).

To make an LPA you need to choose an attorney, complete a form available from the Office of the Public Guardian (OPG), and register the form with the OPG. The OPG is there to help you decide if a lasting power of attorney is right for you.

After reading the information on advance decisions and lasting power of attorney, you may feel that the process is both complicated and off-putting. If this is true in your case, you will be pleased to know that there are several organisations that can guide you through the process and, if necessary, support you to find a solicitor with the relevant legal expertise. Contact details can be found in the 'Useful Websites' section at the end of this chapter.

What follows are some examples of situations you might find yourself in:

- **You have been diagnosed with Alzheimer's disease and/or other neurologic problems that may eventually leave you with little or no mental function.** These conditions generally are not life-threatening, at least not for many years. However, other things can happen to you that can be life-threatening, such as pneumonia and heart attacks. Therefore, you need to decide how much treatment you want. For example, do you

want antibiotics if you get pneumonia? Do you want to be resuscitated if your heart stops? Do you want a feeding tube if you are unable to feed yourself? Remember, it is your choice as to how you answer each of these questions. You may not want to be resuscitated but may want a feeding tube. If you want aggressive treatment, you might want to have all means possible used to sustain life. On the other hand, you might not want any special means to be used to sustain life. For example, you may want to be fed but may not want to be placed on life-support equipment.

- **You have very bad lung function that will not improve.** If you become unable to breathe on your own, do you want to be placed in an intensive care unit on a mechanical ventilator (a breathing machine)? Remember, in this case you will not improve. To say that you never want ventilation is very different from saying that you don't want it if it is used to sustain life if improvement is unlikely. Obviously, mechanical ventilation can be life-saving in cases such as a severe asthma attack, when it is used for a short time until the body can regain its normal function. In this case, the issue is not whether to use mechanical ventilation ever but rather when you want to use it.

- **You have a heart condition that cannot be improved with surgery.** Imagine you are in the cardiac intensive care unit. If your heart stops functioning, do you want to be resuscitated? As with artificial ventilation, the question is not, 'Do you ever want to be resuscitated?' but rather, 'Under what conditions do you or do you not want resuscitation?'

From these examples you can begin to identify some of the directions that you might want to give in your **advance decision** or **Lasting Power of Attorney (LPA) for health and welfare**.

In summary, there are several decisions you need to make in directing your attorney on how to act on your behalf:

■ Generally, how much treatment do you want? This can range from the very aggressive – that is, doing many things to keep you alive – to the very conservative, which means doing almost nothing to keep you alive except to keep you clean and comfortable.

■ Given the types of life-threatening events that are likely to happen to people with your condition, what sorts of treatment do you want and under what conditions do you want them?

■ If you become mentally incapacitated, what sorts of treatment do you want for other illnesses, such as pneumonia?

Sharing Your Wishes About End-of-Life Issues with Friends and Family

Writing down your wishes and having your advance decisions for healthcare in place and a lasting power of attorney for health and welfare is not the end of your job. A good self-manager must do more than just write a memo; a good self-manager must see that the memo gets delivered. If you want your wishes carried out, you must share your wishes with your attorneys, family, and healthcare team. Often, this is not an easy task.

Before you can have this conversation, everyone involved needs to have copies of your LPA for health and welfare. Once you have completed these documents, have them witnessed and signed. In some places you can have your LPA for health and welfare notarised

(by having it certified as a true copy of the original by a professional person, like a solicitor) instead of having it witnessed. Make several copies. You will need copies for your attorney, family members, and hospital doctors. Also, give one to your solicitor if you have one. The Office of the Public Guardian can guide you through these steps.

Now you are ready to talk about your wishes. People don't like to discuss their own death or that of a loved one. Therefore, it should not surprise you that when you bring up this subject, the response may be, 'Oh, don't think about that', or 'That's a long time off', or 'Don't be so morbid; you're not that sick.' Unfortunately, this is usually enough to end the conversation.

Your job is to keep the conversation open. There are several ways to do this. First, plan on how you will have this discussion. Here are some suggestions:

- Prepare your LPA for health and welfare and give copies to the appropriate family members or friends. Ask them to read it and then set a specific time to discuss it. If they give you one of the avoidance responses, explain that you understand that this is a difficult topic but that you must discuss it with them. This is a good time to practice the 'I' messages discussed in Chapter 11, *Communicating with Family, Friends, and Healthcare Professionals*. For example, say, 'I understand that death is a difficult thing to talk about. However, it is very important to me that we have this talk.'

- Another strategy is to get blank copies of the LPA for health and welfare form for all your family members and suggest that you each fill one out and share them. This could even be part of a family get-together. Present this as an important aspect of being mature adults and family members. Making this a family project involving everyone may make it easier to discuss. Besides, it will help clarify everyone's values about death and dying. Even teenagers can be part of this discussion.

- If these two suggestions seem too difficult or for some reason are impossible, you can write a letter or e-mail or prepare a video to send to family members. Talk about why you feel your death is an important topic to discuss and that you want them to know

your wishes. Then state your wishes. Give reasons for your choices. At the same time, send them a copy of your LPA for health and welfare. Ask that they respond in some way or that you set aside some time to talk in person or on the phone.

As mentioned before, when deciding on your attorney, it is key that you choose someone with whom you can talk freely and exchange ideas. If your chosen attorney is not willing to or is unable to talk to you about your wishes, you have probably chosen the wrong person. Remember, the fact that someone is very close to you does not mean that this person really understands your wishes or would be able to carry them out. This topic should not be left to an unspoken understanding unless you don't mind if your attorney goes against your wishes. For this reason, you may want to choose someone who is not as emotionally close to you. If you do choose someone outside of close family members, make sure your family knows who you have appointed and why.

Talking About End-of-Life Issues with Your Doctor

From our research, we have learned that people often have a more difficult time talking with their doctors about their wishes than they do talking with their families about end-of-life issues. In fact, only a very small percentage of people who have written LPAs for health and welfare or other advance decisions ever share these with their doctor.

Even though it is difficult, you should talk with your doctor. You need to be sure that your doctor's values are like yours. If you and your doctor do not have the same values, it may be difficult for your doctor to carry out your wishes. Second, your doctor needs to know what you want. This allows your doctor to take appropriate actions such as writing orders to resuscitate or not to use mechanical resuscitation. Third, your doctor needs to know who your attorney is and how to contact this person. If an important decision must be made and your wishes are to be followed, the doctor must talk with your attorney.

Be sure to give your GP a copy of your LPA for health and welfare so that it can become a permanent part of your medical record. As mentioned earlier, there is another advance decision called a DNACPR (do not attempt cardiopulmonary resuscitation – CPR). The DNACPR decision is a written instruction to medical staff not to attempt to bring you back to life if your heart stops beating or you stop breathing. The decision is usually recorded on a special DNACPR form, completed by a doctor. The form makes it easy for healthcare professionals to quickly recognise a DNACPR decision in an emergency. Your DNACPR form needs to be available in an emergency so that any professionals caring for you know it exists. If you're in hospital, the form will be kept with your notes. If you're sent home, you should give a copy to your GP to keep with your records. You should also tell family members or carers about it and where it's kept. This helps to avoid conflict between medical professionals and family members.

You can also ask for a DNACPR to be recorded in your emergency care plan (ECP),

if you have one. ECPs are drawn up by medical professionals in discussion with you. They are designed to provide easily accessible, brief clinical recommendations for use in an emergency. They are usually put in place for people with complex health needs, life-limiting conditions, or illnesses that can suddenly deteriorate or cause heart failure.

As surprising as it may seem, many doctors also find it hard to talk to their patients about end-of-life wishes. After all, doctors are in the business of keeping people alive and well. They don't like to think about their patients dying. On the other hand, most doctors want their patients to have a lasting power of attorney for health and welfare (and sometimes a DNACPR). These documents relieve both you and your doctor from added stress and worry.

If you wish, plan a time with your GP when you can discuss your wishes. This should not be a side conversation at the end of a regular visit. Rather, start a visit by saying, 'I want a few minutes to discuss my wishes in the event of a serious problem or impending death.' When put this way, most doctors will make time to talk with you. If the GP says that there is not enough time to talk with you, ask when you can make another appointment. This is a situation where you might need to be a little assertive. Sometimes a doctor, like your family members or friends, might say, 'Oh, you don't have to worry about that; let me do it', or 'We'll worry about that when the time comes.' Again, you must take the initiative, using an 'I' message to communicate that this is important to you and that you do not want to put off the discussion.

Sometimes doctors do not want to worry you. They think they are doing you a favour by not describing all the unpleasant things that might happen in case of serious problems. You can help your doctors by telling them that having control and making some decisions about your future will ease your mind. Not knowing or not being clear on what will happen is more worrisome than being faced with the facts, unpleasant as they may be, and dealing with them.

Even if you know all this information, it is still sometimes hard to talk with your GP. Therefore, it might also be helpful to bring your attorney to this discussion. The attorney can facilitate the discussion and at the same time make your doctor's acquaintance. This also gives everyone a chance to clarify any misunderstandings. It opens the lines of communication so that if your attorney and GP must act to carry out your wishes, they can do so with few problems. If you cannot talk with your GP, they should still receive a copy of your LPA for health and welfare for your medical record.

When you go to the hospital, be sure to take a copy of your LPA for health and welfare with you. If you do not take it, be sure your attorney knows to give a copy to the hospital. If you do not have an LPA already prepared, the hospital will ask you to fill out their advance decision form. This is important so that the doctors who oversee your care in the hospital know your wishes.

Do not put your LPA for health and welfare in your safe deposit box – no one will be able to get it when it is needed. And remember, you do not need to see a solicitor to draw up your LPA for health and welfare. You can do this by downloading the form from the GOV.UK website and by seeking the help of the Office of the Public Guardian.

Preparing Yourself and Others

Now that you have done all the important things, the hard work is over. However, remember that you can change your mind at any time. Your attorney may no longer be available, or your wishes might change. Be sure to keep your LPA for health and welfare updated. Like most legal documents, it can be revoked or changed at any time. The decisions you make today are not forever.

Sharing your wishes about how you want to be treated in case of a serious or life-threatening illness is one of the most important self-management tasks. Here are some other steps to help reduce the emotional burden to your family and friends:

■ **Make a Will.** Even if your estate is a small one and your belongings are few, you may have ideas about who should inherit what. If you have a large estate, the tax implications could be significant. A will also ensures that your belongings go where you want them to go. Without a will, some distant or 'long-lost' relative may end up with your estate. You might also want to consider a trust. Your will should include information about what you want done with your financial accounts and give directions about who can access them and how. If you die without a will the law will decide who gets what. You can write your will yourself (by downloading a template from the Internet or buying a will pack from a stationary shop), but you should get advice from a solicitor if your will is not straightforward. You need to get your will formally witnessed and signed to make it legally valid. If you want to update your will, you need to make an official alteration (called a 'codicil') or make a new will. Every October is 'Free Wills Month', during which a group of well-respected charities offer members of the public aged 55 and over the opportunity to have their simple wills written or updated free of charge by participating solicitors in locations across England, Northern Ireland, and Wales.

■ **Plan your funeral.** Write down your wishes or arrange for your funeral. Your grieving family will be very relieved not to have to decide what you would want and how much to spend. Prepaid funeral plans are available. You can purchase your burial space in the location you prefer. Be sure that the people you want to handle things after your death are aware of all they need to know about your wishes. This includes your plans and arrangements, and the location of necessary documents. Talk to them, or at least prepare a detailed letter of instructions. Give the letter to someone you trust to deliver it to the right person at the right time.

■ **Organise your papers.** You can buy (online or at any well-stocked stationery shop) a kit in which you place a copy of your will, your lasting powers of attorney (for health and welfare and for financial and legal matters), other important papers, and information about your financial and personal affairs. If you keep these documents on your computer, be sure others can find your passwords and accounts.

■ **Finish your dealings with the world around you.** Mend any damaged relationships. Pay your debts, both financial and personal. Say what needs to be said to those who need to hear it. Do what needs to be done. Forgive yourself. Forgive others. (By the way, this is a good idea at any time, not just at the end of life.)

■ **Talk about your feelings about your death.** Most family and close friends are reluctant to start this conversation but will appreciate it if you bring it up. You may find that there is much to say to and to hear from your loved ones. If you find that they are unwilling to listen to you talk about your death and the feelings that you have, find someone who will be comfortable and understanding in listening to you. Most hospital and hospice services have chaplains who have these types of conversations daily. You may find it helpful to talk to a person with this experience and training. Your family and friends might be able to listen to you later. Remember, those who love you will also go through the stages of grieving when they think about losing you.

A large part of fear is fear of the unknown: 'What will it be like?' 'Will it be painful?' 'What will happen to me after I die?' Most people who die of an illness are ready to die when the time comes. Painkillers and the disease process weaken body and mind. The awareness of self diminishes without the realisation that this is happening. Most people just 'slip away', with the transition between the state of living and that of no longer living hardly noticeable. Think about how a river meets the ocean. Reports from people who have been brought back to life after being in a state of clinical death indicate that they experienced a sense of peacefulness and clarity and were not frightened.

People who are dying sometimes feel lonely and abandoned. Many people cannot deal with their own emotions when they are around a person they know is dying. They avoid the dying person's company, or they may engage in superficial chitchat, broken by long, awkward silences. This is often puzzling and hurtful to those who are dying, who are seeking companionship and solace from the people they counted on.

You can help by telling your family and friends what you want and need from them – attention, entertainment, comfort, music, practical help, and so on. A person who has something positive to do is more able to cope with difficult emotions. If you can engage your family and loved ones in specific activities, they can feel needed and can relate to you around the activity. This will give you something to talk about, and it will occupy everyone's time in a beneficial way. It helps to define the situation for them and for you.

Considering Palliative Care and Hospice Care

Palliative care and hospice care are available in most parts of the UK. The goal of both palliative and hospice care is to provide comfort. The word *palliative* refers to relieving symptoms such as pain associated with a serious illness and improving quality of life. The word *hospice* refers to care provided for the terminally ill at home or in the community rather than in a hospital. Palliative care can begin at diagnosis and occur at the same time as treatment. Hospice care begins after treatment of the illness is stopped, when it is clear the illness will probably end in death. Whereas the primary aim of hospice is to make the patient more comfortable, hospice professionals also help the family prepare for death with dignity; they help the

surviving family members with emotional and support services during the dying process. This help can extend after a loved one's death.

In everyone's life there comes a time when regular medical care is no longer helpful, and it is time to prepare for death. Today, people often have several weeks or months, and sometimes years, to make these preparations. This is when hospice care is so very useful. In hospice, medical and other care is aimed at making the patient as comfortable as possible and providing a good quality of life. Studies have shown that – at least for some illnesses – people who receive hospice care live longer than those who receive more aggressive treatment. Most hospices only accept people who are expected to die within six months. Rest assured, however, that this does not mean that you or your loved one will be thrown out of hospice care if you live longer. One of our original self-management leaders lived more than two years in hospice care.

Palliative care can take place in a number of hospices:

■ **In a hospice.** Hospices can provide individual care more suited to the person in a calm and peaceful atmosphere. There is no charge for a hospice place because they are charitable organisations. A referral must come from your GP, hospital, or district nurse.

■ **In your own home.** Your GP can arrange for community palliative care nurses, like Macmillan nurses, to support you in the best way possible. They are on call 24 hours a day.

■ **In a care home.** If you are already in a care home, you may find it less distressing to receive the care you need in the home rather than go into a hospital or hospice.

■ **As a day patient in a hospice.** This means you will get the care and support you need without moving away from your own home.

■ **As a day patient in a hospital.** Specialist palliative care teams are available in hospitals. They can advise hospital staff on the best way to control your pain and recommend the most appropriate options for discharge.

One of the problems with hospice care is that people often wait until the last few days before death to ask for it. They somehow see asking for hospice care as 'giving up'. By refusing hospice care, they often put an unnecessary burden on themselves, family, and friends. The reverse is also often true. The carer and family might say they can cope without help. Although this may be true, the patient's life and dying may be much better if hospice cares for all the medical things so that family and friends are free to give love and support to the dying person.

If you, your partner, a family member, or a friend is in the end stage of illness, find and make use of your local hospice. It is a wonderful final gift. Hospice workers are very special people who are kind, thoughtful, and supportive.

■ ■ ■

In closing, we would like to thank you for choosing to become an active self-manager of your health and life and for taking a more active role as the most important member of your healthcare team. Throughout this book, we have tried to give tips and provide tools to make these roles easier for you and for you to continue to live a healthier and more satisfying life with your long-term health condition.

Useful Websites

Age UK (Advance decisions): https://www.ageuk.org.uk/information-advice/money-legal/legal-issues/advance-decisions/

Age UK (Getting legal advice): https://www.ageuk.org.uk/globalassets/age-uk/documents/factsheets/fs43_getting_legal_advice_fcs.pdf

Age UK (Power of attorney): https://www.ageuk.org.uk/information-advice/money-legal/legal-issues/power-of-attorney/

Age UK (Respite services): https://www.ageuk.org.uk/services/in-your-area/carers-support/

Breast Cancer UK: https://www.breastcanceruk.org.uk/

British Red Cross: https://www.redcross.org.uk/get-help/get-support-at-home

Care Inspectorate (Scotland): https://www.careinspectorate.com/index.php/member-of-the-public/5452-who-we-inspect

Care Inspectorate Wales: https://careinspectorate.wales/find-care-service

Care Quality Commission (England): https://www.cqc.org.uk/what-we-do/services-we-regulate/find-care-home

Care Quality Commission (Finding services offering care in the home): https://www.cqc.org.uk/what-we-do/services-we-regulate/find-services-offering-care-home

Citizens Advice (Managing affairs for someone else): https://www.citizensadvice.org.uk/family/looking-after-people/managing-affairs-for-someone-else/

Compassion in Dying (Advance decisions): https://compassionindying.org.uk/making-decisions-and-planning-your-care/planning-ahead/lpa-advance-decision-difference/

Compassion in Dying (Making a lasting power of attorney for health and welfare): https://compassionindying.org.uk/making-decisions-and-planning-your-care/planning-ahead/lasting-power-attorney/making-lpa/

Focus on Disability (Disabled Living Centres UK regional index): https://focusondisability.co.uk/disability-aids-and-equipment-resources/disabled-living-centres-uk-regional-index/

Free Wills Month: https://freewillsmonth.org.uk/

GOV.UK (Certifying a document): https://www.gov.uk/certifying-a-document

GOV.UK (Check if a health condition affects your driving): https://www.gov.uk/health-conditions-and-driving

GOV.UK (Employing someone to work in your home): https://www.gov.uk/au-pairs-employment-law

GOV.UK (Lasting Power of Attorney guide): https://www.gov.uk/government/publications/make
-a-lasting-power-of-attorney/lp12-make-and-register-your-lasting-power-of-attorney-a-guide
-web-version

GOV.UK (Make, register, or end a lasting power of attorney): https://www.gov.uk/power-of-attorney

GOV.UK (Make a will): https://www.gov.uk/make-will

GOV.UK (Pension Tracing Service – find contact details to search for a lost pension):
https://www.gov.uk/find-pension-contact-details

Hospice UK: https://www.hospiceuk.org/

Local Government & Social Care Ombudsman: https://www.lgo.org.uk/

Macmillan Cancer Support (Macmillan nurses): https://www.macmillan.org.uk/cancer
-information-and-support/get-help/macmillan-nurses

Money Advice Service (Choosing a financial adviser): https://www.moneyadviceservice.org.uk/en
/articles/choosing-a-financial-adviser

Money Advice Service (How to fund your long-term care – a beginner's guide):
https://www.moneyadviceservice.org.uk/en/articles/how-to-fund-your-long-term-care
-a-beginners-guide

MS Society: https://www.mssociety.org.uk/

NHS (Advance statements): https://www.nhs.uk/conditions/end-of-life-care/advance-statement/

NHS (Being discharged from hospital): https://www.nhs.uk/using-the-nhs/nhs-services/hospitals
/being-discharged-from-hospital/

NHS (Carers, breaks, and respite): https://www.nhs.uk/conditions/social-care-and-support-guide
/support-and-benefits-for-carers/carer-breaks-and-respite-care/

NHS (Finding a care home): https://www.nhs.uk/conditions/social-care-and-support-guide/care
-services-equipment-and-care-homes/care-homes/

NHS (Finding homecare agencies): https://www.nhs.uk/service-search/other-services/Homecare
/LocationSearch/1833

NHS (Help at home from a carer): https://www.nhs.uk/conditions/social-care-and-support-guide
/care-services-equipment-and-care-homes/homecare/

NHS (Types of talking therapies): https://www.nhs.uk/conditions/stress-anxiety-depression/types
-of-therapy/

NHS (What is a personal health budget?): https://www.nhs.uk/using-the-nhs/help-with-health
-costs/what-is-a-personal-health-budget/

NHS (When the council might pay for your care): https://www.nhs.uk/conditions/social-care-and -support-guide/money-work-and-benefits/when-the-council-might-pay-for-your-care/

NHS (When you need to pay towards NHS care): https://www.nhs.uk/using-the-nhs/help-with -health-costs/when-you-need-to-pay-towards-nhs-care/

Office of Care and Protection (Northern Ireland): https://www.nidirect.gov.uk/articles/managing -your-affairs-and-enduring-power-attorney

Office of the Public Guardian (Scotland): https://www.publicguardian-scotland.gov.uk/general /contact-us

Parkinson's UK: https://www.parkinsons.org.uk/

Regulation and Quality Improvement Authority (Northern Ireland): https://www.rqia.org.uk/what -we-do/inspect/

Resuscitation Council UK: https://www.resus.org.uk/public-resource/cpr-decisions-and-dnacpr

Royal Voluntary Service: https://www.royalvoluntaryservice.org.uk/our-services

Stroke Association: https://www.stroke.org.uk/

UK Homecare Association: https://www.ukhca.co.uk/

Which? (Live-in care): https://www.which.co.uk/later-life-care/home-care/organising-home-care /live-in-care-ab4sl1n154ww

Which? (Personal alarms): https://www.which.co.uk/later-life-care/home-care/technology-to-keep -you-safe/personal-alarms-azbn15v6qmgg

Which? (DNAR decisions): https://www.which.co.uk/later-life-care/end-of-life/end-of-life-care -planning/do-not-attempt-resuscitation-decisions-alvg41p1jzjb

Which? (What are retirement villages?): https://www.which.co.uk/later-life-care/housing-options /retirement-villages/what-are-retirement-villages-aq5g24d82y2c

Index

Note: Page numbers followed by *f* or *t* indicate a figure or table on the designated page

405